T0264148

# Cranial Arteriovenous Malformations (AVMs) and Cranial Dural Arteriovenous Fistulas (DAVFs)

*Guest Editors*

RAFAEL J. TAMARGO, MD
JUDY HUANG, MD

## NEUROSURGERY
## CLINICS OF NORTH AMERICA

www.neurosurgery.theclinics.com

*Consulting Editors*
ANDREW T. PARSA, MD, PhD
PAUL C. McCORMICK, MD, MPH

January 2012 • Volume 23 • Number 1

SAUNDERS an imprint of ELSEVIER, Inc.

**W.B. SAUNDERS COMPANY**
*A Division of Elsevier Inc.*

1600 John F. Kennedy Blvd. • Suite 1800 • Philadelphia, PA 19103-2899

http://www.theclinics.com

**NEUROSURGERY CLINICS OF NORTH AMERICA Volume 23, Number 1**
**January 2012 ISSN 1042-3680, ISBN-13: 978-1-4557-3896-0**

Editor: Jessica McCool
Developmental Editor: Teia Stone

© **2012 Elsevier Inc. All rights reserved.**

This journal and the individual contributions contained in it are protected under copyright by Elsevier, and the following terms and conditions apply to their use:

**Photocopying**

Single photocopies of single articles may be made for personal use as allowed by national copyright laws. Permission of the Publisher and payment of a fee is required for all other photocopying, including multiple or systematic copying, copying for advertising or promotional purposes, resale, and all forms of document delivery. Special rates are available for educational institutions that wish to make photocopies for non-profit educational classroom use. For information on how to seek permission visit www.elsevier.com/permissions or call: (+44) 1865 843830 (UK)/(+1) 215 239 3804 (USA).

**Derivative Works**

Subscribers may reproduce tables of contents or prepare lists of articles including abstracts for internal circulation within their institutions. Permission of the Publisher is required for resale or distribution outside the institution. Permission of the Publisher is required for all other derivative works, including compilations and translations (please consult www.elsevier.com/permissions).

**Electronic Storage or Usage**

Permission of the Publisher is required to store or use electronically any material contained in this journal, including any article or part of an article (please consult www.elsevier.com/permissions). Except as outlined above, no part of this publication may be reproduced, stored in a retrieval system or transmitted in any form or by any means, electronic, mechanical, photocopying, recording or otherwise, without prior written permission of the Publisher.

**Notice**

No responsibility is assumed by the Publisher for any injury and/or damage to persons or property as a matter of products liability, negligence or otherwise, or from any use or operation of any methods, products, instructions or ideas contained in the material herein. Because of rapid advances in the medical sciences, in particular, independent verification of diagnoses and drug dosages should be made.

Although all advertising material is expected to conform to ethical (medical) standards, inclusion in this publication does not constitute a guarantee or endorsement of the quality or value of such product or of the claims made of it by its manufacturer.

*Neurosurgery Clinics of North America* (ISSN 1042-3680) is published quarterly by Elsevier Inc., 360 Park Avenue South, New York, NY 10010-1710. Months of issue are January, April, July, and October. Business and Editorial Offices: 1600 John F. Kennedy Blvd., Suite 1800, Philadelphia, PA 19103-2899. Customer Service Office: 11830 Westline Industrial Drive, St. Louis, MO 63146. Periodicals postage paid at New York, NY, and additional mailing offices. Subscription prices are $346.00 per year (US individuals), $531.00 per year (US institutions), $378.00 per year (Canadian individuals), $649.00 per year (Canadian institutions), $483.00 per year (international individuals), $649.00 per year (international institutions), $170.00 per year (US students), and $233.00 per year (international students). International air speed delivery is included in all *Clinics* subscription prices. All prices are subject to change without notice. **POSTMASTER:** Send address changes to *Neurosurgery Clinics of North America*, Elsevier Periodicals Customer Service, 11830 Westline Industrial Drive, St. Louis, MO 63146. **Customer Service: 1-800-654-2452 (US and Canada). From outside the US and Canada, call: 1-314-453-7041. Fax: 1-314-453-5170. E-mail: JournalsCustomerService-usa@elsevier.com (for print support) and journalsonlinesupport-usa@elsevier.com (for online support).**

*Reprints.* For copies of 100 or more, of articles in this publication, please contact the Commercial Reprints Department, Elsevier Inc., 360 Park Avenue South, New York, NY 10010-1710. Tel. (212) 633-3812; Fax: (212) 462-1935; E-mail: reprints@elsevier.com.

*Neurosurgery Clinics of North America* is covered in *MEDLINE/PubMed (Index Medicus), EMBASE/Excerpta Medica, and Current Contents/Clinical Medicine (CC/CM).*

Cover illustration courtesy of Ian Suk, Johns Hopkins University; with permission.

Printed and bound by CPI Group (UK) Ltd, Croydon, CR0 4YY

Transferred to Digital Print 2012

# Contributors

## CONSULTING EDITORS

**ANDREW T. PARSA, MD, PhD**
Associate Professor, Principal Investigator,
Brain Tumor Research Center, Reza and
Georgianna Khatib Endowed Chair in Skull
Base Tumor Surgery, Department of
Neurological Surgery, University of California,
San Francisco, San Francisco, California

**PAUL C. MCCORMICK, MD, MPH, FACS**
Herbert & Linda Gallen Professor of
Neurological Surgery, Department of
Neurological Surgery, Columbia University
Medical Center, New York, New York

## GUEST EDITORS

**RAFAEL J. TAMARGO, MD, FACS**
Walter E. Dandy Professor of Neurosurgery,
Director, Division of Cerebrovascular
Neurosurgery, Department of Neurosurgery,
The Johns Hopkins Hospital, The Johns
Hopkins University School of Medicine,
Baltimore, Maryland

**JUDY HUANG, MD**
Associate Professor of Neurosurgery, Division
of Cerebrovascular Neurosurgery, Department
of Neurosurgery, The Johns Hopkins University
School of Medicine, Baltimore, Maryland

## AUTHORS

**EDWARD S. AHN, MD**
Assistant Professor of Neurosurgery,
Division of Pediatric Neurosurgery,
The Johns Hopkins Hospital, Baltimore,
Maryland

**ANUBHAV G. AMIN, BS**
Division of Interventional Neuroradiology,
The Johns Hopkins Hospital, Baltimore,
Maryland

**SALAH G. AOUN, MD**
Department of Neurological Surgery,
Northwestern University Feinberg School
of Medicine and McGaw Medical Center,
Chicago, Illinois

**GEOFFREY APPELBOOM, MD**
Postdoctoral Research Scientist, Department
of Neurological Surgery, Columbia University,
New York, New York

**JOHN C. BARR, MD**
Neurosurgical Service, Endovascular and
Neurovascular Neurosurgery, Massachusetts
General Hospital, Boston, Massachusetts

**H. HUNT BATJER, MD, FACS**
Department of Neurological Surgery,
Northwestern University Feinberg School of
Medicine and McGaw Medical Center,
Chicago, Illinois

**BERNARD R. BENDOK, MD, FACS**
Associate Professor of Neurological Surgery
and Radiology, Department of Neurological
Surgery, Northwestern University Feinberg
School of Medicine and McGaw Medical
Center, Chicago, Illinois

**SAMUEL BRUCE, BA**
Administrative Coordinator, Department of
Neurological Surgery, Columbia University,
New York, New York

**KAISORN L. CHAICHANA, MD**
Neurosurgery Resident, Department of
Neurosurgery, The Johns Hopkins University
School of Medicine, Baltimore, Maryland

**JAMES CHEN, BS**
Medical Student, The Johns Hopkins
University School of Medicine, Baltimore,
Maryland

**GEOFFREY P. COLBY, MD, PhD**
Resident, Department of Neurosurgery,
The Johns Hopkins University School of
Medicine, The Johns Hopkins Hospital,
Baltimore, Maryland

**E. SANDER CONNOLLY Jr, MD**
Bennett M. Stein Professor of Neurological
Surgery, Department of Neurological Surgery,
Columbia University, New York, New York

**ALEXANDER L. COON, MD**
Assistant Professor, Department of
Neurosurgery, The Johns Hopkins University
School of Medicine, The Johns Hopkins
Hospital, Baltimore, Maryland

**JASON M. DAVIES, MD, PhD**
Department of Neurological Surgery, University
of California, San Francisco, San Francisco,
California

**PHILIPPE GAILLOUD, MD**
Division of Interventional Neuroradiology, The
Johns Hopkins Hospital, Baltimore, Maryland

**DHEERAJ GANDHI, MBBS, MD**
Director and Professor, Division of
Interventional Neuroradiology, Departments
of Radiology, Neurology and Neurosurgery,
University of Maryland, Baltimore, Maryland

**JUAN GOMEZ, MD**
Division of Interventional Neuroradiology,
The Johns Hopkins Hospital, Baltimore,
Maryland

**LYDIA GREGG, MA, CMI**
Research Associate, Division of Interventional
Neuroradiology, The Johns Hopkins Hospital,
The Johns Hopkins University School of
Medicine, Baltimore, Maryland

**JUHA HERNESNIEMI, MD, PhD**
Department of Neurosurgery, Helsinki
University Central Hospital, Helsinki, Finland

**JUDY HUANG, MD**
Associate Professor of Neurosurgery, Division
of Cerebrovascular Neurosurgery, Department
of Neurosurgery, The Johns Hopkins University
School of Medicine, Baltimore, Maryland

**GEORGE I. JALLO, MD**
Division of Pediatric Neurosurgery, The Johns
Hopkins Hospital, Baltimore, Maryland

**HELEN KIM, PhD**
Department of Anesthesia and Perioperative
Care; Center for Cerebrovascular Research,
University of California, San Francisco, San
Francisco, California

**AKI LAAKSO, MD, PhD**
Department of Neurosurgery, Helsinki
University Central Hospital, Helsinki, Finland

**MICHAEL T. LAWTON, MD**
Department of Neurological Surgery; Center for
Cerebrovascular Research, University of
California, San Francisco, San Francisco,
California

**MICHAEL LIM, MD**
Department of Neurosurgery, The Johns
Hopkins University, Baltimore, Maryland

**CHRISTINA MILLER, MD**
Assistant Professor, Department of
Anesthesiology and Critical Care Medicine,
The Johns Hopkins University School of
Medicine, Baltimore, Maryland

**NEIL R. MILLER, MD, FACS**
Professor of Ophthalmology, Neurology and
Neurosurgery; Frank B. Walsh Professor of
Neuro-Ophthalmology, The Johns Hopkins
Medical Institutions, Baltimore, Maryland

**MAREK MIRSKI, MD, PhD**
Professor, Department of Anesthesiology and
Critical Care Medicine, The Johns Hopkins
University School of Medicine, Baltimore,
Maryland

**MAHMUD MOSSA-BASHA, MD**
Diagnostic Neuroradiology Fellow, Division of
Neuroradiology, Russell H. Morgan
Department of Radiology, The Johns Hopkins
University, Baltimore, Maryland

**CHRISTOPHER S. OGILVY, MD**
Director of Endovascular and Neurovascular
Neurosurgical Service, Robert G. and A. Jean
Ojemann Professor of Neurosurgery,
Massachusetts General Hospital, Boston,
Massachusetts

**ALEXANDRA R. PAUL, MD**
Resident, Division of Neurosurgery, Albany
Medical Center Hospital, Albany, New York

**MONICA PEARL, MD**
Division of Interventional Neuroradiology, The
Johns Hopkins Hospital, Baltimore, Maryland

**GUSTAVO PRADILLA, MD**
Chief Resident, Division of Cerebrovascular
Neurosurgery, Department of Neurosurgery,
The Johns Hopkins University School of
Medicine, Baltimore, Maryland

**MARTIN G. RADVANY, MD**
Assistant Professor, Radiology, Neurosurgery
and Neurology, Division of Interventional
Neuroradiology, The Johns Hopkins University
School of Medicine, Baltimore, Maryland

**GAZANFAR RAHMATHULLA, MD**
Department of Neurosurgery, Cleveland Clinic,
Cleveland, Ohio

**SHAAN RAZA, MD**
Department of Neurosurgery, The Johns
Hopkins University, Baltimore, Maryland

**PABLO F. RECINOS, MD**
Division of Pediatric Neurosurgery, The Johns
Hopkins Hospital, Baltimore, Maryland;
Department of Neurosurgery, Cleveland Clinic,
Cleveland, Ohio

**VIOLETTE RENARD RECINOS, MD**
Department of Neurosurgery, Cleveland Clinic,
Cleveland, Ohio

**ALFRED P. SEE, BS**
Department of Neurosurgery, The Johns
Hopkins University, Baltimore, Maryland

**RAFAEL J. TAMARGO, MD, FACS**
Walter E. Dandy Professor of Neurosurgery,
Director, Division of Cerebrovascular
Neurosurgery, Department of Neurosurgery,
The Johns Hopkins Hospital, The Johns
Hopkins University School of Medicine,
Baltimore, Maryland

**WILLIAM L. YOUNG, MD**
Departments of Anesthesia and Perioperative
Care, Neurological Surgery and Neurology;
Center for Cerebrovascular Research,
University of California, San Francisco,
San Francisco, California

**BRAD E. ZACHARIA, MD**
Resident, Department of Neurological Surgery,
Columbia University, New York, New York

# Contents

> Arteriovenous malformations (AVMs) of the brain are relatively rare congenital developmental vascular lesions. They may cause hemorrhagic stroke, epilepsy, chronic headache, or focal neurologic deficits, and the incidence of asymptomatic AVMs is increasing due to widespread availability of noninvasive imaging methods. Since the most severe complication of an AVM is hemorrhagic stroke, most epidemiologic studies have concentrated on the hemorrhage risk and its risk factors. In this article, the authors discuss the epidemiology, presenting symptoms, and hemorrhage risk associated with brain AVMs.

> Intracranial dural arteriovenous fistulas (DAVFs) are relatively rare lesions consisting of anomalous connections between dural arteries and venous sinuses and/or cortical veins. Their clinical presentation is quite variable, with symptoms dependent on their location and venous drainage pattern. Lesions with cortical venous drainage, however, have the highest risk of causing the most significant morbidity and mortality. This places an emphasis on promptly suspecting and diagnosing these lesions. This review highlights the etiology, epidemiology, clinical presentation, and clinical course of patients with intracranial DAVFs.

> Cerebral arteriovenous malformations and intracranial dural arteriovenous fistulas represent two important classes of intracranial vascular lesions. This article recalls the history on which current technical advances, including diagnoses, characterization, and treatment, is based. It also describes modern therapeutic options, including microsurgical, endovascular, and radiosurgery techniques.

> Imaging plays a major role in the identification, grading, and treatment of cerebral arteriovenous malformations and cerebral dural arteriovenous fistulas. Digital subtraction angiography is the gold standard in the diagnosis and characterization of these vascular malformations, but advances in both magnetic resonance imaging and computed tomography, including advanced imaging techniques, have provided new tools for further characterizing these lesions as well as the surrounding brain structures that may be affected. This article discusses the role of conventional as well as advanced imaging modalities that are providing novel ways to characterize these vascular malformations.

The wide variety of arteriovenous malformation (AVM) anatomy, size, location, and clinical presentation makes patient selection for surgery a difficult process. Neurosurgeons have identified key factors that determine the risks of surgery and then devised classification schemes that integrate these factors, predict surgical results, and help select patients for surgery. These classification schemes have value because they transform complex decisions into simpler algorithms. In this review, the important grading schemes that have contributed to management of patients with brain AVMs are described, and our current approach to patient selection is outlined.

The clinical presentation of dural arteriovenous fistulas (DAVFs), in particular the associated risk of intracranial hemorrhage, shows a strong correlation with their pattern of venous drainage. The two most commonly used and clinically accepted DAVF classifications are the Merland-Cognard classification and the Borden classification, both based on the morphology of the venous drainage. A revised classification that grades DAVFs through a combination of angiographic and clinical features has also been proposed. This article offers a review of these various classification schemes, and discusses their application to treatment decision making.

This article provides management guidelines for arteriovenous malformations (AVMs). Management options include observation, surgical excision, endovascular embolization, and radiosurgery. Each of these can be used individually or combined for multimodal therapy based on the characteristics of the lesion. The article stratifies each lesion based on the AVM and patient characteristics to either observation or a single or multimodal treatment arm. The treatment of an AVM must be carefully weighed in each patient because of the risk of neurologic injury in functional areas of the brain and weighed against the natural history of hemorrhage.

Cranial dural arteriovenous fistulas (DAVFs) represent an important class of cranial vascular lesions. The clinical significance of these lesions is highly dependent on the pattern of venous drainage, with cortical venous reflux being an important marker of an aggressive, high-risk fistula. For asymptomatic benign fistulas, conservative management, consisting of observation with follow-up, is a reasonable option. For symptomatic benign fistulas or aggressive fistulas, treatment is recommended. A variety of treatment modalities are available for DAVF management, including endovascular techniques, open surgery, and radiosurgery. A multimodality approach is often warranted and can offer improved chances of achieving a cure.

Arteriovenous malformations of the brain (AVMs) are a major cause of stroke in young, healthy individuals and present multiple diagnostic and therapeutic challenges, particularly in the acute setting. Although the flow hemodynamics, biology, epidemiology, and natural history of AVMs have been extensively studied, little data have been published on AVM surgery in the acute setting, and acute surgery has been claimed to possibly increase the risk of persistent neurological deficits. Although it is usually preferable to defer AVM surgery for a few weeks or months, acute surgical (open and endovascular) management is essential in specific clinical and radiological settings.

Microsurgical resection remains the treatment of choice for more than half of all patients with arteriovenous malformations (AVMs). It reduces the treatment window to a span of a few weeks and is curative. Careful patient selection, meticulous surgical planning, and painstaking technical execution of surgery are typically rewarded with excellent outcomes. For dural arteriovenous fistulas (DAVFs), microsurgical obliteration is often reserved for cases in which endovascular therapy either cannot be pursued or fails. When performed, however, microsurgical obliteration of DAVFs is associated with excellent outcomes as well. This article reviews the current state of microsurgical treatment of AVMs and DAVFs.

Pial arteriovenous malformations (AVMs) and dural arteriovenous fistulas (DAVFs) are high-flow vascular lesions with abnormal communications between the arterial and venous system. AVMs are congenital lesions, whereas DAVFs are considered acquired lesions. Both can cause significant morbidity and mortality if they rupture and result in intracranial hemorrhage. The primary goal of treatment is to eliminate the risk of bleeding or at least decrease it. Because the epidemiology, clinical presentation, and classification of AVMs and DAVFs have been covered in previous articles in this issue, the authors only briefly touch on these subjects as they relate to endovascular treatment.

Cranial arteriovenous malformations (AVM) and cranial dural arteriovenous fistulas (AVF) carry a significant risk of morbidity and mortality when they hemorrhage. Current treatment options include surgery, embolization, radiosurgery, or a combination of these treatments. Radiosurgery is thought to reduce the risk hemorrhage in AVMs and AVFs by obliterating of the nidus of abnormal vasculature over the course of 2 to 3 years. Success in treating AVMs is variable depending on the volume of the lesion, the radiation dose, and the pattern of vascular supply and drainage. This article discusses the considerations for selecting radiosurgery as a treatment modality in patients who present with AVMs and AVFs.

Arteriovenous malformations (AVMs) are vascular lesions characterized by direct connections between feeding arteries and draining veins without an intervening capillary network. Two hypotheses, normal perfusion pressure breakthrough (NPPB) and occlusive hyperemia, prevail in the literature regarding the occasional development of hemorrhage and edema following AVM resection. The NPPB hypothesis was introduced in 1978. Since the occlusive hyperemia hypothesis was first postulated in 1993, however, a debate has persisted within the cerebrovascular community concerning which hypothesis better explains the complications of edema and hemorrhage seen after AVM resection. Recent advances in cerebrovascular imaging and hemodynamic analysis have allowed a better evaluation of intracerebral changes following AVM resection. It is likely that these 2 hypotheses are not mutually exclusive and perhaps exist in a spectrum of hemodynamic alteration following AVM resection.

The anesthetic considerations for surgical resection of arteriovenous malformations (AVMs) and dural arteriovenous fistulas (DAVFs) incorporate many principles that are common to craniotomies for other indications. However, a high-flow, low-resistance shunt results in chronic hypoperfusion of adjacent brain tissue that is vulnerable to ischemia and at high risk for hyperemia and hemorrhage as resection of the lesion redirects blood flow. A comprehensive understanding of AVM pathophysiology and rapidly titratable anesthetic and vasoactive agents allow the anesthesiologist to alter blood pressure targets as resection evolves for optimal patient outcome. Intensive management is continued post-operatively as the brain acclimatizes to new parameters.

The vein of Galen aneurysmal malformation is a congenital vascular malformation that comprises 30% of the pediatric vascular and 1% of all pediatric congenital anomalies. Treatment is dependent on the timing of presentation and clinical manifestations. With the development of endovascular techniques, treatment paradigms have changed and clinical outcomes have significantly improved. In this article, the developmental embryology, clinical features and pathophysiology, diagnostic workup, and management strategies are reviewed.

Dural arteriovenous fistulas of the cavernous sinus are no longer difficult to diagnose or treat. Specific ocular manifestations allow these fistulas to be diagnosed clinically. Noninvasive imaging techniques can be used to confirm the diagnosis. The most common treatment is endovascular occlusion of the lesion via a transarterial or transvenous route. Manual compression of the ipsilateral internal carotid artery in the neck or radiation therapy is appropriate in selected cases. Regardless of the treatment used, the fistula can be closed completely in most cases, resulting in restoration of normal orbital and intracranial blood flow and resolution of visual deficits.

# Neurosurgery Clinics of North America

**RELATED INTEREST**

*Neuroimaging Clinics of North America,* August 2011 (Volume 21, Issue 3)
**Congenital Anomalies of the Brain, Spine, and Neck**
Hemant A. Parmar, MD, and Mohannad Ibrahim, MD, *Guest Editors*
http://www.neuroimaging.theclinics.com/

**VISIT THE CLINICS ONLINE!**

Access your subscription at:
**www.theclinics.com**

# Preface

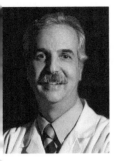 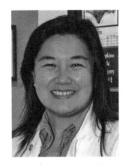

Rafael J. Tamargo, MD            Judy Huang, MD

*Guest Editors*

Brain arteriovenous malformations (AVMs) and dural arteriovenous fistulas (DAVFs) are rare and formidable lesions. The prevalence of AVMs in modern radiographic series is only about 0.2%.[1] The prevalence of DAVFs—which are characteristically difficult to image on CT or MRI and therefore difficult to identify in screening studies—is even more challenging to ascertain, but DAVFs are probably even less common than AVMs.[2] By contrast, intracranial aneurysms have an estimated prevalence of about 3%,[3] which makes aneurysms 15 times more common than AVMs. The rarity of AVMs and DAVFs has frustrated any attempts to study their treatment in prospective randomized trials.[4] Over the past century, however, neurosurgeons, neurointerventional radiologists, and radiosurgeons have made steady progress in the diagnosis and treatment of these complex lesions. This progress is particularly impressive when one considers that current epidemiological and surgical series of AVMs comprise only a few hundred patients. By contrast, contemporary aneurysm series include thousands of patients. Therefore, our current knowledge about AVMs and DAVFs is based and will continue to evolve on empirical evidence derived from a limited number of patients.

At present, the epidemiology of AVMs is fairly well understood, but their etiology and natural history remain enigmatic. Most AVMs can be treated effectively with microsurgical resection, stereotactic radiosurgery, and endovascular embolization. As presented in this issue, our increasingly sophisticated treatment algorithms for AVMs are being rewarded with improved outcomes. Our understanding of DAVFs, which are a more heterogenous group of lesions, is lagging behind that of AVMs. Much remains to be learned about AVMs and DAVFs, but it is apparent that advances are being made.

In this issue of the *Neurosurgery Clinics of North America*, we update our current understanding of the epidemiology, diagnosis, and treatment of cranial AVMs and DAVFs. In the first three articles, we consider the epidemiology of these lesions and review the historical evolution of their surgical, endovascular, and radiosurgical treatments. In the fourth article, we discuss the radiographic evaluation of AVMs and DAVFs, and in the fifth and sixth articles, we describe their classification schemes. The treatment algorithms of AVMs and DAVFs are discussed in the seventh and eighth articles, respectively. In the ninth article, we describe the acute management of hemorrhagic AVMs and DAVFs. Surgery, endovascular therapy, and radiosurgery are discussed in detail in the tenth, eleventh, and twelfth articles, respectively. The clinical and theoretical aspects of occlusive hyperemia and normal perfusion pressure breakthrough are reviewed in article 13. In the fourteenth article, we describe the anesthetic approach to AVM and DAVF patients. Finally, in the last two articles, we consider the epidemiology, diagnosis, and management of the two special forms of AVFs, namely, vein of Galen aneurysmal malformations and carotid cavernous fistulas.

We are indebted to all of our colleagues who have generously contributed their authoritative insights on the management of these lesions. We would like to thank the editorial staff at Elsevier for their invaluable help. In particular, we are most appreciative for the expert guidance and hard work of Jessica McCool (Editor), Teia Stone (Developmental Editor), LeighAnne Helfmann (Journal Manager/Production Editor), and Ruth Malwitz (former Editor). In addition, we would like to thank the Consulting Editors, Dr Andrew Parsa

Neurosurg Clin N Am 23 (2012) xiii–xiv
doi:10.1016/j.nec.2011.10.003
1042-3680/12/$ – see front matter © 2012 Elsevier Inc. All rights reserved.

neurosurgery.theclinics.com

and Dr Paul McCormick, for the opportunity to work on this issue.

Rafael J. Tamargo, MD
Judy Huang, MD

Division of Cerebrovascular Neurosurgery
Department of Neurosurgery
The Johns Hopkins University School of Medicine
Johns Hopkins Hospital
Meyer Building, Suite 8-181
600 North Wolfe Street
Baltimore, MD 21287, USA

E-mail addresses:
rtamarg@jhmi.edu (R.J. Tamargo)
Jhuang24@jhmi.edu (J. Huang)

**REFERENCES**

1. Weber F, Knopf H. Incidental findings in magnetic resonance imaging of the brains of healthy young men. J Neurol Sci 2006;240:81–4.
2. Brown RD Jr, Wiebers DO, Torner JC, et al. Incidence and prevalence of intracranial vascular malformations in Olmsted County, Minnesota, 1965 to 1992. Neurology 1996;46:949–52.
3. Vlak MH, Algra A, Brandenburg R, et al. Prevalence of unruptured intracranial aneurysms, with emphasis on sex, age, comorbidity, country, and time period: a systematic review and meta-analysis. Lancet Neurol 2011;10:626–36.
4. Ross J, Al-Shahi Salman R. Interventions for treating brain arteriovenous malformations in adults. Cochrane Database Syst Rev 2010:CD003436.

# Arteriovenous Malformations: Epidemiology and Clinical Presentation

Aki Laakso, MD, PhD, Juha Hernesniemi, MD, PhD*

## KEYWORDS

- Arteriovenous malformations • Natural history
- Hemorrhagic stroke • Epidemiology
- Intracerebral hemorrhage

Brain arteriovenous malformations (AVMs) are complex vascular lesions in which arterial blood flows directly into draining veins without an intervening capillary bed. The lack of resistance normally created by small diameter arterioles and capillaries and the resulting direct transmission of arterial pressure to venous structures lead to markedly increased blood flow and, eventually, dilatation and tortuous growth of vessels. In addition to anatomic cerebrovascular changes, this process may bring about significant hemodynamic changes in the brain, such as reversal of venous flow, venous hypertension, and hypoperfusion of regions surrounding the AVM.

AVMs are probably congenital lesions that form during either the embryonic or fetal stages of development, but they are usually not hereditary lesions. Their etiology remains unknown. Although brain AVMs are highly heterogeneous and vary greatly in size and angioarchitecture, multiple AVMs in a single patient are rare. The most serious, and the most common, clinical symptom of an AVM is hemorrhagic stroke resulting from its rupture. AVMs may also cause symptoms due to irritation of surrounding cortex, leading to epilepsy, mass effect, and pathologic changes in hemodynamics as mentioned previously. This article reviews the literature concerning the epidemiology of brain AVMs, as well as presenting symptoms, the risk of hemorrhage, and angioarchitectural factors affecting these characteristics.

## EPIDEMIOLOGY

AVMs are rather rare lesions. Although the pathogenesis of AVMs remains unknown, their angioarchitectural characteristics and presentation at any age indicate that they are probably either embryonic or fetal. Despite this, most AVMs seem not to be of hereditary origin, although rare cases of familial occurrence have been reported.[1] Interestingly, AVMs have sometimes been observed to spontaneously disappear, or recur after angiographically complete obliteration.[2–6]

The reported incidence rates of newly diagnosed AVMs have varied in different population-based studies from 0.89 to 1.34 cases per 100,000 person–years.[7–10] The tendency for higher incidence rates in more recent studies reflects increased availability of noninvasive brain imaging, and is accompanied with increased proportion of unruptured and even asymptomatic AVMs in the patient population. Prevalence of AVMs has rarely been estimated; a community-based retrospective study from Scotland reported a prevalence of 18 cases in 100,000 people (ie, <0.02%).[11] At the other end of the prevalence estimate continuum, a German study in over 2500 healthy young men (applicants for the military service in German Air Force) undergoing cranial magnetic resonance imaging (MRI) found a prevalence of 0.2% for incidental brain AVMs.[12] In their neurosurgical unit in Helsinki, the authors are responsible for treating

Department of Neurosurgery, Helsinki University Central Hospital, PO Box 266, Topeliuksenkatu 5, 00260 Helsinki, Finland
* Corresponding author.
E-mail address: juha.hernesniemi@hus.fi

Neurosurg Clin N Am 23 (2012) 1–6
doi:10.1016/j.nec.2011.09.012
1042-3680/12/$ – see front matter © 2012 Elsevier Inc. All rights reserved.

the cerebrovascular anomalies of a southern Finnish population of over 2 million people, and they have been treating annually approximately 25 AVM patients and 300 intracranial aneurysm patients. Considering that the prevalence of aneurysms is well established to be around 3%,[13] the authors' experience conforms very well with the prevalence of the German study, suggesting that prevalence of AVMs is 10- to 15-fold lower than aneurysms (ie, in the range of 0.2%). The total prevalence of AVMs, including all the asymptomatic lesions, is nevertheless extremely difficult to estimate reliably due to the rarity of the disease. The most common age of presentation is the third or fourth decade of life, but AVMs may become symptomatic at any age (**Fig. 1**). There is no consistently observed gender predominance.

Although AVMs may remain asymptomatic for life in many carriers, they are by no means benign lesions. Overall annual mortality rates have varied from 0.7% to 2.9% in different study populations,[7,14–19] but the mortality rates have usually not been compared with the background population. The authors have recently reported that AVM patients have significant excess mortality as compared with matched general population.[20] The authors' study population of 623 AVM patients from Finland also included a subset of 155 untreated patients. In patients with untreated AVMs, the overall annual mortality rate was 3.4% during a median follow-up period of 18.9 years. AVM-related (due to either acute case fatality or chronic sequelae of AVM-related morbidity) annual mortality rate in the same group was 1.6% (ie, almost 50% of mortality was explained by AVMs). AVM patients were compared with the general population using relative survival ratio

(RSR) (ie, the survival of the patient population was compared with the survival of the whole population of Finland, matched for age, sex and historical era). Cumulative RSR in untreated AVM patients 30 years after presentation was 0.49 (ie, 51% excess in mortality compared with general population). In contrast, in AVM patients in whom the AVM was completely obliterated, the cumulative RSR had decreased to only 0.87 after 30 years. Untreated AVM patients thus seem to have a poor long-term prognosis.

## PRESENTING SYMPTOMS

Traditionally, most AVMs come into clinical attention because of hemorrhage, with epilepsy coming far behind as the second most common type of presentation. This pattern is gradually changing, however. Increasing availability of noninvasive imaging methods, mainly MRI, have led to more and more frequent detection of unruptured and even incidental AVMs. A few decades ago, over 70% of AVMs presented with hemorrhage,[15,19] whereas more recent patient series report a hemorrhagic presentation rate of less than 50%.[21,22] Despite this trend, hemorrhagic stroke still remains the most common type of symptom leading to diagnosis, and 45% to 72% (median 52%) of patients have presented with hemorrhage in 10 large AVM series.[15,17,19,22–27]

Although AVMs cause only 2% of all and 4% of hemorrhagic strokes, the victims are often younger than most other stroke patients, and AVMs explain one-third of hemorrhagic strokes in young adults.[28] Hemorrhage from AVM is generally considered less hazardous than the rupture of an intracranial aneurysm or spontaneous hypertensive intracranial hemorrhage, but AVM rupture with associated intraparenchymatous hemorrhage often results in significant neurologic disability. Observed case fatality rates and risk of permanent disability caused by AVM hemorrhage vary widely in different reports, but are usually in the range of 5% to 25% and 10% to 40%, respectively.[19,28–34]

Various anatomic factors associated with hemorrhagic presentation have been identified. Independent risk factors for hemorrhagic presentation according to multivariate analyses include small size,[21,22,25] deep venous drainage,[21,22,25,35] deep,[22,36] nonborder zone (watershed)[22] and infratentorial[37] locations, associated aneurysms,[22] hypertension,[21] small number of draining veins,[36] venous ectasias,[36] and high feeding artery pressure.[35] Although some characteristics of AVMs, such as small size, are undoubtedly more common in AVMs presenting with rupture, it should be noted that factors associated with hemorrhagic

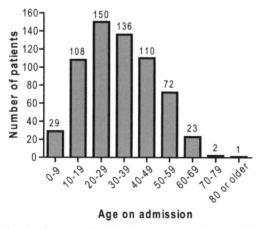

**Fig. 1.** The age distribution on admission in 631 arteriovenous malformations (AVM) patients from Helsinki AVM database (1942–2005).

presentation are not necessarily the same as independent risk factors predicting future AVM rupture. Small AVM size is probably the most obvious example; it is found consistently to associate with hemorrhagic presentation, whereas large AVM size seems to increase the risk for hemorrhage during the follow-up after the initial diagnosis. This is most likely due to the fact that small AVMs are not easily diagnosed unless they bleed, whereas large AVMs may cause a variety of symptoms leading to diagnosis before they rupture. In other words, this apparent discrepancy also suggests that significant proportion of small, unruptured AVMs remain unnoticed and undiagnosed for the whole lifetimes of their carriers.

The second most common form of AVM presentation is symptomatic epilepsy, with 18% to 35% (median 26%) of patients diagnosed because of seizures.[15,17,19,22–27] However, less than 1% of all first episodes of unprovoked seizures are caused by AVMs according to a Swedish prospective, population-based study.[38] Reported anatomic AVM characteristics associated with epileptic presentation have included large size,[39] cortical location of the nidus or the feeders,[39,40] and location of the AVM in the middle cerebral artery territory.[40] Less common presenting symptoms are chronic headache (unrelated to bleeding) in 6% to 14% of patients, and focal neurologic deficit (temporary, fixed or progressive) due to mass effect or hemodynamic disturbances in 3% to 10% of patients. The proportion of patients with incidentally found AVMs has increased from less than 2% in early studies to 10% in contemporary series.

## RISK OF HEMORRHAGE FROM UNTREATED AVMs

Since hemorrhagic stroke is the most severe consequence of harboring an AVM, it is understandable that major efforts have been undertaken to identify risk factors predicting AVM rupture. This is all the more important considering that the treatment of complex AVMs is associated with significant risks of morbidity and mortality, and these should not, naturally, exceed the estimated lifetime risk of harboring an untreated lesion. Establishing the probability of rupture and possible anatomic and demographic factors affecting this risk requires long-term follow-up studies in large cohorts of patients with untreated AVMs, desirably with as little selection bias favoring the lack of treatment as possible. **Table 1** reviews published long-term follow-up studies using Kaplan-Meier life table analyses and univariate or multivariate models to identify risk factors predicting AVM rupture during follow-up. The average annual

AVM rupture rate is approximately 2% to 4% in most of these cohorts, but the rate varies highly depending on various risk factors. When estimating the lifetime risk of hemorrhage from an untreated AVM based on these figures, it is important to remember that the annual risk of rupture should not be multiplied with the (estimated) remaining years at risk; the proper formula for the cumulative probability of hemorrhage is $1-(1-p)^t$, where $p$ = the annual probability of hemorrhage and $t$ = time at risk in years, given that the risk remains constant over time. Unfortunately, to make things more complicated, the risk of rupture in untreated AVMs seems not to be stable over the years. Many studies with sufficiently long average follow-up times suggest a change in the hemorrhage rate over time, the rate being highest during the first years after the diagnosis.[17,22,27,41] This observation also explains why studies with short follow-up durations generally report higher average annual rupture rates than those with longer follow-up periods (see **Table 1**). This phenomenon is not likely explained by drop-out bias during long follow-ups, since it was also observed in the authors' cohort with almost no patients lost to follow-up during the average observation period of 13.5 years (up to 53 years; the follow-up data were 98.7% complete in a cohort of 238 patients).[41] One hypothetical explanation is some kind of hemodynamic destabilization of the AVM around the time it becomes symptomatic.

Previous rupture has been the most consistent factor predicting AVM rupture during follow-up,[15,16,22,24,26,27,41] although even this is not a universal finding.[18,36,42] In the authors' series, hemorrhagic presentation tripled the risk of hemorrhage during the first 5 years after the diagnosis as compared with unruptured AVMs.[41] Deep and infratentorial AVM locations, sometimes together with deep venous drainage pattern, are consistently observed risk factors for subsequent hemorrhage,[22,23,27,36] and they have also been found as independent risk factors in multivariate models.[22,36,41] AVM size is a particularly interesting case. As mentioned previously, small AVM size is commonly associated with hemorrhagic presentation, which does not automatically imply that it predicts future hemorrhage as well. In fact, small AVM size has not predicted hemorrhage in any study using multivariate models. In contrast, large AVM size has been a risk factor for subsequent rupture in 4 different cohorts.[18,36,41,43] On the other hand, many groups have not found AVM size to have any effect.[15,22,24,26,27,44] Age and sex have been inconsistently reported to influence the rupture frequency,[17,22,27,41] and their role remains obscure at present.

**Table 1**
**Follow-up studies estimating the risk of arteriovenous malformations rupture using Kaplan-Meier analysis and univariate and/or multivariate statistical models to find out various risk factors for subsequent hemorrhage**

| Follow-Up (Mean, Years) | Follow-Up (Total Person-Years) | N | Cohort Nationality | Average Annual Rupture Rate | Risk Factors for Hemorrhage (Univariate Analysis) | Risk Factors for Hemorrhage (Multivariate Models) | Reference |
|---|---|---|---|---|---|---|---|
| 13.5 | 3222 | 238 | Finnish | 2.4% | Young age, previous rupture, deep location, infratentorial location, deep venous drainage | Previous rupture, deep location, infratentorial location, large size (>5 cm) | 41 |
| 10.5 | 578 | 55 | Japanese | 2.3% | Large size, deep or infratentorial location | N/A | 18 |
| 10.4 | 217 | 2257 | UK | 2% | Previous rupture, old age | N/A | 15 |
| 4.0 | 3156 | 790 | US | 2.1% | Previous rupture | Previous rupture | 24 |
| 3.1 | 1205 | 390 | Canadian | 3.2% | Deep location, large size (>3 cm), deep venous drainage, deep feeders, associated aneurysms, single draining vein | Deep location, large size (>3 cm) | 36 |
| 2.9 | 892 | 305 | Japanese | 4.7% | Previous rupture; only in previously ruptured: young age, female sex, deep location | Only in previously ruptured: young age, female sex, deep location | 27 |
| 2.8 | 1932 | 678 | Canadian | 4.6% | Previous rupture, deep venous drainage, associated aneurysms | Previous rupture | 30 |
| 2.3 | 1412 | 622 | US | 2.8% | Old age, previous rupture, deep location, deep venous drainage | Old age, previous rupture, deep location, deep venous drainage | 22 |
| 0.9 | 239 | 281 | US | 8.8% | Previous rupture | Previous rupture, male sex, deep venous drainage | 26 |

The cohorts are listed according to the mean length of follow-up.

## SUMMARY

Brain AVMs are rare vascular lesions, with the incidence rate of approximately 1 case per 100,000 person–years, although the incidence of unruptured and asymptomatic AVMs seems to be gradually increasing as the availability of noninvasive imaging is becoming more widespread. The most common form of presentation of an AVM, however, is still hemorrhagic stroke, followed by epileptic seizures, headache, and focal neurologic deficits. Although intracranial hemorrhage caused by an AVM may be somewhat less dangerous than most other forms of hemorrhagic stroke, AVM hemorrhage typically affects young adults and even children, and untreated AVMs are associated with significant long-term excess mortality. Average annual risk of rupture of an untreated AVM is between 2% and 4%, although the risk is highly variable depending on the characteristics of the lesion. Factors associated with increased risk of hemorrhage include previous rupture, deep and infratentorial location, and possibly large size.

## REFERENCES

1. van Beijnum J, van der Worp HB, Schippers HM, et al. Familial occurrence of brain arteriovenous malformations: a systematic review. J Neurol Neurosurg Psychiatry 2007;78(11):1213–7.
2. Waltimo O. The change in size of intracranial arteriovenous malformations. J Neurol Sci 1973;19(1): 21–7.
3. Pasqualin A, Vivenza C, Rosta L, et al. Spontaneous disappearance of intracranial arteriovenous malformations. Acta Neurochir (Wien) 1985;76:50–7.
4. Kader A, Goodrich JT, Sonstein WJ, et al. Recurrent cerebral arteriovenous malformations after negative postoperative angiograms. J Neurosurg 1996;85(1): 14–8.
5. Lee SK, Vilela P, Willinsky R, et al. Spontaneous regression of cerebral arteriovenous malformations: clinical and angiographic analysis with review of the literature. Neuroradiology 2002;44(1):11–6.
6. Buis DR, van den Berg R, Lycklama G, et al. Spontaneous regression of brain arteriovenous malformations—a clinical study and a systematic review of the literature. J Neurol 2004;251(11):1375–82.
7. ApSimon HT, Reef H, Phadke RV, et al. A population-based study of brain arteriovenous malformation: long-term treatment outcomes. Stroke 2002;33(12): 2794–800.
8. Brown RD Jr, Wiebers DO, Torner JC, et al. Incidence and prevalence of intracranial vascular malformations in Olmsted County, Minnesota, 1965 to 1992. Neurology 1996;46(4):949–52.
9. Hillman J. Population-based analysis of arteriovenous malformation treatment. J Neurosurg 2001; 95(4):633–7.
10. Stapf C, Mast H, Sciacca RR, et al. The New York Island's AVM study: design, study progress, and initial results. Stroke 2003;34(5):e29–33.
11. Al-Shahi R, Fang JS, Lewis SC, et al. Prevalence of adults with brain arteriovenous malformations: a community-based study in Scotland using capture–recapture analysis. J Neurol Neurosurg Psychiatry 2002;73(5):547–51.
12. Weber F, Knopf H. Incidental findings in magnetic resonance imaging of the brains of healthy young men. J Neurol Sci 2006;240:81–4.
13. Vlak MH, Algra A, Brandenburg R, et al. Prevalence of unruptured intracranial aneurysms, with emphasis on sex, age, comorbidity, country, and time period: a systematic review and meta-analysis. Lancet Neurol 2011;10:626–36.
14. Abad JM, Alvarez F, Manrique M, et al. Cerebral arteriovenous malformations. Comparative results of surgical vs conservative treatment in 112 cases. J Neurosurg Sci 1983;27(3):203–10.
15. Crawford PM, West CR, Chadwick DW, et al. Arteriovenous malformations of the brain: natural history in unoperated patients. J Neurol Neurosurg Psychiatry 1986;49(1):1–10.
16. Forster DM, Steiner L, Håkanson S. Arteriovenous malformations of the brain. A long-term clinical study. J Neurosurg 1972;37(5):562–70.
17. Itoyama Y, Uemura S, Ushio Y, et al. Natural course of unoperated intracranial arteriovenous malformations: study of 50 cases. J Neurosurg 1989;71(6):805–9.
18. Mine S, Hirai S, Ono J, et al. Risk factors for poor outcome of untreated arteriovenous malformation. J Clin Neurosci 2000;7(6):503–6.
19. Ondra SL, Troupp H, George ED, et al. The natural history of symptomatic arteriovenous malformations of the brain: a 24-year follow-up assessment. J Neurosurg 1990;73(3):387–91.
20. Laakso A, Dashti R, Seppänen J, et al. Long-term excess mortality in 623 patients with brain arteriovenous malformations. Neurosurgery 2008;63(2): 244–53 [discussion: 253–5].
21. Langer DJ, Lasner TM, Hurst RW, et al. Hypertension, small size, and deep venous drainage are associated with risk of hemorrhagic presentation of cerebral arteriovenous malformations. Neurosurgery 1998;42(3):481–6 [discussion: 487–9].
22. Stapf C, Mast H, Sciacca RR, et al. Predictors of hemorrhage in patients with untreated brain arteriovenous malformation. Neurology 2006;66(9):1350–5.
23. Fults D, Kelly DL Jr. atural history of arteriovenous malformations of the brain: a clinical study. Neurosurgery 1984;15(5):658–62.
24. Halim AX, Johnston SC, Singh V, et al. ongitudinal risk of intracranial hemorrhage in patients with

arteriovenous malformation of the brain within a defined population. Stroke 2004;35(7):1697–702.

25. Kader A, Young WL, Pile-Spellman J, et al. The influence of hemodynamic and anatomic factors on hemorrhage from cerebral arteriovenous malformations. Neurosurgery 1994;34(5):801–7 [discussion: 807–8].

26. Mast H, Young WL, Koennecke HC, et al. Risk of spontaneous haemorrhage after diagnosis of cerebral arteriovenous malformation. Lancet 1997; 350(9084):1065–8.

27. Yamada S, Takagi Y, Nozaki K, et al. Risk factors for subsequent hemorrhage in patients with cerebral arteriovenous malformations. J Neurosurg 2007; 107(5):965–72.

28. Al-Shahi R, Warlow C. A systematic review of the frequency and prognosis of arteriovenous malformations of the brain in adults. Brain 2001;124:1900–26.

29. van Beijnum J, Lovelock CE, Cordonnier C, et al. Outcome after spontaneous and arteriovenous malformation-related intracerebral haemorrhage: population-based studies. Brain 2009;132:537–43.

30. da Costa L, Wallace MC, Ter Brugge KG, et al. The natural history and predictive features of hemorrhage from brain arteriovenous malformations. Stroke 2009;40(1):100–5.

31. Brown RD Jr, Wiebers DO, Torner JC, et al. Frequency of intracranial hemorrhage as a presenting symptom and subtype analysis: a population-based study of intracranial vascular malformations in Olmsted Country, Minnesota. J Neurosurg 1996; 85(1):29–32.

32. Choi JH, Mast H, Sciacca RR, et al. Clinical outcome after first and recurrent hemorrhage in patients with untreated brain arteriovenous malformation. Stroke 2006;37(5):1243–7.

33. Hartmann A, Mast H, Mohr JP, et al. Morbidity of intracranial hemorrhage in patients with cerebral arteriovenous malformation. Stroke 1998;29(5):931–4.

34. Laakso A, Dashti R, Juvela S, et al. Risk of hemorrhage in patients with untreated Spetzler-Martin grade IV and V arteriovenous malformations: a long-term follow-up study in 63 patients. Neurosurgery 2011;68(2):372–7 [discussion: 378].

35. Duong DH, Young WL, Vang MC, et al. Feeding artery pressure and venous drainage pattern are primary determinants of hemorrhage from cerebral arteriovenous malformations. Stroke 1998;29(6):1167–76.

36. Stefani MA, Porter PJ, terBrugge KG, et al. Large and deep brain arteriovenous malformations are associated with risk of future hemorrhage. Stroke 2002;33(5):1220–4.

37. Khaw AV, Mohr JP, Sciacca RR, et al. Association of infratentorial brain arteriovenous malformations with hemorrhage at initial presentation. Stroke 2004; 35(3):660–3.

38. Forsgren L. Prospective incidence study and clinical characterization of seizures in newly referred adults. Epilepsia 1990;31(3):292–301.

39. Crawford PM, West CR, Shaw MD, et al. Cerebral arteriovenous malformations and epilepsy: factors in the development of epilepsy. Epilepsia 1986; 27(3):270–5.

40. Turjman F, Massoud TF, Sayre JW, et al. Epilepsy associated with cerebral arteriovenous malformations: a multivariate analysis of angioarchitectural characteristics. AJNR Am J Neuroradiol 1995; 16(2):345–50.

41. Hernesniemi JA, Dashti R, Juvela S, et al. Natural history of brain arteriovenous malformations: a long-term follow-up study of risk of hemorrhage in 238 patients. Neurosurgery 2008;63(5):823–9 [discussion: 829–31].

42. Graf CJ, Perret GE, Torner JC. Bleeding from cerebral arteriovenous malformations as part of their natural history. J Neurosurg 1983;58(3):331–7.

43. Guidetti B, Delitala A. Intracranial arteriovenous malformations. Conservative and surgical treatment. J Neurosurg 1980;53(2):149–52.

44. Brown RD Jr, Wiebers DO, Forbes G, et al. The natural history of unruptured intracranial arteriovenous malformations. J Neurosurg 1988;68(3):352–7.

# Dural Arteriovenous Fistulas: Epidemiology and Clinical Presentation

Kaisorn L. Chaichana, MD, Alexander L. Coon, MD,
Rafael J. Tamargo, MD, Judy Huang, MD*

## KEYWORDS

- Dural arteriovenous fistulas (DAVF)
- Dural arteriovenous malformations (DAVM) • Endovascular
- Epidemiology • Surgery

Dural arteriovenous fistulas (DAVFs) are anomalous connections between dural arteries and venous sinuses and/or cortical veins.[1,2] These relatively rare arteriovenous shunts can occur within the spine or intracranially.[1,2] Intracranial DAVFs can cause ischemic deficits and/or hemorrhage, which can lead to significant morbidity and mortality.[1,3,4] These potentially severe consequences that are associated with a subset of these lesions underscore the need for understanding the natural history, prompt diagnosis, and treatment of these lesions to improve patient outcomes.[2,4] This review aims to characterize the etiology, epidemiology, clinical presentation, diagnostic evaluation, and clinical course of patients with intracranial DAVFs.

## HISTORICAL PERSPECTIVE

The concept of a DAVF has evolved over more than a century. In 1873, Rizzoli described the presence of a cranial DAVF.[5] He described the presence of a dural-based "arteriovenous aneurysm" that passed through the wall of the skull in a 9-year-old girl with symptoms of seizures and pulsatile occipital swelling.[5] The girl's postmortem examination revealed direct communication between the hypertrophic branches of the occipital artery and the transverse sinus.[5] In 1931, Sachs and Tonnis were the first to describe the angiographic

appearance of a DAVF[6]; they described the presence of direct connections between the meningeal arteries and the venous system within the dura.[6]

These lesions were considered congenital, benign lesions until the 1970s. In the late 1970s, Castaigne and Djindjian proposed an acquired etiology, suggesting that DAVFs develop from the opening of microshunts and/or angiogenesis within the dura between meningeal arteries and veins.[7] The putative benign nature of these lesions was challenged principally by Cognard and colleagues,[8–10] who proposed that the nature of these lesions depended on the degree of cortical venous drainage.[8–10] Since these early studies there have been numerous studies describing the angiographic and magnetic resonance imaging (MRI) features, clinical characteristics, and clinical course of DAVFs.[11–14] The literature contains reports using dural arteriovenous malformation (AVM) as the terminology for these lesions, to distinguish them from pial AVMs. Here, the authors use the term DAVF rather than dural AVM or DAVM, as they have a distinct pathophysiology from parenchymal AVMs.

## EPIDEMIOLOGY

DAVFs present at a mean age of 50 to 60 years, but individual presentation is highly heterogeneous.[9,15,16] In the past, DAVFs were relatively

Financial disclosures/conflicts: None.
Cerebrovascular Neurosurgery, The Johns Hopkins Hospital, Department of Neurosurgery, Johns Hopkins University School of Medicine, 600 North Wolfe Street, Meyer 8-181, Baltimore, MD 21287, USA
* Corresponding author.
E-mail address: jhuang24@jhmi.edu

neurosurgery.theclinics.com

uncommon, but are now being diagnosed with increased frequency.[17,18] This increased frequency of incidentally diagnosed DAVFs has been attributed to the wide availability of MRI.[17,18] These lesions account for approximately 10% to 15% of intracranial vascular malformations.[14,17] Among supratentorial and infratentorial vascular malformations, they account for 6% and 35% of lesions, respectively.[14,17] These lesions seem to have no gender preponderance, but several studies have reported an increased incidence of hemorrhage in men in comparison with women.[19] No linkages to family history or genetics have been identified.

## ETIOLOGY

The cause of DAVFs is not always clear. Most of these lesions are believed to initiate from thrombosis of a dural venous sinus.[2,10,20–22] This occlusion causes venous congestion and subsequent venous hypertension.[2,21] Over time, this increased venous pressure dilates small capillaries, which open direct shunts between dural arteries and veins.[21,23,24] This creates DAVFs.[21,23,24] These fistulas will initially drain into larger venous sinuses.[2,23,24] However, with increased venous pressure, the veins will undergo remodeling with hyaline deposition and intimal proliferation.[2,23,24] This remodeling will cause blood to reflux into the cortical veins instead of solely flowing into the venous sinuses.[2,23,24] With progressive remodeling, drainage into the venous sinuses will be completely obstructed and will rely on cortical venous reflux for drainage.[2,23,24]

Increased cortical venous reflux in a retrograde direction will lead to cortical venous hypertension and subsequent cortical venous remodeling.[21] This process can result in intracranial hemorrhage (ICH) or parenchymal ischemia.[3,4,25] ICH is thought to occur from rupture of fragile parenchymal veins. These veins become fragile because of the increased pressure from retrograde venous reflux. Parenchymal ischemia is thought to occur from venous congestion.[4,26,27] This congestion and venous hypertension prevents adequate arterial delivery of oxygen and removal of metabolic byproducts within the surrounding parenchyma.[4,26,27] In exceedingly rare circumstances, venous hypertension can cause venous stasis within the DAVF.[4] This stasis can lead to secondary venous thrombosis, which can spontaneously obliterate the draining vein and resolve the DAVF.[4]

Several antecedent events have been cited as causing the development of DAVFs. Besides incidentally, the most commonly referenced preceding event is head trauma, which can occur with or without skull fractures.[19,23,24] Other preceding events that have been reported include craniotomy,

acupuncture, cerebral infarction, hormonal alterations observed in pregnancy and menopause, increased systemic thrombotic activity, otitis, sinusitis, and tumors, especially meningiomas.[19,23,24] Regardless of the actual antecedent event, decreased flow within a dural venous sinus or vein seems to play a critical role in the development of DAVFs.[19,23,24]

Carotid-cavernous fistulas (CCFs) are typically considered distinct from most other intracranial DAVFs, and are discussed by Pradilla and colleagues elsewhere in this issue.[28] CCFs are typically divided into direct or indirect fistulas.[1] Direct or high-flow fistulas are caused by either trauma (blunt or penetrating) or rupture of an intracavernous carotid artery aneurysm.[1] These events create a direct communication between the cavernous carotid artery and the cavernous sinus. Indirect or low-flow fistulas typically occur spontaneously or by occlusion of the cavernous sinus.[28] These events create a connection typically between branches of the external carotid artery and the cavernous sinus via dural arteries and veins.[28] This creates an indirect connection between the carotid artery and the cavernous sinus.[28] Indirect CCFs behave similarly to the intracranial DAVFs discussed here.[28]

## CLINICAL CHARACTERISTICS
### Presentation

Patients with DAVFs typically present with symptoms at a mean age of 50 to 60 years.[1,9,19] In recent years, with the widespread availability of MRI, there has been an increased frequency of incidentally discovered DAVFs. Nonetheless, most DAVFs are discovered when patients develop symptoms related to their fistula.[1,4,19] Symptoms associated with DAVFs highly depend on the characteristics of the venous outflow.[1,16,19,29] These symptoms can be due to either increased dural sinus drainage or the development of cortical venous hypertension.[1,4,16,19,30]

Symptoms associated with increased dural sinus drainage depend on the location of venous drainage.[1,9,16,19] Anterior fossa lesions are typically supplied by ethmoidal arteries and drain into the cavernous sinus.[1,16,31,32] Because of their proximity to the orbit, these DAVFs therefore typically present with ocular symptoms including proptosis, chemosis, ophthalmoplegia, decreased visual acuity, or retro-orbital pain.[1,4,16,31,32] Middle fossa lesions commonly drain into the transverse or sigmoid sinus, which is in close proximity to the auditory apparatus.[1,16,31,32] These fistulas typically cause symptoms of pulsatile tinnitus.[1,16,31,32] Fistulas that drain into the superior sagittal sinus or deep venous system produce symptoms of global venous congestion and long-term intracranial hypertension, and may manifest with symptoms of hydrocephalus, papilledema, seizures, or dementia.[4,8,9,33–35] Brainstem DAVFs, though less common than the other locations, can present with cranial neuropathies and/or quadriparesis.[4,36]

Besides location of sinus drainage, patient presentation highly depends on whether cortical venous hypertension is present.[1,9,16,25,29,37] The presence of cortical venous hypertension typically causes more severe symptoms, including ICH and neurologic deficits.[1,9,25,29] ICH typically occurs within the parenchyma and can also occur in the subarachnoid or subdural space.[25,37] ICH is believed to result from rupture of fragile parenchymal veins that have been arterialized secondary to cortical venous reflux and hypertension.[25,37] Blood will be distributed within the parenchyma, or subdural and/or subarachnoid spaces, depending on where the vein ruptures.[25,37] The overall hemorrhage rate has been documented as being 2% per year but depends on the degree of cortical venous reflux.[25,37] In addition to ICH, neurologic deficits can occur in patients with DAVF and cortical venous hypertension.[4,29] These deficits include progressive dementia, seizures, parkinsonism, and other focal neurologic deficits including aphasia, alexia, weakness, paraesthesias, and ataxia.[4,8,34,35] In more severe cases, signs of increased intracranial pressure may be present including headaches, papilledema, upgaze palsy, and mental status changes.[4,8,29,33] These neurologic deficits are believed to result from the effects of venous congestion and cerebral ischemia from progressively arterialized cortical venous drainage.[26,27,29] Iwama and colleagues[26] and Kuroda and colleagues[27] performed positron emission tomography (PET) to evaluate the hemodynamics and metabolic patterns in patients with DAVFs before and after treatment. Both these studies demonstrated decreased blood flow and increased oxygen extraction ratios in the regions surrounding the site of cortical venous drainage. These PET findings consistent with cerebral ischemia improved in most patients after either surgical or endovascular treatment of their DAVF.[26,27]

## Clinical Course

DAVFs typically follow a progressive clinical course,[9,10,16] depending on the presence and development of progressive cortical venous reflux.[4,9,10,37] DAVFs without cortical venous reflux usually present incidentally or with signs of increased dural drainage, such as tinnitus.[1,16,31,32] These fistulas typically have a benign natural history.[3,38] Satomi and colleagues[38] performed the largest study thus far in patients without cortical venous drainage. Among 68 patients without cortical venous drainage who were conservatively followed, only 1 (1%) patient suffered an ICH and no patients developed neurologic deficits at a mean follow-up time of 27.9 months.[38] In addition, 50 patients had follow-up catheter angiography at last follow-up, and only 2 (4%) developed cortical venous drainage.[38] This and other studies have shown that DAVFs without cortical venous drainage on digital subtraction angiography at the time of diagnosis have a low risk of causing ICH or neurologic deficits.[38] However, a small subset of these lesions, albeit extremely rarely, can develop cortical venous drainage and subsequent venous stenosis, thrombosis, increased arterial flow, and/or de novo fistula formation.[10,38] This progression has a higher risk of ICH or neurologic deficits.[4,10]

DAVFs with cortical venous drainage have a higher propensity to cause ICH or neurologic deficits (Fig. 1).[3,4,9,10,25,30,37] In 1999 Duffau and colleagues[39] were the first to document a high risk of bleeding for patients with DAVFs and cortical venous drainage. These investigators evaluated 20 patients who presented with ICH secondary to DAVFs and venous reflux, and found that 35% of these patients incurred ICH at a mean time of 20 days after diagnosis.[39] More recently in 2002, van Dijk and colleagues[30] described 20 patients with partially treated or conservatively followed DAVFs with cortical venous drainage for a mean period of 4.3 years. At last follow-up, 16 (80%) patients developed ICH (25%) or ischemic deficits (66%).[30] An annual risk of 8.1% was calculated for ICH and 6.9% for neurologic deficits.[30] DAVFs that occur along the tentorium make up the greatest percentage of lesions with cortical venous reflux.[40] Not surprisingly, these tentorially located DAVFs are also thought to have the highest risk of hemorrhage.[40] Awad and colleagues[41] performed a meta-analysis on 360 tentorial DAVFs, and 31 of 32 cases with cortical venous drainage presented with hemorrhage or nonhemorrhagic stroke. Besides cortical venous drainage and tentorial location, other risk factors predisposing to ICH or neurologic deficit include presence of a venous varix and lesions involving the deep drainage system.[3,42]

It is well known that among patients with DAVFs, patients with cortical venous reflux have an increased risk of hemorrhage or nonhemorrhagic neurologic deficits.[9,10,19,25,30,37] However, among patients with cortical venous drainage, there may be a heterogeneous risk of incurring an ICH or neurologic deficit.[39,43] Patients who present with ICH or neurologic deficits have an even higher risk of developing recurrent hemorrhage or progressive

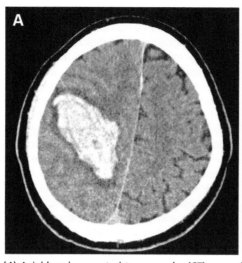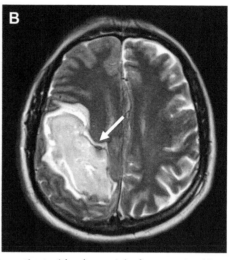

Fig. 1. (A) Axial head computed tomography (CT) scan of a patient with a large right frontoparietal intraparenchymal hematoma, which was later found to be caused by a dural arteriovenous fistula (DAVF). (B) Axial T2-weighted magnetic resonance image (MRI) of the same patient. This image also demonstrates a large inatraparenchymal hematoma; however, there is now a prominent flow void on the medial portion of the hematoma (arrow).

deficits.[25,43] Soderman and colleagues[2] evaluated 85 patients with a DAVF and varying degrees of cortical venous reflux. Patients who presented with ICH had a significant higher annual risk of hemorrhage in comparison with patients without ICH (7.4% vs 1.5%). Strom and colleagues[43] analyzed 28 patients with partially treated or untreated DAVF with cortical venous drainage. Eleven patients presented with symptoms of cortical venous hypertension (ICH or neurologic deficits), whereas 17 patients presented incidentally or with symptoms of increased sinus drainage.[43] Patients presenting with symptoms of cortical venous hypertension had an annual hemorrhage risk of 7.6%, whereas patients without these symptoms had an annual risk of 1.4%.[43] Furthermore, patients with symptomatic venous hypertension had an annual deficit risk of 11.4% as compared with 0% for patients without symptoms.[43] The annual mortality rate was 3.8% for patients with symptomatic venous hypertension whereas it was 0% for patients without symptoms.[43] All these comparisons were statistically significant.[43] Iwama and colleagues[26] and Kuroda and colleagues[27] independently showed that patients with hemodynamic impairments on PET imaging are more likely to have presented with ICH or neurologic deficits.

## Classification Schemes

Several classification schemes have been devised to depict DAVFs. Arguably the most commonly used classification systems are the Borden-Shucart and Cognard systems (**Table 1**).[9] The

Borden-Shucart grading scale is based on the site of venous drainage (dural sinus and/or cortical vein) if cortical venous drainage is present. In this classification system (types I–III), type I DAVFs drain directly into the dural sinus without cortical venous reflux. Type II DAVFs drain into a dural sinus and also have cortical venous drainage.

Table 1
Most commonly used classification schemes for patients with dural arteriovenous fistulas

| Borden-Shucart Classification | Cognard Classification |
| --- | --- |
| Venous drainage into | Venous drainage into |
| Type I: DVS or MV | Type I: DVS with antegrade flow |
| Type II: DVS with CVR | Type IIa: DVS with retrograde flow |
| Type III: CVR only | Type IIb: DVS with antegrade flow and CVR |
| | Type IIa+b: DVS with retrograde flow and CVR |
| | Type III: CVR only (no ectasia) |
| | Type IV: CVR only (ectasia) |
| | Type V: CVR only (spinal) |

Abbreviations: CVR, cortical venous reflux; DVS, dural venous sinus; MV, meningeal vein.

Type III lesions drain completely into a cortical vein. Patients with a single fistula are subclassified as subtype a, while patients with multiple fistulas are subclassified as subtype b. Patients with type II and III DAVFs in this scheme are at highest risk of ICH and/or neurologic deficits.[16,39]

The Cognard grading scale (type I–V) is based on the direction of dural sinus drainage (antegrade or retrograde), presence of cortical venous drainage (present or absent), and venous outflow architecture (nonectactic cortical vein, ectactic cortical vein, and spinal perimedullary vein).[9] In this grading scale, type I lesions drain antegrade into a dural sinus without cortical venous drainage.[9] Type IIa lesions drain retrograde into a dural sinus without cortical venous drainage, type IIb lesions drain antegrade into a dural sinus with cortical venous drainage, and type IIa+b drain retrograde into a dural sinus with cortical venous drainage.[9] Type III, IV, and V DAVFs all have absent dural sinus drainage, present cortical venous drainage, and varying degrees of venous architecture.[9] Type III, IV, and V DAVFs have nonectactic, ectactic, and spinal perimedullary venous outflow architecture, respectively.[9] In the Cognard system, type IIb to V DAVFs are at highest risk of ICH and/or neurologic deficits.[9,16,39]

It is well documented that patients with high-grade DAVFs (Borden-Shucart type II–III and Cognard IIb–V) have an increased risk of developing symptomatic lesions.[9,39] However, these classification systems do not necessarily identify those at highest risk among those with high-grade lesions.[18] Zipfel and colleagues[18] argue that patients who present with symptomatic DAVFs (ICH or neurologic deficit) have a more aggressive DAVF within these high-risk Borden-Shucart and Cognard groups. These classifications have been given a subgroup classification of being symptomatic if they present with ICH or neurologic deficits and asymptomatic if they are discovered incidentally or present with signs of increased dural sinus drainage.[18] Patients with symptomatic lesions may have a higher risk stratification of causing hemorrhage or ischemic deficits independent of Borden-Shucart or Cognard classification.[18]

## DIAGNOSTIC CRITERIA

The gold standard for diagnosing and classifying DAVFs is catheter angiography.[4,25] Angiography is typically done with conventional 4-vessel injections as well as injection of external carotid arteries depending on DAVF location (**Fig. 2**).[13,25] In most cases, the angiogram will reveal several dural arterial feeders with early drainage into a dural sinus or cortical vein.[4,25] Cerebral angiograms will also assess the degree of cortical venous reflux and venous architecture, which is necessary for classifying DAVFs.[25]

Other modalities besides catheter angiography have been used including computed tomography (CT), CT angiography, MRI, and MR angiography (see **Fig. 1**).[44,45] CT is often used as the initial neuroimaging modality.[44,45] CT is not ideal at identifying DAVFs, but can identify ICH and sometimes areas of ischemia or edema.[44,45] CT angiography is better for identifying DAVFs.[44,45] CT angiography can reveal a dilated vessel in relation to an ICH or calcification with chronically congested veins.[44,45] MRI, especially T2-weighted sequences, can reveal flow voids from draining veins and show

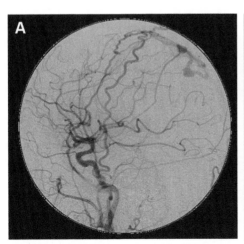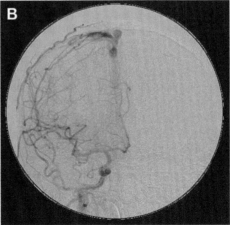

**Fig. 2.** (*A*) Lateral and (*B*) anterior-posterior angiogram after an internal carotid artery (ICA) injection. This angiogram demonstrates a right frontoparietal convexity DAVF with arterial supply from divisions of the middle meningeal artery and transosseous branches from the superficial temporal artery. The drainage is primarily within a lateral parietotemporal vein, consistent with a Borden grade III DAVF.

areas of restricted diffusion or prior infarcts caused by venous hypertension.[44,45] MR angiography, like CT angiography, can reveal dilated vessels.[44,45] Both CT and MR angiography are useful adjuncts to catheter angiography because they can reveal the location of the DAVF in relation to normal brain structures.[44,45] This ability makes these modalities useful for surgical planning as well as for intraoperative navigation, if required.[46] Despite the utility of these less-sensitive modalities, catheter angiography remains the most effective at identifying and classifying DAVFs.[4,25] In fact, there are several case reports documenting catheter angiogram–positive but MRI-negative DAVFs.[4,25]

## SUMMARY

Intracranial DAVFs are relatively uncommon lesions that are assumed to develop from venous thrombosis. Despite their etiology, they represent treatable lesions that can cause significant morbidity and mortality. Their presentation is variable depending on their drainage pattern, degree of cortical venous reflux, and the presence of symptomatic lesions. Patients who have signs of cortical venous drainage and/or already symptomatic from an ICH or nonhemorrhagic deficit are at heightened risk of developing further events. Prompt identification of these clinical and radiographic features remains critical for minimizing the morbidity and mortality of these lesions.

## REFERENCES

1. Kim MS, Han DH, Kwon OK, et al. Clinical characteristics of dural arteriovenous fistula. J Clin Neurosci 2002;9(2):147–55.
2. Soderman M, Pavic L, Edner G, et al. Natural history of dural arteriovenous shunts. Stroke 2008;39(6):1735–9.
3. Brown RD Jr, Wiebers DO, Nichols DA. Intracranial dural arteriovenous fistulae: angiographic predictors of intracranial hemorrhage and clinical outcome in nonsurgical patients. J Neurosurg 1994;81(4):531–8.
4. Lasjaunias P, Chiu M, ter Brugge K, et al. Neurological manifestations of intracranial dural arteriovenous malformations. J Neurosurg 1986;64(5):724–30.
5. Perrini P, Nannini T, Di Lorenzo N. Francesco Rizzoli (1809-1880) and the elusive case of Giulia: the description of an "arteriovenous aneurysm passing through the wall of the skull". Acta Neurochir (Wien) 2007;149(2):191–6 [discussion: 196].
6. Aminoff MJ. Vascular anomalies in the intracranial dura mater. Brain 1973;96(3):601–12.
7. Castaigne P. Rene Djindjian, 1918-1977. Rev Neurol (Paris) 1977;133(12):736–8 [in French].
8. Cognard C, Casasco A, Toevi M, et al. Dural arteriovenous fistulas as a cause of intracranial hypertension due to impairment of cranial venous outflow. J Neurol Neurosurg Psychiatry 1998;65(3):308–16.
9. Cognard C, Gobin YP, Pierot L, et al. Cerebral dural arteriovenous fistulas: clinical and angiographic correlation with a revised classification of venous drainage. Radiology 1995;194(3):671–80.
10. Cognard C, Houdart E, Casasco A, et al. Long-term changes in intracranial dural arteriovenous fistulae leading to worsening in the type of venous drainage. Neuroradiology 1997;39(1):59–66.
11. Brown RD Jr, Wiebers DO, Forbes G, et al. The natural history of unruptured intracranial arteriovenous malformations. J Neurosurg 1988;68(3):352–7.
12. Brown RD Jr, Wiebers DO, Forbes GS. Unruptured intracranial aneurysms and arteriovenous malformations: frequency of intracranial hemorrhage and relationship of lesions. J Neurosurg 1990;73(6):859–63.
13. Houser OW, Baker HL Jr, Rhoton AL Jr, et al. Intracranial dural arteriovenous malformations. Radiology 1972;105(1):55–64.
14. Newton TH, Cronqvist S. Involvement of dural arteries in intracranial arteriovenous malformations. Radiology 1969;93(5):1071–8.
15. Brown RD Jr, Flemming KD, Meyer FB, et al. Natural history, evaluation, and management of intracranial vascular malformations. Mayo Clin Proc 2005;80(2):269–81.
16. Davies MA, TerBrugge K, Willinsky R, et al. The validity of classification for the clinical presentation of intracranial dural arteriovenous fistulas. J Neurosurg 1996;85(5):830–7.
17. Wiebers DO, Whisnant JP, Huston J 3rd, et al. Unruptured intracranial aneurysms: natural history, clinical outcome, and risks of surgical and endovascular treatment. Lancet 2003;362(9378):103–10.
18. Zipfel GJ, Shah MN, Refai D, et al. Cranial dural arteriovenous fistulas: modification of angiographic classification scales based on new natural history data. Neurosurg Focus 2009;26(5):E14.
19. Chung SJ, Kim JS, Kim JC, et al. Intracranial dural arteriovenous fistulas: analysis of 60 patients. Cerebrovasc Dis 2002;13(2):79–88.
20. Houser OW, Campbell JK, Campbell RJ, et al. Arteriovenous malformation affecting the transverse dural venous sinus—an acquired lesion. Mayo Clin Proc 1979;54(10):651–61.
21. Mullan S. Reflections upon the nature and management of intracranial and intraspinal vascular malformations and fistulae. J Neurosurg 1994;80(4):606–16.
22. Pierot L, Chiras J, Duyckaerts C, et al. Intracranial dural arteriovenous fistulas and sinus thrombosis. Report of five cases. J Neuroradiol 1993;20(1):9–18.
23. Chaudhary MY, Sachdev VP, Cho SH, et al. Dural arteriovenous malformation of the major venous sinuses: an acquired lesion. AJNR Am J Neuroradiol 1982;3(1):13–9.

24. Meyer X, Berthezene Y, Ongolo P, et al. Diagnosis of a post-thrombophlebitic dural fistula using MR angiography. J Neuroradiol 1996;23(2):69–73 [in French].

25. Lanzino G, Jensen ME, Kongable GL, et al. Angiographic characteristics of dural arteriovenous malformations that present with intracranial hemorrhage. Acta Neurochir (Wien) 1994;129(3–4):140–5.

26. Iwama T, Hashimoto N, Takagi Y, et al. Hemodynamic and metabolic disturbances in patients with intracranial dural arteriovenous fistulas: positron emission tomography evaluation before and after treatment. J Neurosurg 1997;86(5):806–11.

27. Kuroda S, Furukawa K, Shiga T, et al. Pretreatment and posttreatment evaluation of hemodynamic and metabolic parameters in intracranial dural arteriovenous fistulae with cortical venous reflux. Neurosurgery 2004;54(3):585–91 [discussion: 591–2].

28. Pollock BE, Nichols DA, Garrity JA, et al. Stereotactic radiosurgery and particulate embolization for cavernous sinus dural arteriovenous fistulae. Neurosurgery 1999;45(3):459–66 [discussion: 466–7].

29. Hurst RW, Bagley LJ, Galetta S, et al. Dementia resulting from dural arteriovenous fistulas: the pathologic findings of venous hypertensive encephalopathy. AJNR Am J Neuroradiol 1998;19(7):1267–73.

30. van Dijk JM, terBrugge KG, Willinsky RA, et al. Clinical course of cranial dural arteriovenous fistulas with long-term persistent cortical venous reflux. Stroke 2002;33(5):1233–6.

31. Hashiguchi A, Mimata C, Ichimura H, et al. Venous aneurysm development associated with a dural arteriovenous fistula of the anterior cranial fossa with devastating hemorrhage–case report. Neurol Med Chir (Tokyo) 2007;47(2):70–3.

32. Ito J, Imamura H, Kobayashi K, et al. Dural arteriovenous malformations of the base of the anterior cranial fossa. Neuroradiology 1983;24(3):149–54.

33. Hasumi T, Fukushima T, Haisa T, et al. Focal dural arteriovenous fistula (DAVF) presenting with progressive cognitive impairment including amnesia and alexia. Intern Med 2007;46(16):1317–20.

34. Hirono N, Yamadori A, Komiyama M. Dural arteriovenous fistula: a cause of hypoperfusion-induced intellectual impairment. Eur Neurol 1993;33(1):5–8.

35. Lee PH, Lee JS, Shin DH, et al. Parkinsonism as an initial manifestation of dural arteriovenous fistula. Eur J Neurol 2005;12(5):403–6.

36. Lagares A, Perez-Nunez A, Alday R, et al. Dural arteriovenous fistula presenting as brainstem ischaemia. Acta Neurochir (Wien) 2007;149(9):965–7 [discussion: 967].

37. Malik GM, Pearce JE, Ausman JI, et al. Dural arteriovenous malformations and intracranial hemorrhage. Neurosurgery 1984;15(3):332–9.

38. Satomi J, van Dijk JM, Terbrugge KG, et al. Benign cranial dural arteriovenous fistulas: outcome of conservative management based on the natural history of the lesion. J Neurosurg 2002;97(4):767–70.

39. Duffau H, Lopes M, Janosevic V, et al. Early rebleeding from intracranial dural arteriovenous fistulas: report of 20 cases and review of the literature. J Neurosurg 1999;90(1):78–84.

40. Thompson BG, Doppman JL, Oldfield EH. Treatment of cranial dural arteriovenous fistulae by interruption of leptomeningeal venous drainage. J Neurosurg 1994;80(4):617–23.

41. Awad IA, Little JR, Akarawi WP, et al. Intracranial dural arteriovenous malformations: factors predisposing to an aggressive neurological course. J Neurosurg 1990;72(6):839–50.

42. Willinsky R, Goyal M, terBrugge K, et al. Tortuous, engorged pial veins in intracranial dural arteriovenous fistulas: correlations with presentation, location, and MR findings in 122 patients. AJNR Am J Neuroradiol 1999;20(6):1031–6.

43. Strom RG, Botros JA, Refai D, et al. Cranial dural arteriovenous fistulae: asymptomatic cortical venous drainage portends less aggressive clinical course. Neurosurgery 2009;64(2):241–7 [discussion: 247–8].

44. Meckel S, Maier M, Ruiz DS, et al. MR angiography of dural arteriovenous fistulas: diagnosis and follow-up after treatment using a time-resolved 3D contrast-enhanced technique. AJNR Am J Neuroradiol 2007;28(5):877–84.

45. Noguchi K, Melhem ER, Kanazawa T, et al. Intracranial dural arteriovenous fistulas: evaluation with combined 3D time-of-flight MR angiography and MR digital subtraction angiography. AJR Am J Roentgenol 2004;182(1):183–90.

46. Guo WY, Pan DH, Wu HM, et al. Radiosurgery as a treatment alternative for dural arteriovenous fistulas of the cavernous sinus. AJNR Am J Neuroradiol 1998;19(6):1081–7.

# Historical Perspective of Treatments of Cranial Arteriovenous Malformations and Dural Arteriovenous Fistulas

Geoffrey P. Colby, MD, PhD, Alexander L. Coon, MD,
Judy Huang, MD, Rafael J. Tamargo, MD*

## KEYWORDS

- Intracranial vascular lesions • Arteriovenous malformations
- Dural arteriovenous fistulas

Cerebral arteriovenous malformations (AVMs) and intracranial dural arteriovenous fistulas (DAVFs) represent two important classes of intracranial vascular lesions. This article recalls the history on which current technical advances, including diagnoses, characterization, and treatment, is based. It also describes modern therapeutic options, including microsurgical, endovascular, and radiosurgery techniques.

## INTRODUCTION TO AVMs

Cerebral AVMs are complex, congenital arteriovenous shunts that consist of feeding arteries, an abnormal nidus of vessels, and draining veins. The true pathogenesis of AVMs is unknown and there is currently no animal model that accurately represents the histologic features of human cerebral AVMs. The two main hypotheses for AVM pathogenesis include (1) embryonic agenesis of the capillary system and (2) the retention of a primordial connection between arteries and veins.[1] AVMs are thought to be dynamic and biologically active lesions, rather than static congenital vascular abnormalities. The high-flow state of the lesion also predisposes to arterialization of veins, vascular recruitment, and gliosis of brain tissue within and adjacent to the lesion.[1]

The goal of definitive treatment of cerebral AVMs is complete obliteration of the nidus with preservation of normal neurologic function and elimination of the risk of future hemorrhage. AVM therapy has undergone many changes since the early descriptions of this pathologic entity in the 1700s and 1800s. Modern AVM management requires a multidisciplinary treatment approach. The main three treatment approaches are microsurgery, endovascular embolization, and stereotactic radiosurgery. These treatment options have been used as stand-alone therapies or in combination. The treatments available for AVMs today are based on the development and trialing of numerous techniques and technologies, the history of which is described in this article.

## HISTORICAL PERSPECTIVE OF TREATMENT OF AVMs (PRE-1900)

John Hunter[2] (1728–1793), the Scottish scientist and surgeon, described the clinical characteristics of extracranial AVMs in the mid-1700s, but it was not until Rudolf Virchow[3] (1821–1902), the German

Department of Neurosurgery, The Johns Hopkins University School of Medicine, 600 North Wolfe Street, Baltimore, MD 21287, USA
* Corresponding author.
E-mail address: rtamarg@jhmi.edu

Neurosurg Clin N Am 23 (2012) 15–25
doi:10.1016/j.nec.2011.10.001
1042-3680/12/$ – see front matter © 2012 Elsevier Inc. All rights reserved.

pathologist, in 1863 published *Die Krankhaften Geschwülste*, his three-volume masterpiece on blood vessels, that many of the common intracranial vascular pathologic entities, including AVMs, were described and differentiated. Virchow's book is considered the first landmark in the understanding of AVMs. The first clinicopathological correlate of AVMs likely came in 1888, 25 years after Virchow's publication, when D'Arcy Power[4] (1855–1941), the British surgeon, reported a 20-year-old patient with a right hemiplegia who subsequently died and was found on autopsy to have a left sylvian AVM with an associated massive hemorrhage. The first report of palliative treatment of a true cerebral AVM by ligation of a left parietal feeding artery was by Davide Giordano[5] (1864–1954), the Italian surgeon, in 1889, 26 years after Virchow's publication. Although cerebral AVMs were identified and occasionally treated before 1900, the tools for modern diagnosis, characterization, and treatment of these lesions came about almost exclusively during the 20th century,[6] concurrent with the birth and formalized establishment of cerebrovascular neurosurgery.

### Early Surgical AVM Treatment

In 1928, both Walter Dandy[7] (1886–1946), the American pioneer neurosurgeon, and his mentor Harvey Cushing (1869–1939), the American surgeon and pioneer of neurosurgery, and Percival Bailey[8] (1892–1973), the American neuropathologist and surgeon, independently reported series of AVMs treated before the introduction of angiography, with primarily catastrophic results in both series. In the 1928 article, Dandy described his treatment of eight cases of "arteriovenous aneurysms" at the Johns Hopkins Hospital during surgery for approximately 600 brain tumors during a 5-year span between 1922 and 1926. No successful radical AVM resection was reported out of the 16 cases of Cushing and Bailey or the eight cases of Dandy (**Fig. 1**). At this time, Cushing was quoted as saying that surgical Cushing excision of an AVM was essentially unthinkable secondary to the significant risk of hemorrhage with even surgical exposure of the lesion.[9]

Early surgical management of AVMs consisted of primarily decompressive procedures with goals of relieving elevated intracranial pressure. Ligation of feeding vessels was the next step in AVM surgery. Ligation of the internal carotid artery was reported and thought to result in some patient improvement, although this was only a palliative measure at the time.[7,10] Extracranial vessel ligation was attempted first, and then abandoned for intracranial ligation. Intracranial vessel ligation

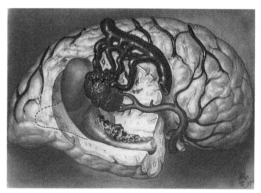

**Fig. 1.** Resection of an AVM performed by Walter Dandy in 1925; drawn by Dorcas Hager Padget. (*From* Dandy WE. Arteriovenous aneurysm of the brain. Arch Surg 1928;17:190–243; with permission. Copyright © 1928 American Medical Association. All rights reserved.)

had mixed results as a sole treatment modality, but it did give rise to the concept for embolization procedures.

Ultimately, Herbert Olivecrona (1891–1980), the surgeon regarded as the founder of Swedish neurosurgery, developed the surgical techniques that rendered AVM excision a reasonable treatment option for small to midsize AVMs that did not involve eloquent areas of brain. He was the first to successfully remove a cerebellar AVM on May 5, 1932, in a 37 year-old male. By 1954, Olivecrona had operated on 125 patients with intracranial AVMs.[11] He achieved complete resection in 81 of these cases, with a remarkably low mortality rate of 9%. He introduced the technique of ligating superficial feeding vessels and then working in a circumferential fashion until the deep portion of the AVM was dissected and separated from the brain. The AVM draining veins were ligated as a final step. Gazi Yasargil[9] (born 1925), the Turkish scientist and neurosurgeon, subsequently compiled information from the literature on 500 AVM patients who were treated between 1932 and 1957, and reported that operative mortality for "small" AVMs was 5% and for "moderate-size" AVMs was 10%. Surgeons such as Wilder Penfield (1891–1976) and Theodore Erickson (1906–1986), Lyle French (1915–2004) and Shelley Chou (1924–2001), and Charles Drake (1920–1998) all reported good early results with AVM surgery,[6] each with some modifications of the techniques introduced by Olivecrona.

## DEVELOPMENT OF NEUROIMAGING

Diagnosis of AVMs before the introduction of cerebral angiography was essentially happenstance.

There were no opportunities for the physician to clinically diagnose an AVM other than a jacksonian seizure and this finding was clearly not specific to AVMs. AVMs were discovered in some patients taken to the operating room for intracerebral hemorrhage or elevated intracranial pressure, but this finding was unexpected at the time of surgery. The subsequent advances in AVM treatment beyond surgery depended on the ability to visualize these lesions radiologically with angiography and tomography.

In the 1920s, Antonio Caetano de Abreu Freire Egas Moniz (1874–1955), the Portuguese neurologist, attempted visualization of intracranial vessels by injecting bromides into the carotid artery of patients. In his sixth patient, the intracranial vessels were barely visualized for the first time; however, the patient developed carotid thrombosis and subsequently died.[12] Following this adverse outcome, Egas Moniz consulted with his staff and, after great debate, continued his investigations but used iodides rather than bromides.[12] On the third case in June of 1927, Egas Moniz was able to visualize portions of the internal carotid artery in the sylvian fissure, thus performing the first successful cerebral angiogram.[13] Once the technique was further refined with better tolerated contrast agents and better imaging systems, cerebral angiography was a major advance for the diagnosis and understanding of AVMs. Today this technique is crucial for the direct and accurate visualization of normal and abnormal cerebral blood vessels in patients with AVMs and other cerebral vascular lesions.

The era of modern neuroimaging was launched in the 1970s with the invention of the noninvasive modalities CT scanning and MRI. The first clinical CT scan on a patient was performed on October 1, 1971, at Atkinson Morley's Hospital in England and the first clinical MRI on July 3, 1977, at Downstate Medical Center in New York. These imaging techniques are essential tools for determining the anatomic location of an AVM. In the 1990s, the development of functional MRI and diffusion tensor imaging further advanced cerebral AVM management by helping to map eloquent areas of brain and their relationship to the lesion.[14–16] Given that sensorimotor and speech centers can be translocated from typical locations in patients with AVMs,[1] these preoperative functional mapping studies are important. All of these imaging modalities can be of great clinical value in the pretreatment assessment of patients with AVMs and they should be used to predict and avoid postoperative deficits.

Intraoperative imaging is also of importance to the neurosurgeon during the resection of an AVM. Intraoperative digital subtraction angiography is an established adjunct tool during the microsurgical treatment of cerebral AVMs.[1,17–21] Intraoperative angiography can evaluate for complete extirpation of the lesion, localize small AVMs, find missing or "hidden" feeding vessels, detect AVM in a patient undergoing evacuation of a hematoma, and evaluate the real-time hemodynamics of the lesion. Unexpected residual AVM is shown in 3.7% to 27.3% of intraoperative digital subtraction angiograms during AVM resection cases.[22] Intraoperative fluorescence video angiography using indocyanine green (ICG) is another technique used in recent years to assist in AVM microsurgical resection.[22–24] ICG is a safe, rapid, and noninvasive tool that is helpful for intraoperative evaluation of blood vessels visible in the surgical field. For AVMs, ICG is used to distinguish AVM vessels from normal vessels and arteries from veins.

### The Birth of Microsurgery

Microsurgical extirpation of cerebral AVMs is an often lengthy and highly choreographed surgical process that requires meticulous and extensive dissection. The introduction of the operative microscope in 1960s and the resulting development of microsurgical instruments and microsurgical techniques significantly advanced the efficacy and safety of AVM surgery. In 1966, J. Lawrence Pool (1906–2004) the American neurosurgeon, and R.P. Colton,[25] reported the first use of the operating microscope in an aneurysm patient. In 1969, Yasargil[26] reported a series of AVM resections in 14 patients using microsurgical techniques. This was the first microsurgical AVM series, and his results were excellent. Surgeons, including Hans Pia (1921–1986), Charles Wilson (born 1929), Leonard Malis (1919–2005), Bennett Stein (born 1931), Dwight Parkinson (1916–2005), Thoralf Sundt (1930–1992), and Helge Nornes (born 1930), are other standout pioneers who further developed the microsurgical treatment of AVMs.[6] During the ensuing decades, up to the modern time, dedicated cerebrovascular surgeons have advanced AVM microsurgery surgery so that small-to-medium size AVMs, particularly those in noneloquent cortex, can be excised with little to no morbidity and mortality.[6,27,28] In addition to enhancing the surgeon's operative ability to perform the AVM resection, the microscope also improved the learning curve for the neurosurgical trainees.[6]

Another important development in surgical instrumentation that assisted the treatment of AVMs was the introduction of bipolar coagulation by Leonard Malis (1919–1995).[29] The availability of improved aneurysm clips, which can be used for temporary clipping, feeding vessel ligation, and obliteration of feeding vessels aneurysms, also advanced AVM surgery.[6]

## THE DEVELOPMENT OF AVM CLASSIFICATION SCHEMES AND THE NATURAL HISTORY OF AVMs

The significant variability of their gross appearance and the complex structure of the vessels in AVMs made early attempts at classification and description of these lesions difficult and confusing. Cushing and Bailey[8] described these "angiomatous malformations" as venous or arterial in nature, primarily based on whether the surface of the lesion appeared more like a tangle of veins or arteries. Dandy[7] preferred the term "arteriovenous aneurysm."

The development of useful classification schemes became important for the preoperative selection of patients with AVMs, particularly with regard to surgical risk. Alfred Luessenhop (1926–2009) and Thomas Gennarelli[30] formulated an early anatomic grading scheme to correspond to the degree of surgical difficulty for total obliteration. This scheme was based on the number of named arterial feeders—those with "anatomic constancy and size to have acquired a generally accepted nomenclature."[30] The investigators mentioned the importance of the AVM location, but this was not considered a major surgical risk factor. Robert Spetzler and Neil Martin[27] developed the next important AVM classification scheme based on lesion size, venous drainage, and eloquence of involved brain. It is currently the most widely used system for predicting the surgical risk of AVM treatment.[31–33] Various modifications of the scheme by Spetzler and Martin have been reported.[31–33] These modifications are described by Dr Lawton elsewhere in this issue.

Understanding the natural history of AVMs, particularly the risk of hemorrhage, has helped guide the indications for therapeutic management of AVMs over the years. In the first half of the 1900s, not much was known about the natural history of these lesions, and they were usually only discovered after a bleed or a seizure. In 1966, George Perret and Hiro Nishioka[34] reported an analysis of 545 cases of cerebral AVMs and fistulae from the Cooperative Study of Intracranial Aneurysms and Subarachnoid Hemorrhage, and found a hemorrhage rate of 1.5% per year. Numerous later series, such as those by Crawford and colleagues,[35] John Jane Sr, and colleagues.[36] Robert Wilkins,[37] and Stephen Ondra and colleagues[38] suggested

that the annualized risk of hemorrhage is between 2% to 4% per year. The study by Ondra and Troupp[38] was particularly useful because it included a single population of patients with centralized medical care and the mean follow-up was 23.7 years. The studies by Ondra[38] and Crawford[35] also demonstrated that 6 months after a bleed, the risk of hemorrhage is the same for patients with prior hemorrhage and for patients who have never had a hemorrhage. This information, plus the data that a 10% to 15% mortality rate and an additional 20% to 30% risk of serious morbidity exists with each hemorrhage,[39] provides an impetus to thoroughly evaluate and consider treatment of all patients with AVM, regardless of rupture status.[6] Currently, the annual hemorrhage risk of all AVMs is estimated to be 2.4%, based on the work of Juha Hernesniemi and colleagues,[40] from Helsinki, Finland.

### Endovascular Techniques and AVM Treatment

Much of the groundbreaking early work on endovascular intracranial embolization was geared toward the treatment of aneurysms, although these techniques were subsequently adapted to the treatment of AVMs and other intracranial vascular pathologies.[41] Endovascular techniques for treatment of AVMs largely developed in the early 1960s, with Luessenhop and William Spence (1908–1992)[42] conceptualizing the blockage of hypertrophied, abnormal feeding vessels. This "artificial embolization," as it was called, relied on the embolic material obstructing the enlarged feeding vessels but not penetrating the smaller vessels of the AVM nidus.

Early embolization procedures relied on open surgical approaches and direct puncture of target vessels to introduce catheters and embolic material. As such, they were fraught with the same morbidity and mortality of the open neurosurgical procedures of that time.[41,43] The development of small, flexible catheters was a major technological advance because this allowed the introduction of these instruments and embolic agents from distal sites, obviating direct punctures. Catheters were initially navigated to their target location largely by flow,[41] as is the case with balloon catheters. Balloon catheterization and occlusion of intracranial vessels was described by the Russian neurosurgeon Fedor Serbinenko[44] (1928–2002) in 1974. In 1976, Charles Kerber[45] described a calibrated leak balloon system for flow-directed catheter guidance and administration of contrast and cyanoacrylate embolic material. This idea of using the relatively high flow of abnormal AVM feeding vessels to direct catheters and embolic material was a driving force behind early endovascular AVM treatment.

Most modern catheter navigation relies on a torqueable guidewire system, in which a catheter is advanced over a wire to its target and the curve of the wire and catheter tip determine its steerability. Although guidewires were initially designed in the mid 1970s, the Tracker catheter system was the first guidewire and catheter system to achieve mass production in 1986.[41] Advances in material science and engineering have subsequently led to an explosion in the development and widespread availability of various guidewires and catheters. Advances include radiopaque markers for better angiographic visualization, shaped tips for improved guidance, and construction with various materials for improved hydrophilic properties and tolerance to different embolic agents.

Embolic agents used for the endovascular management of AVMs, as with catheters and microwires, have undergone many advances over the years. Early attempts at AVM embolization were performed with numerous materials delivered by flow-directed catheters positioned proximal to the actual feeding vessels. Examples include methyl methacrylate spherules (2.5–4.2 mm),[42] silk suture attached to Silastic emboli,[46] gelatin particles, autologous blood clots, and Avitene (C.R. Bard, Inc, Murray Hill, NJ, USA).[41] These early materials were limited by difficulty to control during embolization, high rates of vessel recanalization, and, in some cases, vasculitis. The adaption of acrylic tissue adhesives for embolization, as well as concurrent advances in catheter delivery systems, brought AVM embolization much closer to its current state.

Isobutyl 2-cyanoacrylate is an early generation tissue adhesive that was used for embolization because it polymerizes on contact with blood. However, of the rapid polymerization rate of isobutyl 2-cyanoacrylate led to complications including adhesion and incorporation of the catheter to the glue cast in the feeding artery, and this agent was replaced by N-butyl cyanoacrylate (NBCA). NBCA is currently a popular choice for AVM embolization. Onyx (ev3, Plymouth, MN), a combination of ethylene-vinyl alcohol copolymer and dimethyl sulfoxide, is another agent widely used for the treatment of AVMs.[47] This agent is less adhesive and generally polymerizes slower than NBCA. Platinum coils are also used for AVM embolization to obstruct large feeding vessels.

The ultimate goal of endovascular AVM embolization is angiographic obliteration. However, this is often not achieved, despite attempted staged embolizations, and it may be contraindicated because of the high rate of complications. Many AVMs contain numerous small feeding vessels that cannot be safely catheterized for superselective embolization. In such cases, embolization is used as an adjunct tool before microsurgical resection or radiosurgery. Preoperative embolization can decrease the size of the AVM, reduce intraoperative blood loss, and target blood vessels that might not be surgically accessible. Before radiosurgery, the goals of embolization are to shrink the size of the AVM, particularly at the periphery; address feeding vessel aneurysms and other high-risk features; and, ultimately, to reduce the size of the radiation field required for treatment.

### Radiotherapy for AVMs

The goal of radiotherapy for AVMs is complete obliteration of the AVM by delivering a high radiation dose to the AVM nidus while minimizing the radiation exposure to the surrounding normal brain. Various forms of radiation delivery have been developed over the years and used for AVM treatment. These include external beam x-rays from x-ray tubes or linear accelerators (LINAC), gamma rays from a cobalt source, and Bragg peak (proton beam or helium ion) therapy.[48] Each of these radiation forms can be performed with stereotactic targeting (radiosurgery) and most can be done as single fraction or multifraction therapy. It is now known that the vascular changes seen after radiation are similar, regardless of whether x-rays, gamma rays, or proton beams are used. The limitations of these therapies are nonobliteration of lesions on angiogram, the risk of hemorrhage, and radiation-induced brain injury.

Vilhelm Magnus (1871–1929), Norway's pioneering neurosurgeon, was likely the first to treat cerebral AVMs with radiation in 1914,[6] using conventional fractionated radiation. Cushing and Bailey[8] treated eight AVM patients with conventional radiation and there was an apparent benefit in three of these patients. One of the patients (Case 8) had complete resection of the AVM approximately 1 year after radiotherapy and, from the pathology specimen, it was first demonstrated that the radiation-induced occlusion of AVM vessels was secondary to intimal hyperplasia.[8] This inflammatory change ultimately results in vessel thrombosis and obliteration. Although never truly popular, conventional fractionated radiotherapy was used for AVM treatment intermittently. R.T. Johnson had the largest series of AVMs treated with conventional radiation, with 100 patients treated over 20 years.[49] Twenty of the patients had follow-up angiography. Complete obliteration was reported in nine patients and reduction in the size of the AVM was reported in five patients. Robert Laing and colleagues[50] reported on the ineffectiveness of conventional fractionated radiotherapy in AVM patients. They demonstrated that the actuarial annual risk of bleeding in the treated patients was 2.3%, and this was similar to the risk in untreated AVMs. Ultimately, conventional radiation for AVMs was replaced by stereotactic radiosurgery.

Radiosurgery was first described in 1951 by Lars Leksell[51] (1907–1986), the Swedish neurosurgeon, using a cyclotron. He subsequently introduced the first Gamma Knife using cobalt sources in 1968. Reports using Gamma Knife began appearing in the early 1970s. Ladislau Steiner,[52–55] Christer Lindquist,[55] and L. Dade Lunsford[56,57] and Douglas Kondziolka[57] were instrumental in improving the Gamma Knife technique and demonstrating its effectiveness. Radiosurgery for AVMs based on the Bragg peak phenomenon (proton beam and helium beam) was advanced by Raymond Kjellberg (1925–1993) and colleagues[6] at Harvard and at Berkeley by Jacob Fabrikant (1928–1993) and colleagues[58] and Richard Levy and colleagues.[59] Radiosurgery using LINAC was introduced by Osvaldo Betti and colleagues,[60] and then it was further improved on by William Friedman and F.J. Bova[61] and other investigators. Radiosurgery using each of these 3 main techniques (Gamma Knife, Bragg peak phenomenon, and LINAC) have all been used successfully for treatment of cerebral AVMs. Current AVM management with radiosurgery results in obliteration in 1 to 3 years from the time of treatment, with obliteration rates of 54% to 92% and the risk of hemorrhage during this time period remaining unchanged from untreated patients.[62] The details of radiotherapy for AVMs are described by Michael Lim elsewhere in this issue.

## INTRODUCTION TO DAVFs

Intracranial DAVFs, also referred to as dural arteriovenous malformations, are abnormal arteriovenous shunts between dural arteries and a dural venous sinus or a cortical vein. These lesions can occur throughout the intracranial space, but are most commonly located near dural venous sinuses. They represent 6% of supratentorial and 35% of infratentorial vascular malformations.[63] Most DAVFs are idiopathic, but they have also been described following trauma (eg, skull fracture), cranial surgery, venous channel stenosis, and venous sinus thrombosis.[64–67] DAVFs can be asymptomatic and present incidentally, or they can present with symptoms related to the location and

severity of altered venous drainage. Approximately 20% to 33% of symptomatic DAVFs present with intracranial hemorrhage.[64,68] Other presentations include pulsatile tinnitus (or bruit), visual changes, proptosis, headaches, altered mental status, seizure, cranial nerve palsy, myelopathy, and motor or sensory deficits.

### Imaging

The significance of DAVFs was not well understood until cerebral angiographic techniques were developed and refined. In 1931, Ernest Sachs, Sr[69] (1879–1958), the New York born neurosurgeon who trained under Sir Victor Horsley, reported the original angiographic description of a DAVF. Thomas Newton (1925–2010) and Sten Cronqvist[63] (died 2004) published a good, early angiographic description in 1969. Cerebral angiography with selective injection of both the external and the internal carotid artery remains the gold standard for diagnosis and characterization of these lesions. MRI and CT scan technologies can detect these lesions if a dilated vein s present in the appropriate location. Improvements in CT angiography and MR angiography[70] technology have made these noninvasive modalities more attractive. However, they are far from replacing conventional cerebral angiography for accurate diagnosis, classification, and treatment planning. Furthermore, the introduction of DynaCT (Siemens, Erlangen, Germany) angiography within the past several years has been of great utility in the diagnosis, characterization, and treatment of DAVFs.[71,72] This technique can delineate the fistulous connection, the arterial feeders, the draining veins, and their relationship to the surrounding osseous structures.

### Development of DAVF Classification Schemes and Insights into the Natural History and Prognosis

Much of the important history of DAVF treatment is based on milestones in understanding the natural history of these lesions and in developing classification schemes to guide treatment. Rene Djindjian (1918–1977), the French neuroradiologist, and J.J. Merland[73] published an early classification scheme based on the location of the fistula, meaning the dural sinus to which it drained. Two angiographic classification schemes that are widely used are the Borden-Shucart system, named after Jonathan Borden and William Shucart,[74] and the Cognard system, named after Christophe Cognard.[75] The Borden classification system groups DAVFs into three main types based on the location of venous drainage (dural sinus and/or cortical vein) and on whether cortical venous reflux (CVR) is present or absent.[74] The Cognard classification system groups DAVFs into five main types based on the direction of venous sinus drainage (anterograde or retrograde), the presence or absence of CVR, and the type of venous outflow (eg, nonecstatic vs ecstatic cortical vein).[75]

Both the Borden and the Cognard systems highlight the importance of CVR because this is considered directly related to the clinical symptomatology and prognosis. DAVFs without CVR are generally considered benign.[75] However, DAVFs with persistent CVR are much more aggressive, with an annual mortality of 10.4% and annual risk of hemorrhage or nonhemorrhagic neurologic deficit of 8.1% and 6.9%, respectively.[68]

Recent studies by Michael Soderman and colleagues[76] and Russell Strom and colleagues[77] report that the natural history of DAVFs depends on the angiographic presence of CVR as well as on the mode of presentation. Patients presenting with nonhemorrhagic neurologic deficit or intracranial hemorrhage (ICH) (defined as symptomatic CVR) have a greater neurologic risk and death than patients with asymptomatic CVR (defined as presenting incidentally or with symptoms of increase dural sinus drainage). These reports prompted Gregory Zipfel and colleagues[78] to propose a modification of the DAVF angiographic classification systems to include clinical information about whether the CVR is symptomatic or not. Neurologic risk increases from lesions without CVR or lesions with asymptomatic CVR (1.4%–1.5% annual risk of ICH) to lesions with symptomatic CVR (7.4%–7.6% annual risk of ICH). This new grading system has important implications for treatment algorithms of high-grade DAVFs, suggesting that patients with symptomatic CVR require immediate treatment via an endovascular or open surgical approach. Stereotactic radiosurgery is not suitable for these patients because of the delayed therapeutic efficacy of this treatment option. Exceptions include patients unable to undergo an endovascular or surgical procedure secondary to comorbidities or extremely high procedural risk secondary to the complexity of the lesion. Conversely, patients with asymptomatic CVR may be treated on a elective basis because of their lower risk annual risk of ICH or nonhemorrhagic neurologic deficit.

## Treatment of DAVFs

DAVFs can be treated by open surgery, endovascular embolization, a combination of surgical and endovascular techniques, or by radiation therapy. Carotid-cavernous fistulas (CCFs) were likely the first type of DAVF to be recognized and treated because these lesions presented with striking clinical findings (pulsatile exophthalmos, bruit, visual loss, and eye redness) that did not require advanced imaging to formulate a diagnosis. Unilateral ligation of the common carotid artery was first performed for a CCF by Benjamin Travers (1783–1858), the British surgeon, in England in 1809. Wallace Hamby (1903–1999), the American neurosurgeon, was the first to ligate the intracranial internal carotid as part of the first trapping procedure for a CCF in 1932.[79] The next advance in CCF treatment was muscle embolization. This method, incorrectly credited to Barney Brooks (1884–1952), was first performed by Hamby and W. James Gardner (1898–1987) in 1933, and it represented the origins of neurointerventional surgery.[80] Ultimately, it was Fedor Serbinenko who introduced the miniballoon catheter technique in 1974 and, with it, he opened a new chapter in CCF treatment and significantly advanced endovascular embolization.[44] In 1995, Neil Miller and colleagues[81] reported the combined microsurgical-endovascular treatment of CCFs using the superior ophthalmic vein for access into the cavernous sinus.

The primary treatment modality for many non-CCF cranial DAVFs in the late 1970s and 1980s was an open surgical procedure to disrupt the fistula connection and even resect the associated dura and venous sinus.[82–84] Such procedures were often technically challenging and included significant risk of substantial blood loss, venous stroke, and other morbidity. As with AVM surgery, open surgery for DAVFs benefitted from the development and refinement of the operative microscope, microinstruments, and microsurgical techniques. Surgical intervention is still an important option for modern treatment of DAVFs; however, the first therapeutic attempt for DAVFs at most institutions is endovascular embolization. Surgery is often reserved for patients with continued symptoms and angiographic CVR despite maximal endovascular intervention. Surgery can be a first-line therapy for lesions with difficult arterial access and with drainage through a single cortical vein. Fistulas of the anterior cranial fossa and of the superior petrosal sinus with single cortical draining veins are examples of such surgically treated fistulas.[6,78]

As with surgical procedures for AVM treatment, intraoperative angiography is also important during surgery for DAVFs. Paritosh Pandey and colleagues[85] reported a series of 29 patients (31 DAVFs) treated surgically with adjunct intraoperative angiography and, in 11 patients (37.9%), the results of the intraoperative angiogram resulted in further surgical treatment. Intraoperative ICG angiography is also used successfully for treatment of DAVFs to identify components of the fistula and confirm its obliteration.[86–88]

Advances in endovascular technology and techniques over the past 3 decades (described above for AVMs) have fueled the popularity and widespread use of embolization for DAVF treatment. For example, improvements in microcatheters and microwires have allowed for navigation closer to the fistulous connection, ultimately resulting in more direct and selective embolization. The goal of embolization is to obliterate the fistula connection and to limit adverse outcomes, such as unintentional worsening of cortical venous flow, closing external to internal carotid artery anastomoses, and embolizing external carotid artery branches with arterial supply to cranial nerves. DAVFs can be treated endovascularly by a transarterial, a transvenous, or a combined approach. Liquid embolic agents (eg, NBCA and Onyx) and coils are commonly used for these cases. These techniques are described in detail elsewhere in this issue by Martin Radvany. In many instances, endovascular management can achieve cure as a primary treatment modality.

Radiation therapy, including radiosurgery, is another available treatment modality for DAVFs. Radiosurgery was first used for DAVFs in the early 1980s.[89] Today, radiosurgery can be used as a primary treatment modality, in combination with embolization, or as a salvage strategy for DAVFs that are refractory to embolization and/or surgery. Complete obliteration rates for DAVFs treated exclusively with radiosurgery vary widely, with rates raging from 50% to 100% for indirect CCFs and from 20% to 100% for non-CCF DAVFs.[89]

## SUMMARY

AVMs and DAVFs represent two important classes of intracranial vascular lesions. Numerous technical advances over the past century have dramatically improved our ability to diagnose, characterize, and treat these distinct pathologic entities. Historical progress paved the way for modern therapeutic options, which include microsurgical, endovascular, and radiosurgery techniques. As our understanding of AVMs and DAVFs improves, the future promises to further build on these techniques, as well as introduce novels approaches for treating these lesions.

## REFERENCES

1. Hashimoto N, Nozaki K, Takagi Y, et al. Surgery of cerebral arteriovenous malformations. Neurosurgery 2007;61(Suppl 1):375–87 [discussion: 387–9].
2. Hunter W. Observations on arteriovenous malformations. Med Obser Enquir 1762.
3. Virchow R. Die Krankhaften Geschwülste: Dreissig Vorlesungen, gehalten während des Wintersemesters 1862–1863 an der Universität zu Berlin. Berlin: Hirschwald; 1863 [in German].
4. Power D. Angioma of the cerebral membranes. Trans Path Soc Lond 1888;39(5).
5. Giordano D. Contributo alla cura della lesioni traumatiche ed alla trepanazione del cranio. Gazz Med Ital 1890;61(5) [in Italian].
6. Heros RC, Morcos JJ. Cerebrovascular surgery: past, present, and future. Neurosurgery 2000;47(5):1007–33.
7. Dandy W. Arteriovenous aneurysm of the brain. Arch Surg 1928;17:190.
8. Cushing H, Bailey P. Tumours arising from the blood vessels of the brain: angiomatous malformations and hemangioblastomas, vol. 3. Springfield (IL): Charles C Thomas; 1928.
9. Yasargil M. Microneurosurgery: AVM of the brain, history, embryology, pathological considerations, hemodynamics, diagnostic studies, microsurgical anatomy. In: Yasargil M, editor. A short history of the diagnosis and treatment of cerebral AVMs. Stuttgart (Germany): Georg Thieme; 1987. p. 3–21.
10. Ray BS. Cerebral arteriovenous aneurysm. Surg Gynecol Obstet 1941;73:615.
11. Olivecrona H, Riives J. Arteriovenous aneurysms of the brain: their diagnosis and treatment. Arch Neurol Psychiatry 1948;59:567–603.
12. Doby T. Cerebral angiography and Egas Moniz. AJR Am J Roentgenol 1992;159(2):364.
13. Moniz E. L'encephalographie artérielle: son importance dans la localisation des tumeurs crérébrales. Rev Neurol (Paris) 1927;2:72–90.
14. Filler A. The history, development and impact of computed imaging in neurological diagnosis and neurosurgery: CT, MRI, and DTI. Nature Precedings; 2009. Available at: http://dx.doi.org/10.1038/npre.2009.3267.5. Accessed July 13, 2009.
15. Okada T, Miki Y, Kikuta K, et al. Diffusion tensor fiber tractography for arteriovenous malformations: quantitative analyses to evaluate the corticospinal tract and optic radiation. AJNR Am J Neuroradiol 2007;28(6):1107–13 [in French].
16. Yamada K, Kizu O, Ito H, et al. Tractography for arteriovenous malformations near the sensorimotor cortices. AJNR Am J Neuroradiol 2005;26(3):598–602.
17. Anegawa S, Hayashi T, Torigoe R, et al. Intraoperative angiography in the resection of arteriovenous malformations. J Neurosurg 1994;80(1):73–8.
18. Barrow DL, Boyer KL, Joseph GJ. Intraoperative angiography in the management of neurovascular disorders. Neurosurgery 1992;30(2):153–9.
19. Bartal AD, Tirosh MS, Weinstein M. Angiographic control during total excision of a cerebral arteriovenous

malformation. Technical note. J Neurosurg 1968;29(2): 211–3.

20. Bauer BL. Intraoperative angiography in cerebral aneurysm and AV-malformation. Neurosurg Rev 1984;7(2–3):209–17.

21. Germanwala AV, Thai QA, Pradilla G, et al. Simple technique for intraoperative angiographic localization of small vascular lesions. Neurosurgery 2010; 67(3):818–22 [discussion: 822–3].

22. Killory BD, Nakaji P, Gonzales LF, et al. Prospective evaluation of surgical microscope-integrated intraoperative near-infrared indocyanine green angiography during cerebral arteriovenous malformation surgery. Neurosurgery 2009;65(3):456–62 [discussion: 462].

23. Hanggi D, Etminan N, Steiger HJ. The impact of microscope-integrated intraoperative near-infrared indocyanine green videoangiography on surgery of arteriovenous malformations and dural arteriovenous fistulae. Neurosurgery 2010;67(4):1094–103 [discussion: 1103–4].

24. Takagi Y, Kikuta K, Nozaki K, et al. Detection of a residual nidus by surgical microscope-integrated intraoperative near-infrared indocyanine green videoangiography in a child with a cerebral arteriovenous malformation. J Neurosurg 2007;107(Suppl 5):416–8.

25. Pool JL, Colton RP. The dissecting microscope for intracranial vascular surgery. J Neurosurg 1966; 25(3):315–8.

26. Yasargil M. Microsurgery applied to neurosurgery. Stuttgart (Germany): Georg Thieme; 1969.

27. Spetzler RF, Martin NA. A proposed grading system for arteriovenous malformations. J Neurosurg 1986; 65(4):476–83.

28. Yasargil M. Microneurosurgery: AVM of the brain, clinical considerations, general and special operative techniques, surgical results, nonoperated cases, cavernous and venous angiomas, neuroanesthesia, vol. III B. Stuttgart (Germany): Georg Thieme; 1988.

29. Malis L. Arteriovenous malformations of the spinal cord. In: Youmans JR, editor. Neurological surgery. Philadelphia: W.B. Saunders; 1982. p. 1850–74.

30. Luessenhop AJ, Gennarelli TA. Anatomical grading of supratentorial arteriovenous malformations for determining operability. Neurosurgery 1977;1(1):30–5.

31. de Oliveira E, Tedeschi H, Raso J. Multidisciplinary approach to arteriovenous malformations. Neurol Med Chir (Tokyo) 1998;38(Suppl):177–85.

32. Lawton MT. Spetzler-Martin Grade III arteriovenous malformations: surgical results and a modification of the grading scale. Neurosurgery 2003;52(4): 740–8 [discussion: 748–9].

33. Lawton MT, Kim H, McCulloch CE, et al. A supplementary grading scale for selecting patients with brain arteriovenous malformations for surgery. Neurosurgery 2010;66(4):702–13 [discussion: 713].

34. Perret G, Nishioka H. Report on the cooperative study of intracranial aneurysms and subarachnoid hemorrhage. Section VI. Arteriovenous malformations. An analysis of 545 cases of cranio-cerebral arteriovenous malformations and fistulae reported to the cooperative study. J Neurosurg 1966;25(4):467–90.

35. Crawford PM, West CR, Chadwick DW, et al. Arteriovenous malformations of the brain: natural history in unoperated patients. J Neurol Neurosurg Psychiatry 1986;49(1):1–10.

36. Jane JA, Kassell NF, Torner JC, et al. The natural history of aneurysms and arteriovenous malformations. J Neurosurg 1985;62(3):321–3.

37. Wilkins RH. Natural history of intracranial vascular malformations: a review. Neurosurgery 1985;16(3): 421–30.

38. Ondra SL, Troupp H, George ED, et al. The natural history of symptomatic arteriovenous malformations of the brain: a 24-year follow-up assessment. J Neurosurg 1990;73(3):387–91.

39. Samson D, Batjer HH. Preoperative evaluation of the risk/benefit ratio for arteriorvenous malformations of the brain. In: Wilkins RH, Rengachary SS, editors. Neurosurgery Update II. New York: McGraw-Hill; 1991. p. 121–33.

40. Hernesniemi JA, Dashti R, Juvela S, et al. Natural history of brain arteriovenous malformations: a long-term follow-up study of risk of hemorrhage in 238 patients. Neurosurgery 2008;63(5):823–9 [discussion: 829–31].

41. Bristol RE, Albuquerque FC, McDougall CG. The evolution of endovascular treatment for intracranial arteriovenous malformations. Neurosurg Focus 2006;20(6):E6.

42. Luessenhop AJ, Spence WT. Artificial embolization of cerebral arteries. Report of use in a case of arteriovenous malformation. J Am Med Assoc 1960;172: 1153–5.

43. Kanaan Y, Kaneshiro D, Fraser K, et al. Evolution of endovascular therapy for aneurysm treatment. Historical overview. Neurosurg Focus 2005;18(2):E2.

44. Serbinenko FA. Balloon catheterization and occlusion of major cerebral vessels. J Neurosurg 1974; 41(2):125–45.

45. Kerber C. Balloon catheter with a calibrated leak. A new system for superselective angiography and occlusive catheter therapy. Radiology 1976;120(3): 547–50.

46. Luessenhop AJ, Velasquez AC. Observations on the tolerance of the intracranial arteries to catheterization. J Neurosurg 1964;21:85–91.

47. Taki W, Yonekawa Y, Iwata H, et al. A new liquid material for embolization of arteriovenous malformations. AJNR Am J Neuroradiol 1990;11(1):163–8.

48. Ogilvy CS. Radiation therapy for arteriovenous malformations: a review. Neurosurgery 1990;26(5): 725–35.

49. Johnson RT. Radiotherapy of cerebral angiomas with a note on some problems in diagnosis. In: Pia HW, Gleave JRW, Grok W, et al, editors. Cerebral angiomas: advances in diagnosis and therapy. Berlin: Springer-Verlag; 1975. p. 256–9.

50. Laing RW, Childs J, Brada M. Failure of conventionally fractionated radiotherapy to decrease the risk of hemorrhage in inoperable arteriovenous malformations. Neurosurgery 1992;30(6):872–5 [discussion: 875–6].

51. Leksell L. The stereotaxic method and radiosurgery of the brain. Acta Chir Scand 1951;102(4):316–9.

52. Steiner L. Radiosurgery in cerebral arteriovenous malformations. In: Fein JM, Flamm ES, editors. Cerebrovascular surgery. New York: Springer-Verlag; 1984. p. 1161–215.

53. Steiner L, Leksell L, Forster DM, et al. Stereotactic radiosurgery in intracranial arterio-venous malformations. Acta Neurochir (Wien) 1974;(Suppl 21): 195–209.

54. Steiner L, Leksell L, Greitz T, et al. Stereotaxic radiosurgery for cerebral arteriovenous malformations. Report of a case. Acta Chir Scand 1972;138(5):459–64.

55. Steiner L, Lindquist C, Adler JR, et al. Clinical outcome of radiosurgery for cerebral arteriovenous malformations. J Neurosurg 1992;77(1):1–8.

56. Lunsford LD, Flickinger J, Lindner G, et al. Stereotactic radiosurgery of the brain using the first United States 201 cobalt-60 source gamma knife. Neurosurgery 1989;24(2):151–9.

57. Lunsford LD, Kondziolka F, Flickinger JC, et al. Stereotactic radiosurgery for arteriovenous malformations of the brain. J Neurosurg 1991;75(4):512–24.

58. Fabrikant JI, Levy RP, Steinberg GK, et al. Stereotactic charged-particle radiosurgery: clinical results of treatment of 1200 patients with intracranial arteriovenous malformations and pituitary disorders. Clin Neurosurg 1992;38:472–92.

59. Levy RP, Fabrikant JI, Frankel KA, et al. Stereotactic heavy-charged-particle Bragg peak radiosurgery for the treatment of intracranial arteriovenous malformations in childhood and adolescence. Neurosurgery 1989;24(6):841–52.

60. Betti OO, Galmarini D, Derechinsky V. Radiosurgery with a linear accelerator. Methodological aspects. Stereotact Funct Neurosurg 1991;57(1–2):87–98.

61. Friedman WA, Bova FJ. The University of Florida radiosurgery system. Surg Neurol 1989;32(5): 334–42.

62. Starke RM, Komotar RJ, Hwang BY, et al. A comprehensive review of radiosurgery for cerebral arteriovenous malformations: outcomes, predictive factors, and grading scales. Stereotact Funct Neurosurg 2008;86(3):191–9.

63. Newton TH, Cronqvist S. Involvement of dural arteries in intracranial arteriovenous malformations. Radiology 1969;93(5):1071–8.

64. McConnell KA, Tjoumakaris SI, Allen J, et al. Neuroendovascular management of dural arteriovenous malformations. Neurosurg Clin N Am 2009;20(4): 431–9.

65. Nabors MW, Azzam CJ, Albanna FJ, et al. Delayed postoperative dural arteriovenous malformations. Report of two cases. J Neurosurg 1987;66(5):768–72.

66. Sakaki T, Morimoto T, Nakase H, et al. Dural arteriovenous fistula of the posterior fossa developing after surgical occlusion of the sigmoid sinus. Report of five cases. J Neurosurg 1996;84(1):113–8.

67. Watanabe A, Takahara Y, Ibuchi Y, et al. Two cases of dural arteriovenous malformation occurring after intracranial surgery. Neuroradiology 1984;26(5): 375–80.

68. van Dijk JM, terBrugge KG, Willinsky RA, et al. Clinical course of cranial dural arteriovenous fistulas with long-term persistent cortical venous reflux. Stroke 2002;33(5):1233–6.

69. Sachs E. The diagnosis and treatment of brain tumors. St Louis (MO): Mosby; 1931.

70. Meckel S, Maier M, Ruiz DS, et al. MR angiography of dural arteriovenous fistulas: diagnosis and follow-up after treatment using a time-resolved 3D contrast-enhanced technique. AJNR Am J Neuroradiol 2007; 28(5):877–84.

71. Hiu T, Kitagawa N, Morikawa M, et al. Efficacy of DynaCT digital angiography in the detection of the fistulous point of dural arteriovenous fistulas. AJNR Am J Neuroradiol 2009;30(3):487–91.

72. Lim SP, Lesiuk H, Sinclair J, et al. Preoperative or preembolization lesion targeting using rotational angiographic fiducial marking in the neuroendovascular suite. J Neurosurg 2011;114(1):140–5.

73. Djindjian R, Merland JJ. Superselective arteriography of the external carotid artery. New York: Springer-Verlag; 1978.

74. Borden JA, Wu JK, Shucart WA. A proposed classification for spinal and cranial dural arteriovenous fistulous malformations and implications for treatment. J Neurosurg 1995;82(2):166–79.

75. Cognard C, Gobin YP, Pierot L, et al. Cerebral dural arteriovenous fistulas: clinical and angiographic correlation with a revised classification of venous drainage. Radiology 1995;194(3):671–80.

76. Soderman M, Pavic L, Edner G, et al. Natural history of dural arteriovenous shunts. Stroke 2008;39(6): 1735–9.

77. Strom RG, Botros JA, Refai D, et al. Cranial dural arteriovenous fistulae: asymptomatic cortical venous drainage portends less aggressive clinical course. Neurosurgery 2009;64(2):241–7 [discussion: 247–8].

78. Zipfel GJ, Shah MN, Refai D, et al. Cranial dural arteriovenous fistulas: modification of angiographic classification scales based on new natural history data. Neurosurg Focus 2009;26(5):E14.

79. Pool JL. The development of modern intracranial aneurysm surgery. Neurosurgery 1977;1(3):233–7.

80. Vitek JJ, Smith MJ. The myth of the Brooks method of embolization: a brief history of the endovascular treatment of carotid-cavernous sinus fistula. J Neurointerv Surg 2009;1:108–11.

81. Miller NR, Monsein LH, Debrun GM, et al. Treatment of carotid-cavernous sinus fistulas using a superior ophthalmic vein approach. J Neurosurg 1995; 83(5):838–42.

82. Brown RD Jr, Flemming KD, Meyer FB, et al. Natural history, evaluation, and management of intracranial vascular malformations. Mayo Clin Proc 2005; 80(2):269–81.

83. Hugosson R, Bergstrom K. Surgical treatment of dural arteriovenous malformation in the region of the sigmoid sinus. J Neurol Neurosurg Psychiatry 1974;37(1):97–101.

84. Sundt TM Jr, Piepgras DG. The surgical approach to arteriovenous malformations of the lateral and sigmoid dural sinuses. J Neurosurg 1983;59(1): 32–9.

85. Pandey P, Steinberg GK, Westbroek EM, et al. Intraoperative angiography for cranial dural arteriovenous fistula. AJNR Am J Neuroradiol 2011;32(6):1091–5.

86. Colby GP, Coon AL, Sciubba DM, et al. Intraoperative indocyanine green angiography for obliteration of a spinal dural arteriovenous fistula. J Neurosurg Spine 2009;11(6):705–9.

87. Raabe A, Beck J, Gerlach R, et al. Near-infrared indocyanine green video angiography: a new method for intraoperative assessment of vascular flow. Neurosurgery 2003;52(1):132–9 [discussion: 139].

88. Schuette AJ, Cawley CM, Barrow DL. Indocyanine green videoangiography in the management of dural arteriovenous fistulae. Neurosurgery 2010; 67(3):658–62 [discussion: 662].

89. Loumiotis I, Lanzino G, Daniels D, et al. Radiosurgery for intracranial dural arteriovenous fistulas (DAVFs): a review. Neurosurg Rev 2011;34(3):305–15.

# Imaging of Cerebral Arteriovenous Malformations and Dural Arteriovenous Fistulas

Mahmud Mossa-Basha, MD[a], James Chen, BS[b],
Dheeraj Gandhi, MBBS, MD[c],*

## KEYWORDS

- Arteriovenous malformation • Dural arteriovenous fistula
- Magnetic resonance imaging • Computed tomography
- Advanced imaging

Imaging plays a major role in the identification, grading, and treatment of cerebral arteriovenous malformations (AVMs) and cerebral dural arteriovenous fistulas (DAVFs). Digital subtraction angiography (DSA) is the gold standard in the diagnosis and characterization of these vascular malformations, but advances in both magnetic resonance imaging (MRI) and computed tomography (CT), including advanced imaging techniques, have provided new tools for further characterizing these lesions as well as the surrounding brain structures that may be affected. Advances in MRI techniques have also allowed better noninvasive characterization of these vascular lesions in ways that previously could only be possible with catheter angiography. In this article, the authors discuss the role of conventional as well as advanced imaging modalities that are providing novel ways to characterize these vascular malformations.

## CEREBRAL ARTERIOVENOUS MALFORMATIONS
### General Features

Cerebral AVMs represent congenital vascular abnormalities, in which single or multiple arterial

feeding vessels supply a dysplastic plexiform network of vessels (also known as the nidus) with direct shunting into the venous system. The nidus, which represents a conglomerate of dysplastic, thin-walled vessels, is histologically best characterized as a cluster of arterialized veins. The nidus can be supplied by one vascular distribution, or there can be supply from multiple vascular territories, representing a so-called borderzone AVM.[1] Cerebral AVMs are thought to represent congenital lesions caused by alterations in the vascular modeling process, a theory supported by the vascular complexity of the lesions.[2,3] There is little to no functional brain tissue within the AVM nidus, leading to the assumption that functional brain is displaced to the margins of the lesion.[4]

Micro-AVMs are defined as lesions with a nidus that measures 1 cm or less.[5] These lesions have historically been known as cryptic or occult AVMs because they were not readily seen on imaging studies previously.[5] Nearly 40% to 50% of cerebral AVMs in the setting of hereditary hemorrhagic telangiectasia and 7% of sporadic AVMs are micro-AVMs.[6] These lesions typically have a single normal-sized arterial feeder and a single draining vein. Micro-AVMs are typically

The authors have nothing to disclose.
[a] Division of Neuroradiology, Russell H. Morgan Department of Radiology, Johns Hopkins University, 600 North Wolfe Street, Baltimore, MD 21287, USA
[b] Johns Hopkins University School of Medicine, 733 North Broadway, #100, Baltimore, MD 21205, USA
[c] Departments of Radiology, Neurology and Neurosurgery, University of Maryland, 22 South Greene Street, Baltimore, MD 21201, USA
* Corresponding author.
E-mail address: dgandhi@umm.edu

Neurosurg Clin N Am 23 (2012) 27–42
doi:10.1016/j.nec.2011.09.007
1042-3680/12/$ – see front matter © 2012 Elsevier Inc. All rights reserved.

located superficially, within the cortex or within the subarachnoid space.[5]

Aneurysms are seen in up to 58% of AVMs.[7] Flow-related aneurysms can be found on feeding arteries or within the AVM nidus, which can frequently serve as the focus of AVM rupture. Aneurysms can also occur on arteries remote from the AVM arterial supply. There can be significant varicosity and aneurysmal dilatation of draining venous structures, especially in the setting of high-flow AVM, which also increases the risk of hemorrhage.[8] Direct arteriovenous connections may be present within the lesion and can generally only be identified on superselective microcatheter angiography. Flow-induced angiopathy is often associated and reflective of reactive endothelial hyperplasia; this can result in arterial or venous stenoses.[3] Venous drainage can be superficial, deep, or a combination of the two. The drainage pathway is important to note on imaging studies because of the important role this factor plays in prognostication and in determining the treatment plan.

### Risk of Hemorrhage

The overall estimated likelihood of AVM hemorrhage is between 2% and 4% per year, but can be as low as 0.9% per year without any associated risk factors.[9–11] There is an associated 5% to 17.6% chance of death and 30% to 50% chance of permanent neurologic deficits in the setting of AVM hemorrhage.[10,12] Many factors have been associated with an increased risk of AVM hemorrhage, including small AVM size, high-flow lesions with increased arterial and venous pressure, deep as well as infratentorial locations, and a history of previous AVM hemorrhage.[11,13] In addition, other angiographic characteristics such as intranidal aneurysm(s), flow-related arterial aneurysms, presence of deep venous drainage, and venous stenosis also correlate with increased hemorrhagic risk. The importance of risk factors is, however, somewhat controversial. Duong and colleagues[14] indicate that the most important risk factors for AVM hemorrhage are high arterial input pressure and exclusive deep venous drainage. During a prospective follow-up of 622 patients with AVM for a mean time period of 2.3 years, Stapf and colleagues[11] found that the most important risk factors for hemorrhage of AVM are exclusive deep venous drainage, deep brain location, and history of previous AVM rupture. After an initial hemorrhagic event there is an increased risk of hemorrhage, ranging between 4.5% and 34.4%.[11,15,16] There was an overall 6% rate of hemorrhage in patients who had experienced a previous hemorrhagic event, as compared with

1.3% for patients who did not have a history of AVM rupture.[11] Borderzone location for an AVM, with supply from multiple arterial distributions, appears to be protective against hemorrhage.[1]

### Conventional Imaging: MRI and CT

CT and MRI are the typical initial imaging examinations performed on patients with AVMs, as the most common presentations are not specific for AVM and include intracranial hemorrhage, seizure, headache, and focal neurologic deficit.[17,18] Large AVMs can be readily identified on CT and MRI, but smaller lesions may be more difficult to detect. Noncontrast head CT is usually the initial imaging examination based on the clinical presentation, to evaluate for any hemorrhage. On noncontrast head CT examination, prominent serpentine hyperattenuating structures (**Fig. 1**A, B), representing draining veins, components of the nidus, or dilated arterial feeders, suggest a diagnosis of AVM. Curvilinear or speckled calcifications involving the nidus or the feeding or draining vessels can also be seen. The AVM typically does not cause much mass effect, unless there has been hemorrhage. Instead, there may be hypoattenuation and volume loss in the brain parenchyma surrounding the nidus, relating to gliosis or hemosiderin deposition from previous hemorrhage. Hemorrhage at presentation is seen in 42% to 72% of cases, most commonly parenchymal, followed by subarachnoid and intraventricular hemorrhage.[17–19]

In the absence of a known underlying etiology for parenchymal hemorrhage, CT angiography is frequently the follow-up examination to evaluate for a possible underlying lesion, such as AVM or ruptured aneurysm. CT angiography (CTA) will show the enhancing nidus as well as prominent draining veins, but evaluation is limited on conventional CTA, as temporal flow-related changes are not evaluated. Characteristic features of the AVM, such as feeding arterial and draining venous stenosis, flow-related arterial and intranidal aneurysms, and draining venous aneurysms, may be seen, but are not as well depicted or evaluated as on DSA. Significant venous contamination, if present, limits differentiation between draining veins and normal veins. Even on an excellent quality CTA study, small and micro-AVMs may be difficult to detect. In the setting of hemorrhage, the nidus may be compressed by the hematoma, limiting detection of a small underlying lesion. However, this applies to all imaging modalities, including CTA, MRI/MR angiography (MRA), and even DSA. In the setting of a prominent parenchymal hematoma, it is advised that repeat

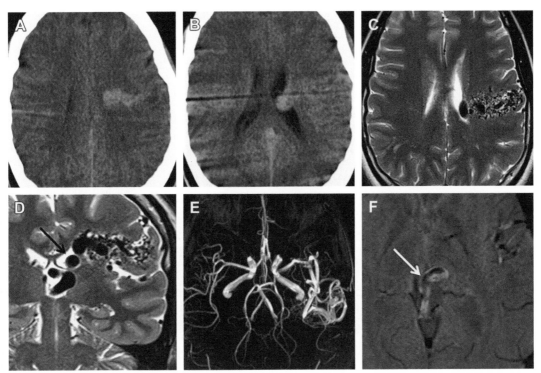

**Fig. 1.** A 16-year-old female patient who initially presented to the emergency department after tonic-clonic seizures. Axial noncontrast CT images (*A* and *B*) show a hyperattenuating serpentine vascular structure coursing from the left corona radiata into the left lateral ventricle. On axial (*C*) and coronal (*D*) T2-weighted sequences, there is a prominent plexiform transmantle perirolandic arteriovenous malformation with a prominent draining terminal vein (*arrow*), which empties deeply into the left basal vein of Rosenthal. Perinidal T2 hyperintensity relates to gliosis. Noncontrast enhanced 3-dimensional time-of-flight magnetic resonance angiography (3D TOF MRA) 3D reformat image in axial plane (*E*) again shows AVM nidus being supplied by multiple distal left middle cerebral artery (MCA) branches. Draining venous structures are not well depicted. Axial susceptibility-weighted image (*F*) shows hyperintense signal within prominent left basal vein of Rosenthal (*arrow*) relating to high-flow arteriovenous shunting.

imaging be performed 4 to 6 weeks after detection of the hematoma. This interval allows time for mass effect related to the hemorrhage to decrease, sometimes permitting for identification of the responsible lesion.

On conventional MRI, dilated arterial feeding arteries, the nidus, and draining veins are represented as flow voids (**Fig. 1**C, D). T2 and FLAIR (fluid-attenuated inversion recovery) hyperintensity involving the adjacent brain parenchyma frequently relates to gliosis (see **Fig. 1**C, D), which is a result of hypoperfusion of portions of the surrounding brain secondary to cerebrovascular steal. There can be T1 and T2 hypointensity and susceptibility on b0 sequences in the adjacent brain structures, relating to hemosiderin from previous hemorrhage. MRI can depict important details of mass effect on adjacent brain structures or involvement of eloquent cortex, which cannot be readily shown on DSA. On postcontrast T1-weighted sequences, there will frequently be enhancement of portions of the AVM nidus. With small AVMs, a small area of cortical and subcortical enhancement may be the only finding on conventional imaging (**Fig. 2**).

MRI in conjunction with MRA can be a useful noninvasive imaging tool in the postradiosurgery setting to evaluate for residual AVM, even though DSA remains the gold standard. The residual nidus is represented as residual flow voids, with persistent feeding arteries and draining veins. On postcontrast sequences, evaluation for AVM-related enhancement is limited, as postradiosurgery patients can frequently have radiation-induced parenchymal enhancement. There was 80% sensitivity (64/80) and 100% specificity (84/84) on conventional MRI for residual AVM postradiosurgery when compared with DSA, according to Pollock and colleagues.[20]

## Susceptibility-Weighted Imaging

Susceptibility-weighted imaging (SWI) relies on exquisite sensitivity to magnetic susceptibility

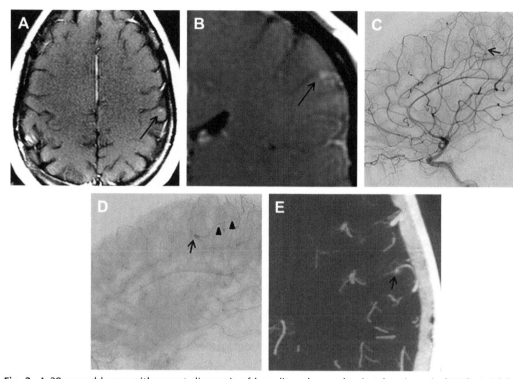

**Fig. 2.** A 28-year-old man with recent diagnosis of hereditary hemorrhagic telangiectasia (HHT). Axial (*A*) and magnified coronal (*B*) T1 postcontrast images of the brain show an enhancing cortical lesion (*long arrow*) involving the left precentral gyrus. Although nonspecific, a lesion like this should raise a suspicion for a micro-AVM in patients with HHT. Micro-AVM nidus (*short arrow*) was confirmed on sagittal digital subtraction angiography (DSA) image in early arterial phase (*C*). Sagittal DSA image in capillary phase (*D*) shows micro-AVM nidus (*short arrow*) with single early draining vein (*arrowheads*). The nidus (*short arrow*) is presented on axial, magnified C-arm cone-beam CT image (*E*).

effects.[21] Sensitivity to magnetic susceptibility is optimized by using long echo time high-resolution flow-compensated 3-dimensional (3D) gradient echo sequences with filtered phase information. This technique relies on the paramagnetic characteristics of deoxyhemoglobin and the resultant phase differences between venous blood and the surrounding brain parenchyma, as well as arterial blood. SWI is very sensitive for the depiction of venous structures as well as extravascular blood.[22]

SWI can provide helpful information in the evaluation of venous structures draining AVMs. Frequently on conventional imaging and time-of-flight (TOF) MRA, differentiation between arterial feeders and draining veins can be difficult.[23] SWI more accurately shows draining venous structures than TOF MRA and conventional MRI. High-flow arteriovenous shunting in AVM can be accurately depicted on SWI as a hyperintense venous signal, which correlates well with findings of arteriovenous shunting on DSA (**Fig. 1**F).[24] This finding relates to rapid wash-in of high-flow oxygenated

blood into draining veins. SWI is accurate in the evaluation of residual arteriovenous shunting after AVM treatment; in the posttreatment setting, residual ectatic veins will have decreased signal due to deoxyhemoglobin, whereas persistent arteriovenous shunting will show a hyperintense venous signal.[24] SWI is advantageous to TOF MR venography because it is more sensitive to slow flow within draining venous structures, and there is no loss of signal in vessels coursing in the imaging plane.[25] SWI can be helpful in depicting micro-AVMs, which may not be depicted on conventional MRI or TOF MRA, by accurately portraying small draining venous structures otherwise not seen.[25] Early identification of micro-AVMs is important, as these lesions have an increased risk of hemorrhage.

### Time-Resolved MRA

Time-resolved MRA is an evolving technique that is showing early promise in its ability to characterize cerebral AVMs. DSA currently remains the gold standard in evaluating the angioarchitecture of cerebral AVMs because of its combination of exquisite spatial and temporal resolution. However, DSA is invasive, expensive, exposes the patient and the operator to ionizing radiation, and has a small but finite risk of associated symptomatic ischemic events. There have been significant advances in contrast-enhanced time-resolved MRA sequences, which allow image acquisition rates of up to 3 frames per second.[26] 3-T MRI units are favored over 1.5-T units because they provide increased signal-to-noise ratio, permitting the use of undersampling techniques, which increases temporal resolution.[27]

Time-resolved MRA can show flow of contrast through each component of the AVM, confirming the suspected findings on conventional MRI/TOF MRA and CT/CTA examinations.[26] Time-resolved contrast-enhanced MRA has been shown to correlate well with DSA in terms of AVM grading, nidus size and location evaluation, venous drainage pattern, and arterial feeders in multiple studies.[28–31] MRA sequences of high spatial resolution and high temporal resolution can be performed as separate sequences during a study to achieve both improved spatial and temporal resolution.[32] At present, however, DSA remains the gold standard in AVM evaluation because at this point, time-resolved MRA cannot match the high spatial and temporal resolution of DSA.

## Time-of-Flight MRA

3D TOF MRA without contrast has remained a first-line diagnostic tool in the evaluation of cerebrovascular disease, including cerebral aneurysms and steno-occlusive disease. TOF MRA is frequently one of the first examinations obtained when there is an initial diagnosis of cerebral AVM, in addition to conventional MRI (see **Fig. 1**). TOF MRA does not typically rely on gadolinium contrast agents, is easy to perform, and provides high-resolution images. The background stationary soft tissues within a slab are saturated with radiofrequency (RF) pulses on TOF imaging. Inflowing blood maintains its signal and appears bright, representing flow-related enhancement.

Contrast-enhanced 3D TOF MRA, when performed in conjunction with conventional MRI, can provide valuable pretreatment information and an overall broad characterization of AVM. While DSA can be used for evaluation of the AVM prior to radiosurgery,[33] contrast-enhanced 3D TOF MRA might provide a more accurate means of delineating the 3D contour and size of the AVM in the pretreatment setting.[34,35] Accurate delineation of the AVM nidus is important for adequate

AVM coverage, which is the most important factor for successful treatment.[33,36,37] Overcoverage can lead to unnecessary irradiation of adjacent brain tissue, and undercoverage will result in inadequate AVM treatment. Because DSA is a 2-dimensional (2D) image, the true nidal size can be obscured or misinterpreted, due to overlapping adjacent vascular structures or inhomogeneous enhancement[35]; this can lead to overestimation of the nidus size and inaccurate delineation of nidal contours.[38] Contrast-enhanced 3D TOF MRA can also be a useful tool in the evaluation for postradiotherapy residual AVM.[39,40] 3D TOF MRA with contrast, as compared with DSA, detected nearly all cases of residual AVM but its specificity was 68% and diagnostic accuracy only 77%, according to Lee and colleagues.[41] The false-positive cases were related to residual ectatic vessels around the thrombosed nidus in combination with radiation-induced parenchymal enhancement.

Unenhanced 3D TOF MRA is limited in the evaluation of feeding arteries and draining veins when compared with DSA. Only 65% of arterial feeders detected on DSA can be seen on 3-T 3D TOF MRA, and only 71% of superficial and 60% of deep draining veins are seen on 3T 3D TOF MRA in comparison with DSA. These percentages are even lower on 1.5-T scans. In addition, it can be difficult to differentiate between arterial feeders and draining veins, especially with complex lesions with multiple feeding arteries and draining veins.[23] Limited visualization of draining veins in part relates to the application of a saturation band, which is applied to suppress venous flow. TOF MRA is limited in its evaluation of turbulent, complex flow, which is frequently seen in AVMs.[26] The turbulent blood flow is saturated by multiple RF pulses. Another limitation of 3D TOF MRA is the evaluation of small AVMs, as frequently the nidus, feeding arteries, and draining veins may not be seen.[42,43] Contrast-enhanced TOF MRA has overcome many of the artifacts that are seen with unenhanced TOF MRA, including loss of flow-related enhancement due to slow, turbulent, or complex flow.[26]

## Diffusion Tensor Imaging

Diffusion tensor imaging relies on directional diffusion (anisotropy) of water molecules along nerve axons and nerve bundles. In normal white matter tracts, myelin sheaths and axonal cell membranes restrict water diffusion in the direction perpendicular to the nerve fibers. The primary direction of water motion is parallel to the orientation of the white matter tract. Tensor maps can be used to generate 3D tractogram maps, which represent the trajectory of the white matter tract.

Diffusion tensor imaging can serve as a valuable noninvasive preoperative and preradiosurgery tool to evaluate for involvement and proximity of cerebral AVMs to white matter tracts.[44] Accurate assessment of white matter tracts can be performed in the setting of adjacent AVMs with or without hemorrhage (**Fig. 3**B, C).[44,45] The proximity of the AVM to eloquent white matter tracts may eliminate surgery as a treatment option, due to the risk of white matter tract injury intraoperatively or secondary to hemorrhage. Diffusion tensor tractography can be useful in determining the radiation dose to the corticospinal tract prior to stereotactic radiosurgery, and thus can help in therapeutic planning, allowing for delivery of an effective dose to the nidus while minimizing the risk of posttreatment complications.[46]

Diffusion tensor imaging and tractography of AVMs can depict fiber tract displacement or disruption, or decreased fiber tract density relating to involvement.[47] Some reports have indicated that there is a strong correlation between involvement of the corticospinal tract by hemorrhage or edema from AVM and contralateral hemiparesis,[44,47] whereas others have not been able to find an association.[45] In the authors' experience with diffusion tensor imaging, there may be the appearance of displacement, compression, or involvement of eloquent white matter tracts, without associated clinical deficits.

There are a few limitations of diffusion tensor imaging and tractography that are important. Hemorrhage or calcifications related to cerebral AVM, surgical clips, or postoperative changes can cause susceptibility artifacts on diffusion tensor imaging, which are problematic because the echo planar imaging technique is typically used.[48] In the setting of edema or involvement of a white matter tract, a drop in fractional anisotropy (FA) values may fall below the preset threshold for

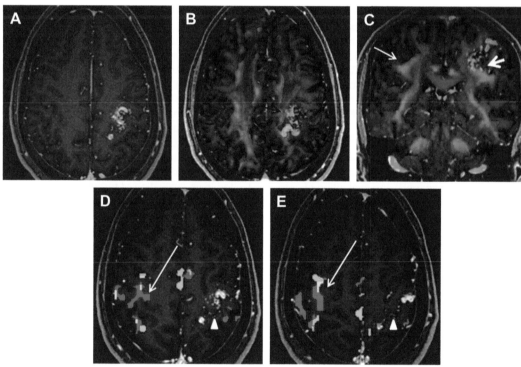

**Fig. 3.** A 40-year-old man who initially presented with right-sided weakness and numbness. Axial postcontrast T1-weighted sequence (*A*) shows left perirolandic arteriovenous malformation. Axial postcontrast T1-weighted sequence with overlaid color fractional anisotropy (FA) map (*B*) shows AVM nidus and prominent draining vein abutting and impressing on the left corticospinal tract (*arrow, surrounding blue white matter tracts*). On coronal postcontrast T1-weighted sequence with overlaid color FA map (*C*), the AVM is abutting and displacing the left superior longitudinal fasciculus (SLF) (*short arrow, green white matter tract*), in comparison with the normal contralateral SLF (*arrow*). Composite motor activation maps (*D* and *E*), with hand (*red*), foot (*blue*), and tongue (*yellow*) task-based BOLD functional MRI maps overlaid on axial T1 postcontrast sequences. There is no task-based activation overlaying the left motor cortex (*arrowhead*), whereas there is normal task-based activation on the right (*long arrow*). On breath-hold cerebrovascular reactivity maps (not shown), there was evidence of neurovascular uncoupling involving the left perirolandic regions.

tractography, leading to the false-positive appearance of disruption of this fiber tract. The FA threshold can be lowered to allow for detection through low-anisotropy regions; however, this may allow for the appearance of spurious white matter tracts. The authors prefer to rely on the color FA maps to evaluate for eloquent white matter tract involvement or displacement, due to the aforementioned limitations of tractography. At their institution the authors typically perform diffusion tensor imaging in conjunction with task-based functional MRI for preoperative planning, mostly in the setting of brain tumors, but occasionally in the setting of AVMs (see **Fig. 3**).

## Functional MRI in the Assessment of Cerebral Arteriovenous Malformation

Blood oxygen level–dependent (BOLD) functional MRI is a noninvasive technique that has developed into an important tool for preoperative planning. This technique relies on changes of susceptibility in regions of brain activated by specific tasks, related to slight changes of blood oxygenation. With neuronal activation there is a change in the microenvironment, leading to vascular dilatation, and an increase in blood oxygenation. Functional MRI allows for eloquent cortical mapping (both lateralization and localization) and evaluation of the spatial relationship of eloquent brain to the pathologic lesions that are being evaluated preoperatively. Frequently structures such as the motor or sensory strips, Broca's area, or Wernicke's area can be displaced, distorted, or involved by pathologic processes such as AVMs. In addition, normal variations of cortical surface anatomy make localization difficult or even impossible without functional imaging.[49] Functional imaging allows for prediction of resectability of a lesion, and identification of the components of a lesion that can be removed without sacrificing eloquent brain structures. Preoperative functional MRI can shorten the surgical time as well as alter the surgical approach.[50] With preoperative functional MRI smaller craniotomies are needed, as limited intraoperative cortical mapping can be used. Negative cortical mapping can be performed with electrical stimulation of the margins of the lesions to evaluate for any eloquent cortex.[51]

Functional MRI can serve as a helpful planning tool in the treatment of AVMs. Damage to eloquent cortex can be avoided before embolization, surgical resection, or radiosurgery of these lesions. Preoperative functional MRI may also alter the clinical plan, from surgery to radiosurgery, depending on the anatomic relationship to eloquent cortex.[51] When considering that AVMs represent congenital

lesions, it is no surprise that intrahemispheric and interhemispheric cortical reorganization can be seen in such patients.[52,53] An important limitation of task-based functional MRI in the evaluation of AVMs, as well as tumors, is neurovascular uncoupling. Functional MRI relies on cerebrovascular dilatation related to increased neuronal activity, leading to increased blood oxygen content. In the setting of cerebrovascular abnormality, such as is seen with AVM and dysplastic vessels supplying tumors, the abnormal vessels do not respond to these stimuli, and there can be diminished or no task-related BOLD activation of normal functioning neurons within the lesion or in the adjacent cortex. Neurovascular uncoupling can simulate cortical reorganization, as the normal cortex will have no task-related BOLD activation (see **Fig. 3**D, E).[54] At their institution, the authors use breath-hold BOLD cerebrovascular reactivity (CVR) maps to qualitatively evaluate for neurovascular uncoupling. Abnormal vessels such as those seen within and around cerebral AVM will not vasodilate in response to increased carbon dioxide levels, and will show absent or diminished activity on the CVR map relative to the rest of the brain.

### MRI Perfusion

First-pass dynamic susceptibility-weighted contrast-enhanced (DSC) MR perfusion imaging is an established perfusion technique used to evaluate relative cerebral blood volume (rCBV), mean transit time (MTT), relative cerebral blood flow (rCBF), and time to peak (TTP). The major clinical use of perfusion imaging is to evaluate ischemic penumbra in the setting of acute stroke and for tumor evaluation.

On MR perfusion examinations in the setting of cerebral AVM, there is increased CBF and CBV across the lesion, as expected, relating to increased transnidal flow. Perfusion of perinidal and remote brain relative to the AVM in the ipsilateral hemisphere is variable.[55] Guo and colleagues[56] reported two dominant patterns of perfusion, both of which showed increased perinidal rCBF and rCBV; this may result from dilatation of the perinidal arteries, which may be adaptive in response to adjacent low-resistance AVM feeding arterial structures, or could relate to angiogenesis in response to hypoperfusion secondary to cerebral steal.[55–57] A third pattern, however, is also discussed, in which there is reduced perinidal rCBV and rCBF, secondary to cerebral steal by the adjacent AVM.[56] After radiosurgery treatment, rCBV and rCBF values of the perinidal and remote brain parenchyma trended toward the normal values of the contralateral brain.[56]

## Digital Subtraction Angiography

Despite advancements in noninvasive imaging modalities, conventional DSA remains the gold standard for evaluation of cerebrovascular disease, including cerebral AVMs. The combination of exceptional spatial (0.2 mm) and temporal resolution (up to 24 frames per second) is unmatched by other imaging modalities.[28] DSA is optimal for the evaluation of AVM angioarchitecture, including improved detection of associated intranidal aneurysms, obstruction of venous outflow, arterial feeder anatomy, and venous drainage patterns (**Fig. 4**). Superselective microcatheter angiography can help further characterize AVM angioarchitecture by allowing targeting of specific feeding arterial branches. DSA is the optimal imaging modality to evaluate for potential risk factors for AVM rupture, including deep venous drainage, venous outflow stenosis or occlusion, intranidal and arterial feeder aneurysms, and high-flow lesions with increased arterial and venous pressure. DSA can be used for preradiosurgery delineation of the AVM nidus.[34] Catheter angiography allows for

planning of endovascular embolization, which is frequently an important component of the treatment strategy.

DSA is the gold standard for preradiosurgery evaluation of nidus size due to its excellent spatial and temporal resolution, allowing for evaluation of the size of the nidus before there is venous filling. However, because DSA is a 2D image depicting a 3D structure, the true nidal size can be inadequately assessed by overlap from adjacent vascular structures or inhomogeneous enhancement.[33] As described later, 3D rotational angiography supplements 2D DSA for the evaluation of the 3D contours of the nidus.

Limitations of DSA include that it is a 2D modality evaluating a 3D structure. Dilated venous varicosities and arterial feeders will overlap with the nidus on 2D DSA, obscuring evaluation of nidal size and contours. 3D rotational DSA (3D RDSA) provides 3D images that use the high spatial resolution of conventional DSA. This technique can provide improved evaluation of the relationship between the nidus, feeding arteries, and venous output. There is better depiction of the

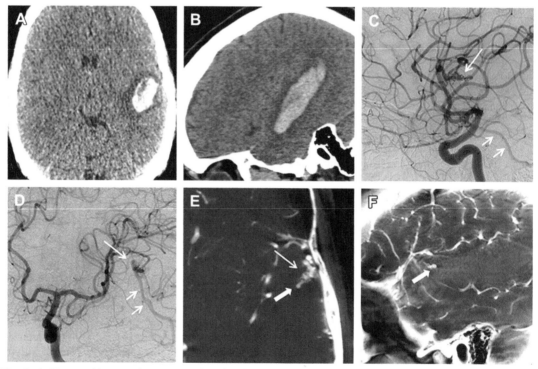

**Fig. 4.** A 40-year-old man who presented with aphasia. Axial (*A*) and sagittal (*B*) noncontrast CT of the head shows a left temporal lobe hematoma. Sagittal (*C*) and anteroposterior (*D*) DSA images during late arterial phase after left internal carotid injection show left temporal arteriovenous malformation nidus (*long arrow*) supplied by left MCA branches, with early draining vein (*short arrows*). C-arm cone-beam CT images in axial (*E*) and sagittal (*F*) planes show small peripheral temporal AVM nidus (*arrow*). There is a small outpouching projecting from the posterior aspect of the nidus (*thick arrow*) representing intranidal aneurysm, which projects into the anterior aspect of the left temporal hematoma. The intranidal aneurysm represented the AVM rupture point.

3D contours of the nidus shape, allowing for superior determination of the radiation target.[33]

Because DSA does not show the relationship and involvement of the adjacent brain parenchyma, conventional imaging modalities are frequently used for this evaluation. With the advent of cone-beam CT technology, some of these limitations of DSA can be overcome. DSA is an invasive procedure, with a small but finite risk of permanent neurologic deficit of approximately 0.1% to 1.0%.[29] Moreover, there are procedural risks associated with exposure to ionizing radiation and iodinated contrast dyes.

## C-Arm Cone-Beam CT

C-arm cone-beam CT (CBCT) represents a 3D C-arm mounted flat-panel detector cone-beam CT system, which produces high-resolution volumetric data acquisition with a single rotation of the C-arm.[58] The system is incorporated into the interventional suite, and high-resolution multiplanar reformats can be quickly generated at an independent workstation. After selecting the vascular structures of interest by catheter-directed interventional procedure, diluted contrast is injected immediately before imaging, thus providing high-resolution, selective cross-sectional 3D images, focusing on the vascular pathology of interest.

The applications of this technology are extensive, including evaluation of intracranial and extracranial vascular abnormalities, including AVMs, DAVFs, and aneurysms. CBCT has also shown the ability to show exquisite detail regarding venous intracranial anatomy, which cannot be achieved with MRA, CTA, or DSA. During intracranial vascular embolization, CBCT can help guide management in the setting of complications by producing high-quality CT scans.[59]

In the setting of cerebral AVM, CBCT provides excellent high-resolution 3D cross-sectional images, allowing for better characterization of the vascular lesion. Feeding arterial and draining venous structures can be better depicted, with cross-sectional images providing the exact point of communication with the nidus. Nidal angioarchitecture can also be better determined. CBCT can provide improved localization and characterization of nidal and flow-related venous and arterial aneurysms (see **Fig. 4**E, F). The relationship of the vascular malformation to adjacent brain structures is better depicted on CBCT than on 2D DSA contrast injections alone. Gupta and colleagues[60] reported a case in which CBCT allowed for better characterization of diffuse basal ganglionic AVM arterial supply, allowing for improved targeted embolization while sparing vascular supply to the intervening internal capsule.

## DURAL ARTERIOVENOUS FISTULAS
### General Features

DAVFs make up 10% to 15% of intracranial vascular malformations,[61] and are abnormal connections between dural arteries and dural venous sinuses, meningeal veins, or cortical veins. The etiopathogenesis remains to be fully elucidated, but DAVFs have been associated with history of trauma, previous craniotomy, or dural venous sinus thrombosis. In the setting of interrupted normal sinus outflow and elevated local venous pressures, it is hypothesized that tiny physiologic shunts may enlarge,[62] or neoangiogenic factors may promote the formation of pathologic connections.[63] Adult DAVFs, which constitute the majority of lesions, are most common at the transverse, sigmoid, and cavernous sinuses.[64] There is also a subset of pediatric lesions that can often involve the torcula, superior sagittal sinus, and large venous lakes.[65] The etiology of pediatric DAVFs is thought to be congenital or related to birth trauma, infection, or in utero venous thrombosis.

Adult intracranial DAVFs present most commonly in the fifth and sixth decades of life. Pulsatile tinnitus is one of the most common symptoms of transverse and sigmoid sinus lesions, and is related to increased flow through the dural venous sinuses. Cavernous sinus DAVFs can cause ophthalmoplegia, proptosis, chemosis, retroorbital pain, and decreased visual acuity.[62,66,67] Additional nonhemorrhagic neurologic deficits (NHND) include seizures, dementia, chronic headache, and cranial nerve abnormalities. Hemorrhage is more common in high-grade lesions, which demonstrate retrograde cortical venous drainage (CVD).

Accurate diagnosis and classification of DAVFs is essential in identifying patients with high-risk lesions and to triage them toward appropriate therapies. The Borden[66] and Cognard[68] classification schemes, which have been well substantiated as predictors of DAVF behavior, both emphasize the relationship between CVD and increased risk of hemorrhage or NHND. The absence of CVD (Borden I; Cognard IIa) is associated with a benign natural history. These patients typically present with pulsatile tinnitus and other signs of increased dural venous drainage, but have a low risk of hemorrhage. The presence of CVD (Borden II, III; Cognard IIb–V) indicates a more aggressive lesion, associated with an annual mortality rate of up to 10.4%, hemorrhage rate of up to 8.1%, and risk of NHND of up to 6.9%.[67] Zipfel and colleagues[69] have further subclassified lesions exhibiting CVD into those that present with hemorrhage or NHND and those that are detected incidentally or present with nonaggressive symptoms (ie, tinnitus, ophthalmologic symptoms). The former group has a higher annual risk of hemorrhage at approximately 7.5% whereas the latter group has lower risk at approximately 1.5%, suggesting that this additional subclassification may improve the accuracy of risk stratification in DAVF patients.[69]

The diagnosis of DAVFs at an early stage may be difficult because of nonspecific clinical and imaging findings. A high index of suspicion is thus necessary when a patient presents with an unexplained constellation of neurologic complaints and deficits. The goal of imaging is not only to determine the presence or absence of a DAVF but also to clarify the pattern of venous drainage. Once the morphology and hemodynamics of the lesion are appropriately delineated, the need to pursue aggressive therapies can be determined.

## Conventional Cross-Sectional Imaging

Although the diagnosis of DAVFs has traditionally been by DSA, many of these lesions are now first detected or suspected on cross-sectional imaging. Noncontrast head CT is often used as an initial screening tool to determine the presence of hemorrhage or edema from venous congestion, but is otherwise limited in its diagnostic contribution. MRI can demonstrate engorged vessels, dilated venous pouches, or abnormal vascular enhancement in the presence of a DAVF. Several of these findings are the result of venous hypertension or retrograde CVD, leading to medullary venous congestion. In a series of 27 patients, Kwon and colleagues[61] demonstrated a significant association between dilated vessels or prominent vascular enhancement with the presence of retrograde CVD. Venous hypertension in high-grade lesions is also thought to contribute to abnormalities such as white matter T2 hyperintensity, intracranial hemorrhage, or venous infarction. Low-grade lesions may exhibit only flow-void clustering, engorged veins, or proptosis. The presence of any suspicious findings on MRI should warrant further imaging evaluation with dynamic CTA, MRA, or DSA for clarification of lesion grade and management decision making.[61]

## MRI Perfusion

DSC MR perfusion can be a very sensitive marker for the evaluation of impaired venous drainage in the setting of cerebral DAVF, and permits for the quantitative evaluation of MTT, CBV, and CBF. In patients with cerebral DAVF with retrograde CVD, there are increased CBV values involving the affected cerebral hemisphere secondary to impaired venous drainage.[70] The correlation of increased parenchymal perfusion to retrograde cortical venous drainage is controversial. According to Noguchi and colleagues,[71] CBV ratios (CBV values of the affected hemisphere relative to the contralateral normal hemisphere) show increased values in the affected cerebral hemisphere with DAVF and retrograde CVD, in comparison with normal control subjects and patients with DAVF without retrograde CVD. CBV ratios in patients with DAVF without retrograde CVD approximated ratios in control subjects.[71] Fujita and colleagues[72] claim that in the setting of DAVF with or without retrograde CVD, there is increased CBV ratio, prolonged transit time, and decreased CBF in the affected cerebral hemisphere, consistent with a pattern-impaired venous outflow. No statistically significant difference was found in perfusion between DAVF with or without retrograde cortical venous drainage.[72] After treatment of DAVF with retrograde CVD, CBV ratios of the affected cerebral hemispheres decreased, trending toward the values seen in normal control subjects.[71]

## Susceptibility-Weighted Imaging

SWI is a technique that allows for improved detection of extravascular blood and better characterization of veins carrying deoxygenated blood. SWI can clearly depict arteriovenous shunting in cerebral DAVF, represented as hyperintense venous signal relating to rapid wash-in of oxygenated blood.[24]

SWI can accurately depict retrograde CVD associated with DAVF. In the setting of DAVF there is impaired venous drainage and increased venous pressure, resulting in cortical venous engorgement, as well as prolonged venous stagnation, leading to increased venous oxygen extraction. These factors are thought to result in increased prominence of cortical veins on SWI in the setting of retrograde CVD with DAVF.[73] According to Noguchi and colleagues,[70] SWI depicts dilated superficial veins involving the ipsilateral cerebral hemisphere in all cases of DAVF with retrograde CVD, whereas conventional MRI sequences depict dilated superficial veins in only 71% of cases. SWI portrays prominent deep draining veins in 64% of the affected cerebral hemispheres, whereas T2-weighted sequences show prominent veins in only 34% of cases.[70] This finding corresponds to the expected increased rCBV values on DSC perfusion sequences of the affected cerebral hemisphere, secondary to impaired venous drainage.[70]

## MR Angiography

3D TOF MRA is limited in the evaluation of DAVFs because of the lack of hemodynamic information, but can suggest the presence of a lesion by abnormal flow enhancement.[74,75] In a series of 11 patients by Kwon and colleagues,[61] MRA demonstrated fistula-site enhancement in 83% of cases, and venous flow-related enhancement in 91% of cases. Fistula-site enhancement was detected only in cases with CVD; this reliance in flow dynamics contributed to the failure in visualization of one DAVF (8%) with slow venous flow. Lesions with smaller and multiple arterial feeders and draining veins, as commonly seen in carotid-cavernous fistulas, are also more difficult to visualize precisely. The dependence of TOF MRA on flow velocity can present a challenge of distinguishing abnormal, fast, or slow shunt flow from normal flow in certain cases.

Dynamic MRA using time-resolved imaging of contrast kinetics (TRICKS) has evolved substantially in recent years and has developed an increasing role in DAVF imaging. The dynamic resolution of this modality is adequate for separating early arterial, arterial, parenchymal, and venous phases. Initial studies using 1.5-T scanners were limited by low spatial resolution, signal-to-noise ratio, and region of coverage, precluding clear identification of feeding arteries and draining veins or the presence of CVD.[75,76] The advent of 3-T scanning technology has offered a solution to many of these issues, and recent studies on whole-head time-resolved MRA (trMRA) have suggested the advantages of this modality as a screening and surveillance tool.[77,78] In a retrospective series of 42 patients (20 of whom harbored DAVFs), comparing the results of trMRA to DSA for presence, location, and classification of DAVFs, Farb and colleagues[77] reported only a 2.4% error rate of diagnosis using trMRA. These errors included 2 cases in which CVD was interpreted on trMRA images, but not demonstrated on DSA, and one case of a Borden I lesion that was missed on trMRA.[77] Nishimura and colleagues[78] reported a prospective series of 18 patients in which DSA and trMRA results were independently interpreted by radiologists who were blinded to the results of the other modality. Intermodality agreement for fistula site and lesion grade, based on venous drainage pattern, was 100%, but for the identification of arterial feeders was 89%. These data reflected the limitations of trMRA spatial resolution compared with DSA (1 × 1 × 1.5 mm vs submillimeter, respectively), which hinders its ability to fully characterize lesions for therapeutic purposes. Despite this limitation, the investigators suggest that trMRA is a suitable modality for primary diagnosis and follow-up evaluations for DAVFs. It must be emphasized, however, that in patients who demonstrate objective clinical signs of a vascular lesion, DSA should still be performed to definitively rule out a DAVF, irrespective of negative MRA findings.

## CT Angiography

CTA can provide a useful adjunct for treatment planning by defining the location of the arteriovenous shunt relative to surrounding brain and skull anatomy. CTA can be performed rapidly, is widely available, and can be easily combined with other CT evaluations. DAVFs, however, can be obscured by overlapping osseous structures on conventional CTA, reducing the sensitivity of the modality to as low as 15.4% in some studies.[79] Several techniques for bone subtraction, including direct subtraction, local subtraction, matched mask bone elimination, and hybrid CTA, have been investigated as potential solutions to these limitations. Hybrid CTA uses reconstruction algorithms to remove bone structures while preserving the appearance of vascular channels, and has demonstrated promising results in recent studies. Lee and colleagues[80] analyzed the diagnostic efficacy of 64-detector-row hybrid CTA in the evaluation of 24 DAVFs, using DSA as the reference standard. The most common findings on CTA were asymmetric sinus enhancement (92%), engorged arteries (79%), and enhancing transosseous vessels (79%).[80] Lesion grade by CTA was confirmed by DSA in 100% of cavernous sinus lesions and 78% to 89% of transverse-sigmoid lesions. Hybrid CTA images were also suitable for treatment planning in most cases. Hybrid CTA lacks dynamic information, and requires further experience before its full role in DAVF evaluation can be determined.[80]

The advent of 320-detector-row CT scanners has also opened investigations into 4-dimensional (4D) dynamic CTA for the evaluation of DAVFs (Fig. 5).[81,82] The appeal of this technology is similar to that of trMRA, as a potential tool to replace DSA for primary diagnosis and follow-up in patients who would otherwise require repeat DSA studies. Willems and colleagues[82] have described their preliminary experience with 4D CTA in the evaluation of 11 DAVFs. DSA and CTA studies were interpreted independently by two blinded observers using a standardized scoring system. Ten of 11 cases were successfully detected on 4D CTA and agreed fully with the Borden classification on DSA. However, one Borden III lesion (9%), which had presented with a hemorrhage, was undetected on 4D CTA as a result of slow flow and low shunt volume. Large arterial feeders were recognized in 6 of 10 cases on 4D CTA, but additional contributors were missed in

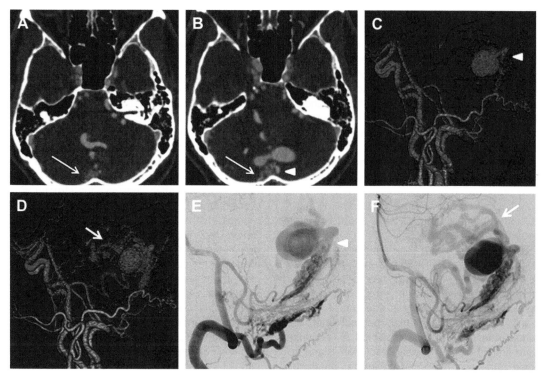

**Fig. 5.** A 56-year-old man with history of chronic progressive headaches. Axial dynamic 320-slice CTA images of the head (*A* and *B*) show high-flow posterior fossa dural arteriovenous fistula with multiple tiny posterior inferior cerebellar artery and posterior meningeal (from vertebral artery) arterial feeding branches (*long arrow*), with arteriovenous fistula point (*arrowhead*). There is a large dilated draining venous varix anterior to the fistula. 3D reformatted sagittal dynamic CT angiography image (*C*) and sagittal DSA image (*E*) in early arterial phase, with multiple arterial feeders, fistulous point (*arrowhead*), adjacent early draining vein, and dilated draining venous varix. 3D reformat sagittal dynamic 320 CTA image (*D*) and sagittal DSA image (*F*) in late arterial phase shows multiple tortuous early draining veins (*short arrows*).

up to 8 of 10 cases on 4D CTA.[82] The investigators concluded that 4D CTA currently lacks the spatial resolution to sufficiently delineate the angioarchitecture of DAVFs, and suggested the continued use of DSA for diagnosis and treatment planning. Of interest, the spatial and temporal resolution achieved on 4D CTA is greater than that of trMRA, but studies have demonstrated superior sensitivity for DAVF detection with trMRA.[77,79] With continued developments in CT scanning technologies and reconstruction algorithms, 4D CTA will undoubtedly continue to advance, and further evaluation of its diagnostic value as an adjunct to DSA is merited. As with any CT-based technology, consideration of radiation dose will also ultimately be important in determining the optimal application of this modality toward patient care.

## 2D DSA and C-Arm Cone-Beam CT

Despite advancements in noninvasive imaging modalities, conventional DSA remains the gold standard for detection and classification of DAVFs

(see **Figs. 5** and **6**). DSA has a submillimeter spatial resolution, allowing detection of small lesions that may be missed by other modalities. The temporal resolution and ability to perform selective injections allow for precise identification of early dural venous sinus filling or cortical venous reflux. Catheter angiography also provides the foundation for endovascular embolization, which has become a first-line therapy for DAVF treatment.

The use of 3D CBCT, also called flat detector CT, as an adjunct to 2D DSA has recently been described for the evaluation of DAVFs. CBCT addresses several of the challenges of DSA: it has a high spatial resolution of 0.1- to 0.4-mm voxels and can clearly delineate venous structures that are often obscured by the effects of contrast dilution or motion artifact on DSA. These advantages allow it to accurately demonstrate fistulous points and visualize even very small arterial feeders or draining veins without the need for additional selective DSA injections (see **Fig. 6**D, E). A series of 14 patients reported by Hiu and colleagues[83] found that CBCT contributed

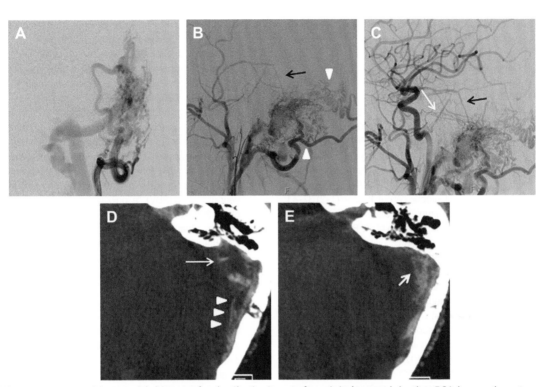

**Fig. 6.** A 54-year-old man with history of pulsatile tinnitus. Left occipital artery injection DSA images in antero-posterior (*A*) and external carotid artery injection in the lateral (*B*) planes, and left common carotid injection DSA image in the lateral plane (*C*) were performed during early arterial phase. Prominent left temporal arteriovenous fistula is present, which is being supplied by multiple left occipital arterial feeding branches (*arrowheads*), left middle meningeal branch (*black arrow*), and left meningohypophyseal branches (*white arrow*), with early filling of the left sigmoid sinus and jugular bulb best seen on image *A*. Axial cone-beam CT images (*D* and *E*) show multiple left occipital branch vessels (*arrowheads*) and left meningohypophyseal branch arterial vessel (*long arrow*) that converge on arteriovenous fistulous point (*short arrow*), which drains into the left sigmoid sinus.

additional findings in 57% of cases compared with corresponding DSA images; the majority of these findings demonstrated the precise fistulous point. Similar evidence for the utility of CBCT has been compiled for the evaluation of spinal DAVFs.[84] In addition to demonstrating fine vascular detail, CBCT also has the advantage of concurrently visualizing the surrounding osseous structures, which can be of particular value for surgical planning. CBCT does not provide a dynamic evaluation, so arterial and venous components are visualized simultaneously and can be challenging to differentiate without corresponding DSA images. Although more experience is needed to further evaluate the utility of CBCT as an adjunct to DSA, preliminary evidence already highlights its potential contributions to the diagnosis and treatment of DAVFs.

## SUMMARY

Imaging of cerebral AVMs and DAVFs is central to the diagnosis, proper characterization, and evaluation of these lesions. Imaging is helpful in pretreatment planning as well as posttreatment evaluation for residual arteriovenous shunting. DSA remains the gold standard for evaluation of AVM and DAVF, and CBCT is providing improved 3D evaluation. CT and MRI applications are complementary, and provide useful information relating to the association of the vascular lesions to the surrounding intracranial structures as well as physiologic information, which cannot always be adequately evaluated with DSA. Significant improvement in imaging techniques has allowed progressive improvement in temporal and spatial resolution for MRA and CTA techniques, thereby allowing for improved noninvasive evaluation of time-dependent characteristics.

## REFERENCES

1. Stapf C, Mohr JP, Sciacca RR, et al. Incident hemorrhage risk of brain arteriovenous malformations located in the arterial borderzones. Stroke 2000; 31(10):2365–8.

2. Lasjaunias P. A revised concept of the congenital nature of cerebral arteriovenous malformations. Interv Neuroradiol 1997;3(4):275–81.

3. Osborn AG. Diagnostic cerebral angiography. 2nd edition. Philadelphia: Lippincott Williams and Wilkins; 1999.

4. Alkadhi H, Kollias SS, Crelier GR, et al. Plasticity of the human motor cortex in patients with arteriovenous malformations: a functional MR imaging study. AJNR Am J Neuroradiol 2000;21(8):1423–33.

5. Willinsky R, Lasjaunias P, Comoy J, et al. Cerebral micro arteriovenous malformations (mAVMs). Review of 13 cases. Acta Neurochir (Wien) 1988;91(1–2):37–41.

6. Berenstein A, Lasjaunias P. Classification of CVMs. Surgical neuroangiography, vol. 4. Berlin: Springer; 1992. p. 25–80.

7. Turjman F, Massoud TF, Vinuela F, et al. Correlation of the angioarchitectural features of cerebral arteriovenous malformations with clinical presentation of hemorrhage. Neurosurgery 1995;37(5):856–60 [discussion: 860–2].

8. Pritz MB. Ruptured supratentorial arteriovenous malformations associated with venous aneurysms. Acta Neurochir (Wien) 1994;128(1–4):150–62.

9. Brown RD Jr, Wiebers DO, Forbes GS. Unruptured intracranial aneurysms and arteriovenous malformations: frequency of intracranial hemorrhage and relationship of lesions. J Neurosurg 1990;73(6):859–63.

10. Graf CJ, Perret GE, Torner JC. Bleeding from cerebral arteriovenous malformations as part of their natural history. J Neurosurg 1983;58(3):331–7.

11. Stapf C, Mast H, Sciacca RR, et al. Predictors of hemorrhage in patients with untreated brain arteriovenous malformation. Neurology 2006;66(9):1350–5.

12. ApSimon HT, Reef H, Phadke RV, et al. A population-based study of brain arteriovenous malformation: long-term treatment outcomes. Stroke 2002;33(12):2794–800.

13. Fleetwood IG, Steinberg GK. Arteriovenous malformations. Lancet 2002;359(9309):863–73.

14. Duong DH, Young WL, Vang MC, et al. Feeding artery pressure and venous drainage pattern are primary determinants of hemorrhage from cerebral arteriovenous malformations. Stroke 1998;29(6):1167–76.

15. Crawford PM, West CR, Chadwick DW, et al. Arteriovenous malformations of the brain: natural history in unoperated patients. J Neurol Neurosurg Psychiatry 1986;49(1):1–10.

16. Mast H, Young WL, Koennecke HC, et al. Risk of spontaneous haemorrhage after diagnosis of cerebral arteriovenous malformation. Lancet 1997; 350(9084):1065–8.

17. Brown RD Jr, Flemming KD, Meyer FB, et al. Natural history, evaluation, and management of intracranial vascular malformations. Mayo Clin Proc 2005; 80(2):269–81.

18. Choi JH, Mohr JP. Brain arteriovenous malformations in adults. Lancet Neurol 2005;4(5):299–308.

19. Hofmeister C, Stapf C, Hartmann A, et al. Demographic, morphological, and clinical characteristics of 1289 patients with brain arteriovenous malformation. Stroke 2000;31(6):1307–10.

20. Pollock BE, Kondziolka D, Flickinger JC, et al. Magnetic resonance imaging: an accurate method to evaluate arteriovenous malformations after stereotactic radiosurgery. J Neurosurg 1996;85(6):1044–9.

21. Reichenbach JR, Jonetz-Mentzel L, Fitzek C, et al. High-resolution blood oxygen-level dependent MR venography (HRBV): a new technique. Neuroradiology 2001;43(5):364–9.

22. Tsui YK, Tsai FY, Hasso AN, et al. Susceptibility-weighted imaging for differential diagnosis of cerebral vascular pathology: a pictorial review. J Neuro Sci 2009;287(1–2):7–16.

23. Heidenreich JO, Schilling AM, Unterharnscheidt F, et al. Assessment of 3D-TOF-MRA at 3.0 Tesla in the characterization of the angioarchitecture of cerebral arteriovenous malformations: a preliminary study. Acta Radiol 2007;48(6):678–86.

24. Jagadeesan BD, Delgado Almandoz JE, Moran CJ, et al. Accuracy of susceptibility-weighted imaging for the detection of arteriovenous shunting in vascular malformations of the brain. Stroke 2011; 42(1):87–92.

25. Essig M, Reichenbach JR, Schad LR, et al. High-resolution MR venography of cerebral arteriovenous malformations. Magn Reson Imaging 1999;17(10): 1417–25.

26. Krings T, Hans F. New developments in MRA: time-resolved MRA. Neuroradiology 2004;46(Suppl 2): s214–22.

27. Cashen TA, Carr JC, Shin W, et al. Intracranial time-resolved contrast-enhanced MR angiography at 3T. AJNR Am J Neuroradiol 2006;27(4):822–9.

28. Eddleman CS, Jeong HJ, Hurley MC, et al. 4D radial acquisition contrast-enhanced MR angiography and intracranial arteriovenous malformations: quickly approaching digital subtraction angiography. Stroke 2009;40(8):2749–53.

29. Griffiths PD, Hoggard N, Warren DJ, et al. Brain arteriovenous malformations: assessment with dynamic MR digital subtraction angiography. AJNR Am J Neuroradiol 2000;21(10):1892–9.

30. Oleaga L, Dalal SS, Weigele JB, et al. The role of time-resolved 3D contrast-enhanced MR angiography in the assessment and grading of cerebral arteriovenous malformations. Eur J Radiol 2010; 74(3):e117–21.

31. Saleh RS, Lohan DG, Villablanca JP, et al. Assessment of craniospinal arteriovenous malformations at 3T with highly temporally and highly spatially resolved contrast-enhanced MR angiography. AJNR Am J Neuroradiol 2008;29(5):1024–31.

32. Saleh RS, Singhal A, Lohan D, et al. Assessment of cerebral arteriovenous malformations with high temporal and spatial resolution contrast-enhanced magnetic resonance angiography: a review from protocol to clinical application. Top Magn Reson Imaging 2008;19(5):251–7.

33. Berger MO, Anxionnat R, Kerrien E, et al. A methodology for validating a 3D imaging modality for brain AVM delineation: application to 3DRA. Comput Med Imaging Graph 2008;32(7):544–53.

34. Bednarz G, Downes B, Werner-Wasik M, et al. Combining stereotactic angiography and 3D time-of-flight magnetic resonance angiography in treatment planning for arteriovenous malformation radiosurgery. Int J Radiat Oncol Biol Phys 2000; 46(5):1149–54.

35. Kondziolka D, Lunsford LD, Kanal E, et al. Stereotactic magnetic resonance angiography for targeting in arteriovenous malformation radiosurgery. Neurosurgery 1994;35(4):585–90 [discussion: 590–1].

36. Flickinger JC, Pollock BE, Kondziolka D, et al. A dose-response analysis of arteriovenous malformation obliteration after radiosurgery. Int J Radiat Oncol Biol Phys 1996;36(4):873–9.

37. Steiner L, Lindquist C, Adler JR, et al. Clinical outcome of radiosurgery for cerebral arteriovenous malformations. J Neurosurg 1992;77(1):1–8.

38. Spiegelmann R, Friedman WA, Bova FJ. Limitations of angiographic target localization in planning radiosurgical treatment. Neurosurgery 1992;30(4):619–23 [discussion: 623–4].

39. Kauczor HU, Engenhart R, Layer G, et al. 3D TOF MR angiography of cerebral arteriovenous malformations after radiosurgery. J Comput Assist Tomogr 1993;17(2):184–90.

40. Morikawa M, Numaguchi Y, Rigamonti D, et al. Radiosurgery for cerebral arteriovenous malformations: assessment of early phase magnetic resonance imaging and significance of gadolinium-DTPA enhancement. Int J Radiat Oncol Biol Phys 1996; 34(3):663–75.

41. Lee KE, Choi CG, Choi JW, et al. Detection of residual brain arteriovenous malformations after radiosurgery: diagnostic accuracy of contrast-enhanced three-dimensional time of flight MR angiography at 3.0 Tesla. Korean J Radiol 2009;10(4):333–9.

42. Mukherji SK, Quisling RG, Kubilis PS, et al. Intracranial arteriovenous malformations: quantitative analysis of magnitude contrast MR angiography versus gradient-echo MR imaging versus conventional angiography. Radiology 1995;196(1):187–93.

43. Murata T, Horiuchi T, Rahmah NN, et al. Three-dimensional magnetic resonance imaging based on time-of-flight magnetic resonance angiography for superficial cerebral arteriovenous malformation–technical note. Neurol Med Chir (Tokyo) 2011;51(2):163–7.

44. Itoh D, Aoki S, Maruyama K, et al. Corticospinal tracts by diffusion tensor tractography in patients with arteriovenous malformations. J Comput Assist Tomogr 2006;30(4):618–23.

45. Okada T, Miki Y, Kikuta K, et al. Diffusion tensor fiber tractography for arteriovenous malformations: quantitative analyses to evaluate the corticospinal tract and optic radiation. AJNR Am J Neuroradiol 2007; 28(6):1107–13.

46. Maruyama K, Kamada K, Shin M, et al. Integration of three-dimensional corticospinal tractography into treatment planning for gamma knife surgery. J Neurosurg 2005;102(4):673–7.

47. Berube J, McLaughlin N, Bourgouin P, et al. Diffusion tensor imaging analysis of long association bundles in the presence of an arteriovenous malformation. J Neurosurg 2007;107(3):509–14.

48. Field AS, Alexander AL. Diffusion tensor imaging in cerebral tumor diagnosis and therapy. Top Magn Reson Imaging 2004;15(5):315–24.

49. Naidich TP, Grant JL, Altman N, et al. The developing cerebral surface. Preliminary report on the patterns of sulcal and gyral maturation–anatomy, ultrasound, and magnetic resonance imaging. Neuroimaging Clin N Am 1994;4(2):201–40.

50. Petrella JR, Shah LM, Harris KM, et al. Preoperative functional MR imaging localization of language and motor areas: effect on therapeutic decision making in patients with potentially resectable brain tumors. Radiology 2006;240(3):793–802.

51. Latchaw RE, Hu X, Ugurbil K, et al. Functional magnetic resonance imaging as a management tool for cerebral arteriovenous malformations. Neurosurgery 1995;37(4):619–25 [discussion: 625–6].

52. Caramia F, Francia A, Mainero C, et al. Neurophysiological and functional MRI evidence of reorganization of cortical motor areas in cerebral arteriovenous malformation. Magn Reson Imaging 2009;27(10): 1360–9.

53. Lazar RM, Marshall RS, Pile-Spellman J, et al. Interhemispheric transfer of language in patients with left frontal cerebral arteriovenous malformation. Neuropsychologia 2000;38(10):1325–32.

54. Ulmer JL, Krouwer HG, Mueller WM, et al. Pseudo-reorganization of language cortical function at fMR imaging: a consequence of tumor-induced neurovascular uncoupling. AJNR Am J Neuroradiol 2003;24(2):213–7.

55. Turski PA. MR evaluation of brain perfusion after radiosurgery of cerebral arteriovenous malformations: a neuroradiologist's perspective. AJNR Am J Neuroradiol 2004;25(10):1631.

56. Guo WY, Wu YT, Wu HM, et al. Toward normal perfusion after radiosurgery: perfusion MR Imaging with independent component analysis of brain arteriovenous malformations. AJNR Am J Neuroradiol 2004; 25(10):1636–44.

57. Quick CM, Leonard EF, Young WL. Adaptation of cerebral circulation to brain arteriovenous malformations increases feeding artery pressure and decreases regional hypotension. Neurosurgery 2002;50(1):167–73 [discussion: 173–5].

58. Orth RC, Wallace MJ, Kuo MD. C-arm cone-beam CT: general principles and technical considerations for use in interventional radiology. J Vasc Interv Radiol 2008;19(6):814–20.

59. Heran NS, Song JK, Namba K, et al. The utility of DynaCT in neuroendovascular procedures. AJNR Am J Neuroradiol 2006;27(2):330–2.

60. Gupta V, Chugh M, Walia BS, et al. Use of CT angiography for anatomic localization of arteriovenous malformation nidal components. AJNR Am J Neuroradiol 2008;29(10):1837–40.

61. Kwon BJ, Han MH, Kang HS, et al. MR imaging findings of intracranial dural arteriovenous fistulas: relations with venous drainage patterns. AJNR Am J Neuroradiol 2005;26(10):2500–7.

62. Chung SJ, Kim JS, Kim JC, et al. Intracranial dural arteriovenous fistulas: analysis of 60 patients. Cerebrovasc Dis 2002;13(2):79–88.

63. Kojima T, Miyachi S, Sahara Y, et al. The relationship between venous hypertension and expression of vascular endothelial growth factor: hemodynamic and immunohistochemical examinations in a rat venous hypertension model. Surg Neurol 2007; 68(3):277–84 [discussion: 284].

64. Kirsch M, Liebig T, Kuhne D, et al. Endovascular management of dural arteriovenous fistulas of the transverse and sigmoid sinus in 150 patients. Neuroradiology 2009;51(7):477–83.

65. Morita A, Meyer FB, Nichols DA, et al. Childhood dural arteriovenous fistulae of the posterior dural sinuses: three case reports and literature review. Neurosurgery 1995;37(6):1193–9 [discussion: 1199–1200].

66. Borden JA, Wu JK, Shucart WA. A proposed classification for spinal and cranial dural arteriovenous fistulous malformations and implications for treatment. J Neurosurg 1995;82(2):166–79.

67. van Dijk JM, terBrugge KG, Willinsky RA, et al. Clinical course of cranial dural arteriovenous fistulas with long-term persistent cortical venous reflux. Stroke 2002;33(5):1233–6.

68. Cognard C, Gobin YP, Pierot L, et al. Cerebral dural arteriovenous fistulas: clinical and angiographic correlation with a revised classification of venous drainage. Radiology 1995;194(3):671–80.

69. Zipfel GJ, Shah MN, Refai D, et al. Cranial dural arteriovenous fistulas: modification of angiographic classification scales based on new natural history data. Neurosurg Focus 2009;26(5):E14.

70. Noguchi K, Kuwayama N, Kubo M, et al. Intracranial dural arteriovenous fistula with retrograde cortical venous drainage: use of susceptibility-weighted imaging in combination with dynamic susceptibility contrast imaging. AJNR Am J Neuroradiol 2010; 31(10):1903–10.

71. Noguchi K, Kubo M, Kuwayama N, et al. Intracranial dural arteriovenous fistulas with retrograde cortical venous drainage: assessment with cerebral blood volume by dynamic susceptibility contrast magnetic resonance imaging. AJNR Am J Neuroradiol 2006;27(6):1252–6.

72. Fujita A, Nakamura M, Tamaki N, et al. Haemodynamic assessment in patients with dural arteriovenous fistulae: dynamic susceptibility contrast-enhanced MRI. Neuroradiology 2002;44(10):806–11.

73. Saini J, Thomas B, Bodhey NK, et al. Susceptibility-weighted imaging in cranial dural arteriovenous fistulas. AJNR Am J Neuroradiol 2009;30(1):E6.

74. Cellerini M, Mascalchi M, Mangiafico S, et al. Phase-contrast MR angiography of intracranial dural arteriovenous fistulae. Neuroradiology 1999;41(7):487–92.

75. Noguchi K, Melhem ER, Kanazawa T, et al. Intracranial dural arteriovenous fistulas: evaluation with combined 3D time-of-flight MR angiography and MR digital subtraction angiography. AJR Am J Roentgenol 2004;182(1):183–90.

76. Akiba H, Tamakawa M, Hyodoh H, et al. Assessment of dural arteriovenous fistulas of the cavernous sinuses on 3D dynamic MR angiography. AJNR Am J Neuroradiol 2008;29(9):1652–7.

77. Farb RI, Agid R, Willinsky RA, et al. Cranial dural arteriovenous fistula: diagnosis and classification with time-resolved MR angiography at 3T. AJNR Am J Neuroradiol 2009;30(8):1546–51.

78. Nishimura S, Hirai T, Sasao A, et al. Evaluation of dural arteriovenous fistulas with 4D contrast-enhanced MR angiography at 3T. AJNR Am J Neuroradiol 2010;31(1):80–5.

79. Cohen SD, Goins JL, Butler SG, et al. Dural arteriovenous fistula: diagnosis, treatment, and outcomes. Laryngoscope 2009;119(2):293–7.

80. Lee CW, Huang A, Wang YH, et al. Intracranial dural arteriovenous fistulas: diagnosis and evaluation with 64-detector row CT angiography. Radiology 2010; 256(1):219–28.

81. Siebert E, Bohner G, Dewey M, et al. 320-slice CT neuroimaging: initial clinical experience and image quality evaluation. Br J Radiol 2009;82(979):561–70.

82. Willems PW, Brouwer PA, Barfett JJ, et al. Detection and classification of cranial dural arteriovenous fistulas using 4D-CT angiography: initial experience. AJNR Am J Neuroradiol 2011;32(1):49–53.

83. Hiu T, Kitagawa N, Morikawa M, et al. Efficacy of DynaCT digital angiography in the detection of the fistulous point of dural arteriovenous fistulas. AJNR Am J Neuroradiol 2009;30(3):487–91.

84. Aadland TD, Thielen KR, Kaufmann TJ, et al. 3D C-arm conebeam CT angiography as an adjunct in the precise anatomic characterization of spinal dural arteriovenous fistulas. AJNR Am J Neuroradiol 2010; 31(3):476–80.

# Classification Schemes for Arteriovenous Malformations

Jason M. Davies, MD, PhD[a], Helen Kim, PhD[b,c],
William L. Young, MD[a,b,c,d], Michael T. Lawton, MD[a,c],*

**KEYWORDS**

- Arteriovenous malformation • Classification
- Grading system • Spetzler-Martin

Judicious patient selection is essential to avoid surgical complications and poor neurologic outcomes with microsurgical resection of brain arteriovenous malformations (AVMs). The wide variety of AVM anatomy, size, location, and clinical presentation makes patient selection for surgery a difficult process. Neurosurgeons have analyzed their surgical experiences to identify factors that determine the risks of surgery to assist them in this selection process. Numerous classification schemes have been developed, each with its own emphasis, accuracy, advantages, and disadvantages. Some are complex and others simple, each striving to predict surgical risk and to achieve bedside applicability. These classification schemes have value because they transform complex decisions into algorithms. In this review, the important grading schemes that have contributed to management of patients with brain AVMs are described, and our current approach to patient selection is outlined.

## PRE–SPETZLER-MARTIN CLASSIFICATION SCHEMES

The first major AVM grading scheme developed by Luessenhop and Gennarelli[1] in 1977 formulated a grade from I to IV based on the number of feeding arteries for which there is standardized nomenclature. The score was determined by counting the number of tertiary arteries feeding the AVM from a single vascular territory, like the middle cerebral artery (MCA), anterior cerebral artery (ACA), or posterior cerebral artery (PCA) territory. When the AVM was supplied by multiple territories, the grade was determined by the vascular territory with the largest number of feeders. No additional grade was assigned for large AVMs with more than 4 arteries, because these lesions were deemed inoperable. There were several exceptions in this scheme: lenticulostriate vessels were counted as named arteries; choroid plexus-based AVMs were deemed grade III because they are supplied by 1 anterior and 2

[a] Department of Neurological Surgery, University of California San Francisco, 505 Parnassus Avenue, M780, San Francisco, CA 94143-0112, USA
[b] Department of Anesthesia and Perioperative Care, University of California San Francisco, 521 Parnassus Avenue, C450, San Francisco, CA 94143-0648, USA
[c] Center for Cerebrovascular Research, University of California San Francisco, 1001 Potrero Avenue, Box-1371, San Francisco, CA 94110, USA
[d] Department of Neurology, University of California San Francisco, 505 Parnassus Avenue, M798, San Francisco, CA 94143-0110, USA
* Corresponding author.
E-mail address: lawtonm@neurosurg.ucsf.edu

Neurosurg Clin N Am 23 (2012) 43–53
doi:10.1016/j.nec.2011.09.002
1042-3680/12/$ – see front matter © 2012 Elsevier Inc. All rights reserved.

posterior choroidal arteries; and corpus callosum AVMs were deemed grade II when supplied by pericallosal arteries and grade III when supplied by the PCA. The investigators made allowances for clinical status to supplement anatomic grading scale, but clear guidelines for integrating clinical and anatomic factors were lacking. Surgical results in 49 patients showed that grade I AVMs were associated with low risk, higher-grade AVMs were associated with increasing risks, and grade IV AVMs were managed nonoperatively.

Luessenhop and Rosa[2] simplified this grading scheme in 1984 by considering only the angiographic size of the AVM, which was believed to be easier than counting arterial feeders. The new grades were assigned based on nidus diameter: grade I, less than 2 cm; grade II, 2 to 4 cm; grade III, 4 to 6 cm; and grade IV, greater than 6 cm. The original classification scheme excluded AVMs in the cerebellum, brain stem, and region of the vein of Galen malformations, whereas the new scheme included cerebellar AVMs. In a surgical series consisting of 90 patients, the investigators showed low morbidity and mortality with grades I and II AVMs, and therefore recommended surgical resection for these lesions, with minimal consideration of nidus location, age, or comorbidities. The investigators recommended more conservative management of patients with high-grade lesions (grade III and IV) and careful consideration of these other anatomic and clinical factors.

Shi and Chen[3] presented an alternative classification scheme in 1986 that considered AVM size, location and depth, arterial supply, and venous drainage. Each of these 4 aspects was divided into 4 grades. Specifically, size was graded as less than 2.5 cm (grade I), 2.5 to 5 cm (grade II), 5 to 7.5 cm (grade III), or greater than 7.5 cm (grade IV). Location and depth were graded as superficial/nonfunctional (grade I), superficial/functional (grade II), deep (grade III), and deep/vital (grade IV). Arterial supply was graded as single superficial branch of MCA or ACA (grade I), multiple superficial branches of MCA or ACA (grade II), PCA branches or deep MCA or ACA branches (grade III), and branches of all 3 cerebral arteries or vertebrobasilar artery (grade IV). Venous drainage was graded as single superficial (grade I), multiple superficial (grade II), deep (grade III), and deep with variceal dilatation (grade IV). The final AVM grade was "matched to the appropriate highest grade when at least 2 criteria are in that grade," or was a mixed or intermediary grade if only one was in the highest grade. Although this classification scheme has 4 grades, this method of grading led to 6 different groupings in the investigators' surgical series of 100 patients. Excellent results were achieved in patients with grade I, to II, and II AVMs, with increasing morbidity/mortality in patients with AVMs grade II to III, III and III to IV. This classification scheme incorporated similar anatomic features as the Spetzler-Martin[4] scheme, but it failed to gain acceptance because of its complexity, with grading within grades and mixed final grades.

## SPETZLER-MARTIN CLASSIFICATION SCHEME

In 1986, Spetzler and Martin[4] published what has become the predominant classification scheme for brain AVMs. After considering a range of factors including size, number of feeding arteries, location, operative accessibility, shunt flow, vascular steal, location, and venous drainage, these investigators settled on a simplified scheme using only size, eloquence of surrounding brain parenchyma, and venous drainage pattern. Simplicity, applicability at the bedside, and accurate outcome prediction were the investigators' principal objectives.

Each factor in the grading scale was scored independently. Size was divided into 3 categories, with small AVMs less than 3 cm assigned 1 point, medium AVMs 3 to 6 cm assigned 2 points, and large AVMs greater than 6 cm assigned 3 points. Venous drainage was considered superficial if it drained into cortical veins and convexity sinuses and assigned 0 points, or deep if it drained into veins that coursed to the vein of Galen (ie, internal cerebral veins, basal veins of Rosenthal, and precentral cerebellar vein) and assigned 1 point. AVM eloquence was assessed anatomically based on the presumed function of surrounding brain tissue, with 1 point assigned to lesions located in sensorimotor cortex, language areas, visual cortex, hypothalamus, internal capsule, brain stem, cerebellar peduncle, or deep cerebellar nuclei. AVMs not in these regions were assigned 0 points for eloquence. The final AVM grade was the sum of points across the 3 domains, with a range from I to V. AVMs that are too complex for resection, like intrinsic brain stem and holohemispheric AVMs, were deemed grade VI.

The Spetzler-Martin grading system was initially evaluated in a retrospective analysis of the investigators' surgical experience in 100 consecutive surgically resected AVMs. Outcomes were categorized as "no deficit," "minor deficit" (including temporary worsening of neurologic function, mild ataxia, or mild increase in brain stem deficit), or "major deficit" (including aphasia, hemianopsia, or hemiparesis). There were no major deficits and only 1 minor deficit in patients with low-grade AVMs (grades I and II, **Table 1**). Patients with

**Table 1**
**Grading scheme of Spetzler and Martin correlated with operative outcome by grade in 100 consecutive patients**

| Grade | Patients (n) | No Deficit (n) | (%) | Minor Deficit (n) | (%) | Major Deficit (n) | (%) | Death (%) |
|-------|--------------|----------------|-----|-------------------|-----|-------------------|-----|-----------|
| I     | 23           | 23             | 100 | 0                 | 9   | 0                 | 0   | 0         |
| II    | 21           | 20             | 95  | 1                 | 5   | 0                 | 0   | 0         |
| III   | 25           | 21             | 84  | 3                 | 12  | 1                 | 4   | 0         |
| IV    | 15           | 11             | 73  | 3                 | 20  | 1                 | 7   | 0         |
| V     | 16           | 11             | 69  | 3                 | 19  | 2                 | 12  | 0         |
| Total | 100          | 86             | 86  | 10                | 10  | 4                 | 4   | 0         |

*Adapted from* Spetzler RF, Martin NA: A proposed grading system for arteriovenous malformations. J Neurosurg 1986;65:476–83.

high-grade AVMs experienced higher rates of both major (grade IV, 7%; and grade V, 12%) and minor deficits (grade IV, 20%; and grade V, 19%). A subsequent prospective analysis by the senior author[5] as well as independent analyses by other groups[6–8] confirmed the accuracy of the grading system to predict operative morbidity and mortality.

This grading system has been widely accepted by neurosurgeons and other clinicians for its simplicity and practicality, quickly providing estimates of surgical risk. Furthermore, its easy applicability has made the grading system an integral part of the description and language of brain AVMs. Experience with this grading has identified 3 distinct groups of patients. Low-grade AVMs (grades I and II) have low morbidity associated with their resection and are frequently treated surgically. High-grade AVMs (grades IV and V) have high morbidity associated with their resection and are frequently managed conservatively. Grade III AVMs have intermediate morbidity associated with their surgical resection, and treatment recommendations require an individualized approach with multimodality treatment.

## MODIFICATIONS OF THE SPETZLER-MARTIN CLASSIFICATION SCHEME

One deficiency of the Spetzler-Martin grading system is its handling of grade III AVMs. A 2-cm thalamic AVM with deep drainage has the same score as a 7-cm right frontal pole AVM with superficial drainage, yet these 2 different lesions have the same grade. Grade III AVMs are the most heterogeneous of the 5 grades, with 4 different combinations of size, venous drainage, and eloquence and one-third of all combinations of these elements of the grading scale. In addition, these AVMs are technically challenging, at the limit

of what many neurosurgeons are willing to accept in terms of technical difficulty and potential morbidity. The Spetzler-Martin grading system groups these diverse lesions together and fails to provide the clarity in management that it does for low-grade and high-grade AVMs.

In an analysis of a consecutive series of 76 grade III AVMs, Lawton[9] confirmed that neurologic outcomes varied according to the subtype of grade III AVM (**Table 2**). Small grade III AVMs, with 1 point assigned for size, deep venous drainage, and eloquence (S1V1E1), were the most common and had the lowest surgical risk (3% morbidity). In contrast, medium-sized/eloquent grade III AVMs (S2V0E1) had the highest surgical risk (15% morbidity). Medium-sized/deep grade III AVMs (S2V1E0) had an intermediate surgical risk (7%). Large grade III AVMs (S3V0E0) are rare, with none in this surgical experience.

Based on these data, grade III AVMs should not be considered a homogeneous group with equivalent risks for all subtypes, as the Spetzler-Martin scheme suggests. Instead, grade III AVMs should be analyzed according to the 4 subtypes defined by the Spetzler-Martin scheme. Lawton proposed a modification to the Spetzler-Martin scheme to emphasize these differences. Small grade III AVMs were designated grade III− because their surgical risk was less than the average grade III lesion, more like a grade II lesion. Medium/eloquent grade III AVMs were designated grade III+ because their surgical risk was more than the average grade III lesion, more like a grade IV lesion. Medium/deep grade III AVMs were designated plain grade III because their surgical risk was the same as the average grade III lesion. Large grade III AVMs were designated grade III* because they are lesions fabricated by the grading system with an incidence so low that their surgical risk is unclear and their clinical relevance minimal.

**Table 2**
**Surgical risk, according to the type of Spetzler-Martin grade III arteriovenous malformation[a]**

| Grade III Type | Total | No. of Patients Improved or Unchanged (Number [%]) | New Deficit or Death | Modified Spetzler-Martin Grade |
|---|---|---|---|---|
| S1V1E1 | 34 | 33 (97.1) | 1 (2.9) | III− |
| S2V1E0 | 14 | 13 (92.9) | 1 (7.1) | III |
| S2V0E1 | 27 | 23 (85.2) | 4 (4.8) | III+ |
| S3V0E0 | 0 | 0 | 0 | III* |
| Overall | 75 | 69 (92.0) | 6 (8.0) | |

[a] Patients lost to follow-up monitoring, for whom outcome data were not available, were excluded from the calculations.
*Adapted from* Lawton MT: Spetzler-Martin Grade III arteriovenous malformations: surgical results and a modification of the grading scale. Neurosurgery 2003;52:740–8 [discussion: 748–9].

Large, superficial AVMs in noneloquent brain can occur only in the frontal or temporal poles; large AVMs in other locations are likely to have a deep draining vein or abut eloquent brain tissue.

This modification to the Spetzler-Martin system facilitates treatment recommendations. Grade III− and III AVMs are typically managed surgically, whereas grade III+ lesions are managed conservatively. This modification improves the capacity of the Spetzler-Martin grading system for bedside decision making.

## NEW AND SUPPLEMENTARY CLASSIFICATION SCHEMES

Although the original Spetzler-Martin classification scheme has become an established part of the AVM literature[5,10–14] Spetzler himself recognized that there was redundancy in the grading system, with low-grade AVMs being managed similarly with surgery and high-grade AVMs managed conservatively. Therefore, Spetzler and Ponce[15] condensed the original 5-tier grading system into 3 tiers: grades I and II were combined into class A; grade III became class B; and grades IV and V became class C. In a compilation of 1476 cases from the literature, the investigators showed by pair-wise comparison that the differences in surgical outcomes were smallest between grades I and II AVMs and again between grades IV and V AVMs. The predictive power, as measured by calculated area under the receiver operating characteristic (ROC) curve, for the 3-tiered system was identical to that for the 5-tiered system (0.713 and 0.711, respectively), supporting this condensed classification system.

Ponce and Spetzler made broad treatment recommendations based on AVM class. Class A

lesions are managed surgically with a goal of complete resection; class B are managed with multimodality treatment that includes endovascular and radiosurgical intervention in addition to surgical resection; and class C lesions are largely deemed nonsurgical, with exceptions made for recurrent hemorrhage, progressive neurologic deficits, steal-related symptoms, and AVM-related aneurysm. Proponents of this simplification of the grading system emphasize that fewer classes group together patients with a rare disorder and that the larger groups correspond more directly with treatment recommendations. Opponents of this simplification argue that it does not simplify the analysis of the AVM because the same scoring steps of the original Spetzler-Martin scale are required with an additional step to reclassify the AVM. Opponents also emphasize that the class-specific recommendations are vague and encumbered with exceptions. For example, the class system does nothing to shed light on the heterogeneous group of grade III lesions. Patient selection is a sophisticated process that requires more complexity, not less.

To counter this trend toward simplification, new and supplementary classification schemes have been proposed. Additional factors are important to patient selection but are not part of the Spetzler-Martin grading scale, including hemorrhagic presentation, age, deep perforating artery supply, and diffuseness. Presentation with hemorrhage not only indicates AVMs with high risk of rehemorrhage but also facilitates surgery. Hematomas help separate AVMs from adjacent brain; evacuation of hematoma creates working space around the AVM that can minimize transgression of normal brain or access a deep nidus that might otherwise have been unreachable; and hemorrhage can obliterate some of the arterial supply of the AVM to reduce its flow during resection. AVM hemorrhage and microsurgery can injure brain tissue, but young age and plasticity can enhance a patient's ability to recover neurologic function. Compact AVMs with tightly woven arteries and veins often have distinct borders that separate cleanly from the adjacent brain, whereas diffuse AVMs with ragged borders and intermixed brain force the neurosurgeon to establish dissection planes that can extend into normal brain. Deep perforating arteries are thin, fragile, and difficult to occlude with cautery. Bleeding during surgery can escape into deep white matter tracts and cause significant deficits. All of these factors (hemorrhagic presentation, young age, compactness, and absence of deep perforator supply) have been identified as predictors of good outcomes after microsurgical resection.[1,2,16–19]

Alternative AVM classification schemes have been proposed since the introduction of the Spetzler-Martin grading system to incorporate these other factors and improve surgical risk prediction and patient selection. Tamaki and colleagues[17] identified age as a significant predictor of outcome, but did not include it in the grading system. They assigned points for size (small or large), number of feeding artery systems (1–2 or ≥3), and location (superficial or deep), stratifying AVMs into 5 grades ranging from 0 to 4 that correlated with surgical difficulty. Their grading system was too similar to the Spetzler-Martin system and they failed to use age in their classification scheme.

After finding that neither AVM size nor venous drainage pattern influenced outcome in their experience, Hollerhage[19] proposed a grading system based on 5 territories of feeding artery supply (ACA, MCA, PCA, Rolandic branches, and anterior communicating artery shunt flow). This grading system was among the first to incorporate a clinical variable in addition to these anatomic variables, assigning 1 point for Hunt and Hess[20] grades I to II and 2 points for Hunt and Hess grades III to V. The Hunt and Hess grade contained within this AVM grading system is a surrogate for hemorrhagic presentation, but Hunt and Hess designed their scale for patients with aneurysm with subarachnoid hemorrhage, and its application to patients with AVM was awkward. Despite the possibility of an AVM grade as high as 7, grades ranged from 1 to 4 in this study and correlated with Glasgow Outcome Scale (GOS) scores. However, by measuring surgical results by final GOS rather than changes in GOS scores, this grading scale failed to recognize the surgical

advantages associated with hemorrhagic presentation.

Perhaps the most comprehensive grading system for AVMs was proposed by Pertuiset and colleagues.[16] In addition to angiographic factors like AVM location and feeding artery supply, this system analyzed AVM sectors, caliber of feeding arteries, nidus volume, and hemodynamic factors including cerebral steal and circulatory velocity of radiolabeled red blood cells. This system included age and previous hemorrhage in its clinical variables. Using elaborate tables, each variable was coded, and these codes were added to generate operability scores ranging between 3 and 69, with AVM scores less than 30 considered operable. The investigators concluded that the score system was too complicated and too impractical for clinical use.

The University of Toronto Brain AVM Study Group[18] developed a discriminative prediction model of neurologic outcomes associated with AVM resection that recognized nidus diffuseness as a critical predictor variable. The Toronto model incorporated just 3 variables, weighted them with rounded odds ratios (eloquence = 4, diffuseness = 3, and deep venous drainage = 2), and added points to form a 9-point stratified risk score. Discrimination of this model for predicting permanent disabling neurologic outcomes was high (area under the ROC curve, 0.79), and better than the Spetzler-Martin scale (area under the ROC curve, 0.69). The grading system of the Toronto group is simple, but it has not been widely applied in the years since its publication because it competes with the Spetzler-Martin grading system, reaffiliating eloquence and venous drainage with the newer scale.

Lawton and colleagues[21] envisioned a grading system that would supplement rather than replace the already entrenched Spetzler-Martin grading system (**Table 3**). This supplementary grading system has its own unique variables separate from the Spetzler-Martin scale. Points were assigned for patient age, hemorrhagic presentation, and AVM diffuseness, analogous to the Spetzler-Martin scoring system. Pediatric patients (age <20 years) were assigned 1 point; adults (age 20–40 years) were assigned 2 points; and older patients (>40 years) were assigned 3 points. Patients presenting with unruptured AVMs were assigned 1 point and ruptured AVMs 0 points. Diffuse AVMs were assigned 1 point and compact AVMs 0 point. These points were added together for a supplementary AVM grade that ranged from 1 to 5. Simplicity is a critical aspect of a popular grading scale, and a supplementary grading scale was designed with this in mind. In addition, the 2

**Table 3**
**Comparison of the Spetzler-Martin grading system and the supplementary grading system**

| Spetzler-Martin | | Points | Supplementary | |
|---|---|---|---|---|
| Size | <3 cm | 1 | Age | <20 y |
| | 3–6 cm | 2 | | 20–40 y |
| | >6 cm | 3 | | >40 y |
| Venous Drainage | Superficial | 0 | Unruptured | No |
| | Deep | 1 | | Yes |
| Eloquence | No | 0 | Diffuse | No |
| | Yes | 1 | | Yes |
| Total | | 5 | | |

*Adapted from* Lawton MT, Kim H, McCulloch CE, et al. A supplementary grading scale for selecting patients with brain arteriovenous malformations for surgery. Neurosurgery 2010;66:702–13 [discussion: 713].

grading systems are analogous in their structure to make the supplementary grading scale memorable. These investigators analyzed a consecutive surgical series of 300 patients to compare the predictive accuracy using the Spetzler-Martin scale and the supplementary scale. The supplementary grading scale had high predictive accuracy (area under the ROC curve, 0.73 vs 0.65 for the Spetzler-Martin grading system) and stratified surgical risk more evenly (**Table 4**).

Lawton and colleagues proposed that this supplementary grading system be used to improve and refine patient selection for AVM surgery. Clinical decisions begin with an analysis of nidus size, venous drainage, location, diffuseness, age, and presentation, generating Spetzler-Martin and supplementary grades. The Spetzler-Martin grade provides an initial risk estimate. The supplementary grade can be considered separately, with supplementary grades ≤3 having an acceptably low risk of AVM resection. It can also be added to the Spetzler-Martin grade, with combined grades ≤6 having an acceptably low surgical morbidity. An analysis of supplementary factors can affect a management decision by confirming the risk predicted by the Spetzler-Martin grade. For example, an AVM with a low Spetzler-Martin grade (grade I–III) may be favorable for microsurgical resection, and a low supplementary grade (I–III) may strengthen the recommendation for surgery. Lawton and colleagues found that 62% of patients had low-grade AVMs according to both grading systems, and 85% of these patients were improved or unchanged after surgery (**Table 5**). Conversely, an AVM with a high Spetzler-Martin grade (IV–V) may be unfavorable for microsurgical resection, and a high supplementary grade (IV–V) may strengthen the recommendation for nonoperative management. In

these cases of matched Spetzler-Martin and supplementary grades, the supplementary grading system has a confirmatory role and may not alter management decisions.

However, in cases of mismatched Spetzler-Martin and supplementary grades, the supplementary grading system may alter management decisions and therefore has a more important role. Lawton and colleagues found that 28% of patients had low Spetzler-Martin grades and high supplementary grades, and 41% of these patients were neurologically worse after surgery (see **Table 5**), which is a higher morbidity than that of Spetzler-Martin grade IV AVMs (31%). Insight provided by the supplementary grade might have discouraged the recommendation for surgery in some of these patients. Similarly, 7% of patients had high Spetzler-Martin grades and low supplementary grades, and 29% of these patients were neurologically worse after surgery (see **Table 5**). This proportion of worsening was lower than the 35% morbidity for the overall group of Spetzler-Martin grade IV and V AVMs, and equivalent to the 30% morbidity seen for grade III AVMs. Again, insight provided by the supplementary grade might have encouraged the recommendation for surgery in some of these patients. Spetzler-Martin grade III AVMs have surgical risks that depend on the subtype, with small grade III− lesions associated with lower risk and medium/eloquent grade III+ lesions associated with higher risk. In addition to considering the grade III subtype, considering the supplementary grade may influence surgical decisions for patients with AVM at the borderline between high and low risk. The University of California at San Francisco experience shows that factors outside the Spetzler-Martin grading system improve the prediction of neurologic outcome after AVM resection, and that a simple

**Table 4**
**Application of the supplementary grading system and combined Spetzler-Martin/supplementary scores**

| | Worse of Dead | | Improved or Unchanged | |
|---|---|---|---|---|
| | N | % | N | % |
| Spetzler-Martin Grade | | | | |
| I | 5 | 8.9 | 51 | 91.1 |
| II | 30 | 24.4 | 93 | 75.6 |
| III | 27 | 30.0 | 63 | 70.0 |
| IV | 9 | 31.0 | 20 | 69.0 |
| V | 2 | 100.0 | 0 | 0.0 |
| Supplemental Grade | | | | |
| I | 1 | 3.7 | 26 | 96.3 |
| II | 8 | 11.9 | 59 | 88.1 |
| III | 25 | 22.1 | 88 | 77.9 |
| IV | 32 | 40.5 | 47 | 59.5 |
| V | 7 | 50.0 | 7 | 50.0 |
| Combined Grade | | | | |
| 1 | 0 | 0.0 | 0 | 0.0 |
| 2 | 0 | 0.0 | 7 | 100.0 |
| 3 | 0 | 0.0 | 21 | 100.0 |
| 4 | 5 | 9.1 | 50 | 90.9 |
| 5 | 19 | 21.1 | 71 | 78.9 |
| 6 | 19 | 27.1 | 51 | 72.9 |
| 7 | 24 | 54.5 | 20 | 45.5 |
| 8 | 4 | 50.0 | 4 | 50.0 |
| 9 | 2 | 40.0 | 3 | 60.0 |
| 10 | 0 | 0.0 | 0 | 0.0 |

*Adapted from* Lawton MT, Kim H, McCulloch CE, et al. A supplementary grading scale for selecting patients with brain arteriovenous malformations for surgery. Neurosurgery 2010;66:702–13 [discussion: 713].

**Table 5**
**Matched and unmatched prediction of risk for morbidity after surgery**

| | Total | | Improved, Unchanged | | Worse, Dead | |
|---|---|---|---|---|---|---|
| | N | % | N | % | N | % |
| Matched Risk Prediction | | | | | | |
| Low-grade, Spetzler-Martin and supplemental scores | 186 | 62 | 158 | 85 | 28 | 15 |
| High-grade, Spetzler-Martin and supplemental scores | 10 | 3 | 5 | 50 | 5 | 50 |
| Mismatched Risk Prediction | | | | | | |
| Low Spetzler-Martin, high supplemental scores | 83 | 28 | 49 | 59 | 34 | 41 |
| High Spetzler-Martin, low supplemental scores | 21 | 7 | 15 | 71 | 6 | 29 |
| | 300 | 100 | 227 | — | 73 | — |

*Adapted from* Lawton MT, Kim H, McCulloch CE, et al. A supplementary grading scale for selecting patients with brain arteriovenous malformations for surgery. Neurosurgery 2010;66:702–13 [discussion: 713].

supplementary grading system can be easily applied at the bedside to refine patient selection for AVM surgery.

## NATURAL HISTORY RISK PREDICTION

Neurosurgeons have focused on the prediction of surgical risk with classification schemes to help them recommend AVM resection. However, the natural alternative to AVM resection is observation, which is particularly important with high-grade AVMs associated with high surgical risks. Therefore, predicting the natural history risk of an AVM is as important in the clinical decision as predicting the surgical risk. An accurate understanding of the hemorrhagic behavior of untreated AVMs is essential when comparing conservative and surgical options.

Ondra and colleagues[22] examined prospectively a cohort of 160 patients with AVM managed nonoperatively over a 33-year period in Finland, drawn from a population that included more than 90% of patients with AVM in that country. These patients presented with hemorrhage (71%), seizures without evidence of hemorrhage (24%), or other symptoms including headaches, asymptomatic bruits, or other neurologic complaints (5%). The annual rate of AVM hemorrhage was 4%, regardless of presentation and constant over a mean follow-up of 23.7 years. The mortality was 1% annually and the combined major morbidity/mortality was 2.7% annually. The mean interval between presentation and subsequent hemorrhagic events was 7.7 years.

Other reports in the literature estimate the annual risk of AVM hemorrhage to be 2% to 4% (**Table 6**).[22–26] The New York Islands AVM Hemorrhage Study,[27,28] a prospective survey of a zip-code–defined population of nearly 10 million inhabitants, found an AVM detection rate of 1.21/100,000 person-years, with incidence of hemorrhage being 0.42/100,000 person-years. The Northern Manhattan Stroke Study[29,30] found the incidence of first-ever AVM hemorrhage to be 0.55/100,000 person-years. These studies offer insight into the clinical and anatomic factors that influence AVM natural history. Data from Columbia AVM Databank[31] showed that deep brain location, exclusively deep venous drainage, and presentation with AVM hemorrhage were all associated with increased risk of new hemorrhage. The hemorrhage risks associated with these factors were additive, with an average annual rupture rate that ranged from 0.9% with no risk factors to 34.4% with all 3. In addition, associated arterial aneurysms increased the risk of hemorrhage, with a relative risk of 2.28 for patients with intranidal aneurysms and 1.88 for patients with feeding artery aneurysms.[32] Stapf and colleagues also reported that borderzone AVMs fed by at least 2 arteries from the circle of Willis had a decreased risk of hemorrhage (27% vs 60%, respectively). Based on a cohort of 705 patients with AVM, Nataf and colleagues[33] identified similar angiographic factors associated with hemorrhage risk: venous recruitment, venous stenosis, venous reflux, deep venous drainage, and intranidal or juxtanidal aneurysms. A classification scheme incorporating these factors showed increasing hemorrhage risk with grade.

Despite these insights, most estimates of untreated AVM rupture risk are crude at best. There are statistical estimates based on the multiplicative law of probability for the lifetime risk of hemorrhage[34]: Rupture risk $= 1 - $ (risk of no hemorrhage)$^{(\text{life expectancy})}$. This formula assumes a constant yearly risk of hemorrhage with independent behavior over all years. This formulaic approach yields an estimate lifetime hemorrhage risk, but is not a practical bedside tool. Simplified formulas are more practical and popular: rupture risk $= 105 - $ patient age.[34,35] The use of simplified formulas and the lack of an accepted natural history grading system show that efforts to define

**Table 6**
**Summary of natural history studies for arteriovenous malformation rupture**

| Author | Study Design | Cases | Follow-up Term (y) | Hemorrhage Rate (%/y) |
|---|---|---|---|---|
| Graf et al,[23] 1983 | Retrospective | 71 | 4.8 | 4.1 |
| Crawford et al,[24] 1986 | Retrospective | 217 | 10.4 | 3.4 |
| Brown et al,[25] 1988 | Retrospective | 168 | 8.2 | 2.3 |
| Ondra et al,[22] 1990 | Retrospective | 160 | 23.7 | 1.7 |
| Mast et al,[26] 1997 | Prospective | 139 | 1.0 | 2.2 |

*Adapted from* http://www.neurosurgery.ufl.edu/residency/images/Vascular_Malformations.pdf.

the risks of observation have lagged behind efforts to define the surgical risks. The importance of such a natural history grading system is clear. As the underlying biology of AVMs and AVM rupture is elucidated, this system will likely include the clinical and anatomic factors discussed earlier but also genetic and hemodynamic factors that influence the ongoing inflammation and angiogenesis inside an AVM nidus.

## CLASSIFICATION SCHEMES FOR NONSURGICAL THERAPIES

AVMs are treated by other modalities besides surgery, and with multimodality strategies. Classification schemes predicting surgical risk say nothing about the risks of these alternative therapies. However, the usefulness of surgical grading systems provided impetus to develop similar radiosurgical and endovascular grading systems.

The factors that are important to AVM obliteration by stereotactic radiosurgery are different from the factors in the Spetzler-Martin grading system. Inoue and colleagues[36] identified size, morphology, and hemodynamics as factors most predictive of radiosurgical outcome. The investigators classified AVM hemodynamics as Moya-type (small-caliber feeding arteries, compact nidus, and veins that drain in the venous phase of the angiogram), shunt type (large-caliber feeding arteries, indistinct nidus, and veins that drain early in the arterial phase), or mixed. AVM morphology was classified as homogeneous or heterogeneous. Radiosurgical results in 30 patients showed that small, homogeneous, Moya-type AVMs had the best obliteration rates, and that other AVMs with shunt and mixed hemodynamics benefit from preradiosurgical embolization.

Pollock and Flickinger[37] developed a more quantitative radiosurgical classification scheme called the radiosurgery-based AVM grading system. Multivariate analysis of data from 220 patients identified 5 variables associated with radiosurgical success, defined as complete nidus obliteration without new or worsening neurologic deficit: AVM volume, age, location, previous embolization, and number of draining veins. The latter 2 factors added little to predictive accuracy and were omitted from the final equation for outcome: AVM score = 0.1 × (volume in cm$^3$) + 0.02 × (patient age in years) + 0.3 × (location of lesion (frontal or temporal = 0; parietal, occipital, intraventricular, corpus callosum, or cerebellar = 1; and basal ganglia, thalamic, or brainstem = 2)). Patients with a composite score of less than 1 had excellent outcomes, whereas only 39% of patients with scores greater than 2 had excellent outcomes. The predictive equation was validated at a different institution using a separate patient cohort of 136 patients. To reduce the complexity of the scheme, the location variable was modified to be 2-tiered, with lesions in the hemispheres, corpus callosum, and cerebellum assigned 0 points, and those in the basal ganglia, thalamus, and brain stem assigned 1 point.[38] This modified equation was validated on an additional 247 patients. Although this grading system was developed at a center using exclusively Gamma Knife (Elekta AB, Sweden) radiosurgery, it has been validated at linear accelerator-based centers as well.[39] The scale was based on outcome data after a single radiosurgery procedure. Radiosurgery has a long latency period, and many radiosurgical patients require repeat radiosurgery or surgery to achieve complete obliteration of the lesion. Therefore, outcome data used for radiosurgical grading scales require diligent follow-up.

Endovascular embolization of AVMs has long been a surgical adjunct rather than a curative therapy. Consequently, there have been few attempts to create an endovascular classification scheme. The Vienna group[40] produced a classification based on AVM size, number of feeding arteries, and pial versus perforating feeding arteries. Low-grade AVMs that were small, had fewer than 2 feeding arteries, and were not supplied by perforators were suitable for endovascular therapy, whereas high-grade AVMs that were large (>4 cm), had more than 4 feeding arteries, and were supplied by perforators were not suitable for endovascular therapy. Improved embolic agents like Onyx (ev3 Endovascular, Inc, Irvine, CA, USA) and more navigable microcatheters have increased the rates of curative AVM embolization. As technology and techniques evolve and obliteration rates increase, there will undoubtedly be additional classification schemes that will help select patients for curative endovascular intervention.

## SUMMARY

The decision to treat a patient's AVM is a complex process that must consider the individual's clinical presentation, anatomy, and biology. A treatment strategy is conceived that may involve 1 or multiple modalities, and the cumulative risks of the overall treatment strategy are estimated. Alternative treatments and strategies are also conceived and analyzed for risk. Grading systems are useful in making these estimations. The grading systems that stand the test of time are simple, applicable, and accurate. Other grading systems that are complex, cumbersome, or inaccurate are quickly discarded. Final recommendations are derived by comparing the therapeutic risks with the natural history risks. It is important to not only individualize recommendations for a particular patient but also to individualize grading systems for a particular neurosurgeon and a particular institution. There is no value in quoting published results if they differ from one's own personal results at one's own institution. Ultimately, grading systems enable clinicians to make management recommendations, but patients have the final say. The decision to embark on AVM treatment is difficult and frightening to most patients, and their individual preferences and feelings should dictate the final decision. Guiding patients through this decision process is an art from that cannot be replaced by grades or outcome data. One of the hardest things for neurosurgeons to accept is their limitations, and grading systems remind us when to say no.

The current crop of grading systems is generally useful, but imperfect and evolving. As the pathophysiology of AVMs is elucidated through research, grading systems will incorporate these advances with genetic information and biologic markers. Hemodynamic data may also become a defining element of rupture risk and future grading scales. Therefore, the work of developing AVM grading systems should be viewed as an ongoing process, and clinicians should be open to reshaping established, proven grading systems.

## REFERENCES

1. Luessenhop AJ, Gennarelli TA. Anatomical grading of supratentorial arteriovenous malformations for determining operability. Neurosurgery 1977;1(1): 30–5.
2. Luessenhop AJ, Rosa L. Cerebral arteriovenous malformations. Indications for and results of surgery, and the role of intravascular techniques. J Neurosurg 1984;60(1):14–22.
3. Shi YQ, Chen XC. A proposed scheme for grading intracranial arteriovenous malformations. J Neurosurg 1986;65(4):484–9.
4. Spetzler RF, Martin NA. A proposed grading system for arteriovenous malformations. J Neurosurg 1986; 65(4):476–83.
5. Hamilton MG, Spetzler RF. The prospective application of a grading system for arteriovenous malformations. Neurosurgery 1994;34(1):2–6 [discussion: 6–7].
6. Deruty R, Pelissou-Guyotat I, Mottolese C, et al. The combined management of cerebral arteriovenous malformations. Experience with 100 cases and review of the literature. Acta Neurochir (Wien) 1993;123(3–4):101–12.
7. Heros RC, Tu YK. Is surgical therapy needed for unruptured arteriovenous malformations? Neurology 1987;37(2):279–86.
8. Steinmeier R, Schramm J, Müller HG, et al. Evaluation of prognostic factors in cerebral arteriovenous malformations. Neurosurgery 1989;24(2):193–200.
9. Lawton MT. Spetzler-Martin Grade III arteriovenous malformations: surgical results and a modification of the grading scale. Neurosurgery 2003;52(4) 740–8 [discussion: 748–9].
10. Ponce FA, Lozano AM. Highly cited works in neurosurgery. Part I: the 100 top-cited papers in neurosurgical journals. J Neurosurg 2010;112(2):223–32.
11. Ponce FA, Lozano AM. Highly cited works in neurosurgery. Part II: the citation classics. J Neurosurg 2010;112(2):233–46.
12. Hartmann A, Stapf C, Hofmeister C, et al. Determinants of neurological outcome after surgery for brain arteriovenous malformation. Stroke 2000;31(10) 2361–4.
13. Heros RC, Korosue K, Diebold PM. Surgical excision of cerebral arteriovenous malformations: late results. Neurosurgery 1990;26(4):570–7 [discussion 577–8].
14. Davidson AS, Morgan MK. How safe is arteriovenous malformation surgery? A prospective, observational study of surgery as first-line treatment for brain arteriovenous malformations. Neurosurgery 2010; 66(3):498–504 [discussion: 504–5].
15. Spetzler RF, Ponce FA. A 3-tier classification of cerebral arteriovenous malformations. Clinical article. J Neurosurg 2011;114(3):842–9.
16. Pertuiset B, Ancri D, Kinuta Y, et al. Classification of supratentorial arteriovenous malformations. A score system for evaluation of operability and surgical strategy based on an analysis of 66 cases. Acta Neurochir (Wien) 1991;110(1–2):6–16.
17. Tamaki N, Ehara K, Lin TK, et al. Cerebral arteriovenous malformations: factors influencing the surgical difficulty and outcome. Neurosurgery 1991, 29(6):856.
18. Anon Arteriovenous malformations of the brain in adults. N Engl J Med 1999;340(23):1812–8.
19. Höllerhage HG. Cerebral arteriovenous malformations: factors influencing surgical difficulty and outcome. Neurosurgery 1992;31(3):604–5.
20. Hunt WE, Hess RM. Surgical risk as related to time of intervention in the repair of intracranial aneurysms. J Neurosurg 1968;28(1):14–20.
21. Lawton MT, Kim H, McCulloch CE, et al. A supplementary grading scale for selecting patients with brain arteriovenous malformations for surgery. Neurosurgery 2010;66(4):702–13 [discussion: 713].
22. Ondra SL, Troupp H, George ED, et al. The natural history of symptomatic arteriovenous malformations of the brain: a 24-year follow-up assessment. J Neurosurg 1990;73(3):387–91.

23. Graf CJ, Perret GE, Torner JC. Bleeding from cerebral arteriovenous malformations as part of their natural history. J Neurosurg 1983;58(3):331–7.
24. Crawford PM, West CR, Chadwick DW, et al. Arteriovenous malformations of the brain: natural history in unoperated patients. J Neurol Neurosurg Psychiatry 1986;49(1):1–10.
25. Brown RD, Wiebers DO, Forbes G, et al. The natural history of unruptured intracranial arteriovenous malformations. J Neurosurg 1988;68(3):352–7.
26. Mast H, Young WL, Koennecke HC, et al. Risk of spontaneous haemorrhage after diagnosis of cerebral arteriovenous malformation. Lancet 1997;350(9084):1065–8.
27. Stapf C, Khaw AV, Sciacca RR, et al. Effect of age on clinical and morphological characteristics in patients with brain arteriovenous malformation. Stroke 2003;34(11):2664–9.
28. Stapf C, Mast H, Sciacca RR, et al. The New York Islands AVM Study: design, study progress, and initial results. Stroke 2003;34(5):e29–33.
29. Stapf C, Mohr JP, Sciacca RR, et al. Incident hemorrhage risk of brain arteriovenous malformations located in the arterial borderzones. Stroke 2000;31(10):2365–8.
30. Stapf C, Labovitz DL, Sciacca RR, et al. Incidence of adult brain arteriovenous malformation hemorrhage in a prospective population-based stroke survey. Cerebrovasc Dis 2002;13(1):43–6.
31. Choi JH, Mast H, Hartmann A, et al. Clinical and morphological determinants of focal neurological deficits in patients with unruptured brain arteriovenous malformation. J Neurol Sci 2009;287(1–2):126–30.
32. Stapf C, Mohr JP, Pile-Spellman J, et al. Concurrent arterial aneurysms in brain arteriovenous malformations with haemorrhagic presentation. J Neurol Neurosurg Psychiatry 2002;73(3):294–8.
33. Nataf F, Meder JF, Ghossoub M, et al. Hemorrhage in arteriovenous malformations: clinical and anatomic data. Neurochirurgie 2001;47(2–3 Pt 2):158–67 [in French].
34. Kondziolka D, McLaughlin MR, Kestle JR. Simple risk predictions for arteriovenous malformation hemorrhage. Neurosurgery 1995;37(5):851–5.
35. Brown RD. Simple risk predictions for arteriovenous malformation hemorrhage. Neurosurgery 2000;46(4):1024.
36. Inoue H, Kohga H, Kurihara H, et al. Classification of arteriovenous malformations for radiosurgery. Stereotact Funct Neurosurg 1995;64(1):110–7.
37. Pollock BE, Flickinger JC. A proposed radiosurgery-based grading system for arteriovenous malformations. J Neurosurg 2002;96(1):79–85.
38. Pollock BE, Flickinger JC. Modification of the radiosurgery-based arteriovenous malformation grading system. Neurosurgery 2008;63(2):239–43 [discussion: 243].
39. Richling B, Killer M, Al-Schameri AR, et al. Therapy of brain arteriovenous malformations: multimodality treatment from a balanced standpoint. Neurosurgery 2006;59(5 Suppl 3):S148–57 [discussion: S3–13].
40. Vinuela F, Duckwiler T, Guglielmi G. Intravascular embolization of brain arteriovenous malformations. In: Maciuna R, editor. Endovascular neurological intervention. Rolling Meadows (IL): The American Association of Neurological Surgeons; 1995. p. 189–99.

# Classification Schemes of Cranial Dural Arteriovenous Fistulas

Juan Gomez, MD, Anubhav G. Amin, BS,
Lydia Gregg, MA, CMI, Philippe Gailloud, MD*

## KEYWORDS

- Vascular malformation • Dural arteriovenous fistula
- Classification • Merland-Cognard • Borden

Dural arteriovenous fistulas (DAVFs) are abnormal arteriovenous communications developed within a venous space contained between the two layers of the dura mater and typically vascularized by meningeal arteries. Rizzoli has been credited with the first anatomic description of a DAVF in 1881,[1] although the lesion seems to have been a scalp arteriovenous fistula, draining intracranially through a torcular emissary vein.[2] Sachs is widely quoted as having offered the first angiographic description of a DAVF in 1931; the origin of this claim is unclear, as angiography is neither mentioned nor illustrated in his monograph on brain tumors.[3] A brief discussion of angiography as an ancillary test and an example of cerebral aneurysm were added to a second edition in 1949.[4] However, one of Sachs' patients may be the earliest reported case of a DAVF,[5] likely a high-grade lesion in which branches of the middle meningeal artery were "found to connect with the vessels of the cortex" (**Fig. 1**). To the authors' knowledge, the first two angiographic demonstrations of DAVFs were published in 1936 by Bergstrand and colleagues.[6] Of particular interest is that one of their cases was also a high-grade DAVF with significant (and possibly exclusive) cortical drainage documented both

by angiography and during surgical exposure (**Fig. 2**). These early observations of DAVFs, made before the era of noninvasive neuroimaging and involving cortical venous drainage, anticipate the link between pial reflux and clinical conspicuity that lies at the base of the DAVF classifications discussed in this article.

DAVFs are said to represent approximately 10% to 15% of all intracranial vascular malformations, most commonly involving the transverse, sigmoid, and cavernous sinuses. While the etiology of DAVFs remains controversial, it is thought that they represent acquired conditions developing in a context of dural sinus thrombosis or venous hypertension. Other associations have been documented, including trauma, prior neurosurgical procedures (eg, craniotomy), and ear infection. The clinical impact of DAVFs ranges from a benign course, including incidentally discovered, asymptomatic lesions, to malignant presentations resulting in profound cognitive impairment, intracranial hemorrhage, and death.

The natural history of DAVFs strongly correlates with their pattern of venous drainage, in particular the presence of reflux into pial veins.[7–10] The venous anatomy of the lesion is therefore a central component of most DAVF classification schemes,

Disclosures: Dr Gailloud is a consultant for Codman Neurovascular and Artventive Medical. The Johns Hopkins Hospital (Division of Interventional Neuroradiology) is the recipient of a research grant from Siemens Medical. The other authors have nothing to disclose.
Division of Interventional Neuroradiology, The Johns Hopkins Hospital, Nelson B100, 600 North Wolfe Street, Baltimore, MD 21287, USA
* Corresponding author.
E-mail address: phg@jhmi.edu

Neurosurg Clin N Am 23 (2012) 55–62
doi:10.1016/j.nec.2011.09.003
1042-3680/12/$ – see front matter © 2012 Published by Elsevier Inc.

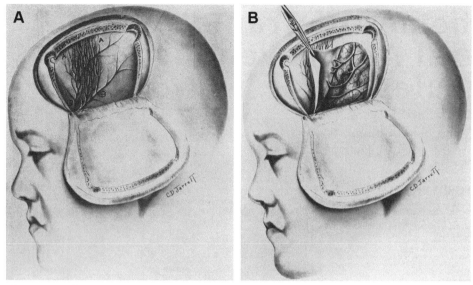

**Fig. 1.** Observation of a probable dural arteriovenous fistula (DAVF) published by Sachs in 1931. The original captions are reproduced here. (*A*) Case VIII, telangiectasis of the dura. In this case the major part of the process was in the dura and affected the middle meningeal artery. (*B*) Case VIII, after the dura was opened, connections between the middle meningeal artery and the cortical arteries [sic] were discovered. These were all doubly ligated and cut. (*From* Sachs E. The diagnosis and treatment of brain tumors. St Louis (MO): Mosby; 1931.)

starting with the first system proposed by Djindjian and colleagues in 1978.[11] Since then, the link between cortical venous drainage and aggressive symptomatology has been confirmed, leading to

continuous refinements in our understanding of DAVFs and their classification schemes.[12–18] In particular, the mode of presentation of a DAVF has recently been shown to influence the risk of

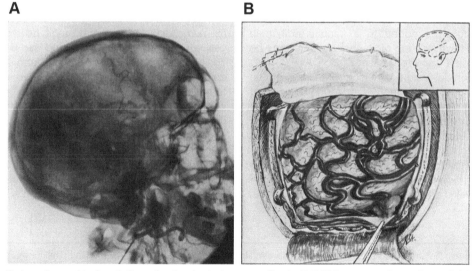

**Fig. 2.** First angiographic description of a dural arteriovenous fistula (DAVF) known to the authors of this article. The captions, translated from the German original, are reproduced here. (*A*) Arteriography of a dural arteriovenous aneurysm (Case 1). Arterial inflow: posterior branch of the middle meningeal artery. Drainage: superficial cerebral veins. (*B*) Surgical illustration of Case 1. The arteriovenous connection between the dural arteries and the superficial cerebral veins can be seen at the bottom right angle of the craniotomy defect. (*From* Bergstrand H, Olivecrona H, Tönnis W. Gefässmissbildungen und Gefässgeschwülste des Gehirns. Leipzig (Germany): Georg Thieme Verlag; 1936.)

subsequent significant clinical event. This new information has led to the proposal of a revised classification that grades DAVFs according to a combination of angiographic and clinical features. This article offers a review of the various classification schemes currently in use, and discusses their application to treatment decision making.

## CLASSIFICATION SCHEMES OF CRANIAL DURAL ARTERIOVENOUS FISTULAS
### *The Merland-Cognard Classification*

Cognard and colleagues[14] proposed a modification of the original Djindjian-Merland classification

scheme based on the clinical presentation of 205 consecutive patients seen over an 18-year period. The Merland-Cognard classification divides DAVFs in 5 types (I–V), with Type II lesions further subdivided into Type IIa, IIb, and IIa+b (**Fig. 3**). Type I and IIa DAVFs drain directly into dural venous sinuses, without pial reflux; in Type I, the venous drainage is antegrade whereas in Type IIa, it is partially or completely retrograde. Retrograde drainage is generally related to outflow impairment, that is, a dural sinus stenosis or occlusion, but can at times also result from high-volume arteriovenous shunting that exceeds the drainage capacity of a normal or even enlarged dural sinus. Type IIb and IIa+b DAVFs have dural and pial

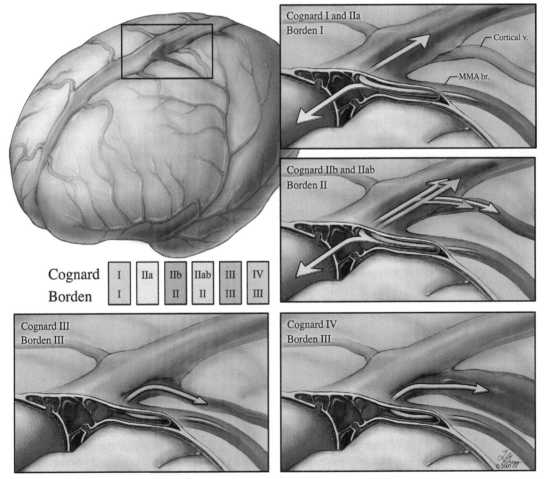

**Fig. 3.** The Merland-Cognard and Borden classifications. The various types of DAVFs are illustrated using a lesion of the middle third of the superior sagittal sinus (*upper left* orientation view). The color-coding shows the correspondence between the two classifications. Merland-Cognard classification: Type I and IIA DAVFs (no pial drainage) are shown in the top right inset, Type IIb and IIa+b (pial and dural drainage) in the middle right inset, and Type III and IV (pial drainage only) in the bottom two insets. Borden classification: Type I DAVF (no pial drainage) is shown in the top right inset, Type II (pial and dural drainage) in the middle right inset, and Type III (pial drainage only) in the bottom two insets. (Copyright © 2007 Lydia Gregg.)

venous drainage; in Type IIb, retrograde drainage occurs into pial vein(s) only, whereas in Type IIa+b both dural and pial retrograde drainage is seen. Type III and IV DAVFs drain only into the pial venous system, either directly or via an isolated dural sinus segment. Note that the pial veins constituting the primary drainage of the DAVF can themselves drain into a dural sinus not directly connected to the lesion. In Type IV, the draining vein is enlarged (venous ectasia). Cognard and colleagues define venous ectasia as a segment larger than 5 mm in diameter or 3 times larger than the diameter of the draining vein. Finally, Type V DAVFs are cranial lesions draining into spinal perimedullary veins, potentially resulting in cervical myelopathy.[19]

The strength of the Merland-Cognard classification lies in the correlation established between the angiographic characteristics of the DAVFs and their clinical presentation, which offers a management tool based on an objective assessment of the risk of adverse clinical event associated with a specific lesion. In their series, 83 of 84 patients with a Type I DAVF presented with nonaggressive symptoms, which included headache, bruit, minimal vertigo, and ocular symptoms not related to intracranial hypertension. Aggressive symptoms, such as intracranial hemorrhage, intracranial hypertension, focal neurologic deficits, and seizures, were found more frequently with higher grades, that is, in 37% of patients with Type IIa, 30% with Type IIb, 66% with Type IIa+b, 76% with Type III, and 97% with Type IV. All 12 patients with a Type V DAVF showed aggressive symptoms. Six of them had progressive myelopathy due to spinal cord venous hypertension. The perimedullary venous drainage extended down to the thoracic or lumbar levels in patients with myelopathy, whereas it was limited to the cervical region in those without myelopathy. Type V DAVFs without myelopathy were associated with subarachnoid hemorrhage in 5 cases and focal neurologic deficit in 1 case. DAVFs without cortical drainage (Type I or IIa) did not present with hemorrhage. The role of pial reflux and venous flow dynamics was further emphasized by the progressive increase in the hemorrhagic risk associated with less favorable venous configurations: 11% in Type IIb and IIa+b (combined pial and dural drainage), 40% in Type III (exclusive pial drainage without ectasia), and 65.5% in Type IV (exclusive pial drainage with ectasia).

## The Borden Classification

The Borden classification scheme[12] also takes inspiration from the morphologic characteristics of the venous drainage. It recognizes 3 principal types of DAVFs (I, II, III) and 2 subtypes (a, b) (see **Fig. 3**). Borden Type I DAVFs drain into dural venous sinuses without pial reflux; they typically have a benign course. Type II DAVFs drain into venous sinuses, but show retrograde flow into a pial vein, with an increased risk of neurologic events from venous hypertension or hemorrhage. Type III DAVFs drain directly into a pial vein (or an isolated dural sinus segment), are associated with significant venous hypertension, and typically present with hemorrhage or severe neurologic symptoms. Each type is further characterized by the complexity of the architecture of the arteriovenous shunt into Subtype A, a simple fistula with a direct, single connection between the feeding artery and the draining vein or sinus, and Subtype B, a complex lesion with multiple fistulous connections (**Fig. 4**).

## Recent Classification Refinements

Although they have shown good correlation with clinical presentations and outcomes, the Borden and Merland-Cognard classification schemes base their characterization of DAVFs solely on angiographic features. It was recently shown that when considering DAVFs with pial venous drainage, symptomatic patients may have a higher risk of future neurologic events than patients with incidentally found, asymptomatic lesions.[16,17] Soderman and colleagues[16] evaluated the annual incidences of intracranial hemorrhage, progressive dementia, and death in 85 patients harboring a DAVF with pial drainage, and found that patients with an initial intracranial hemorrhage had a higher risk of subsequent hemorrhage than patients with other presentations (7.4% vs 1.5%). Strom and colleagues[17] divided 28 cases of DAVFs with pial drainage into asymptomatic cases (ie, patients with incidentally diagnosed DAVFs or presenting with pulsatile tinnitus or orbital symptoms) and symptomatic cases (ie, patients with intracranial hemorrhage or nonhemorrhagic neurologic deficits). Only 1 of the 17 patients in the asymptomatic group suffered an intracranial hemorrhage (5.9%), while none had a nonhemorrhagic neurologic deficit. In the symptomatic group, 2 patients had an intracranial hemorrhage (18%) and 3 (27.3%) experienced new or worsening nonhemorrhagic neurologic deficits. Annual rates for hemorrhage and nonhemorrhagic neurologic deficits were of 7.6% and 11.4% (cumulative 19%) in the symptomatic group, and 1.4% and 0% in the nonsymptomatic group (cumulative 1.4%).

This new evidence suggests that, in addition to the well-established link between pial venous

A                                          B

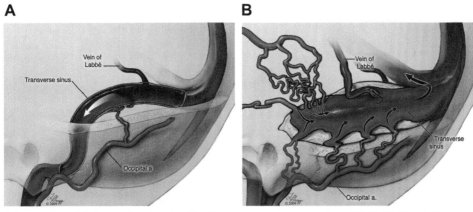

**Fig. 4.** Subtypes A and B for the Borden classification, using a transverse sinus DAVF. (*A*) Simple transverse sinus DAVF with a single feeding artery and antegrade dural drainage (Merland-Cognard Type I, Borden Type Ia). (*B*) Complex transverse sinus DAVF with multifocal arteriovenous shunts, and dural sinus disease with pial and dural retrograde drainage (Merland-Cognard Type IIa+b, Borden Type IIb). (Copyright © 2009 Lydia Gregg.)

drainage and unfavorable natural history, DAVFs that present with intracranial hemorrhage or nonhemorrhagic neurologic deficits have a higher risk of new significant events than asymptomatic fistulas. Zipfel and colleagues[18] have elegantly incorporated this factor into the Borden and Merland-Cognard classification schemes by adding symptomatic and asymptomatic subtypes. Their modified Type 1 DAVFs drain into dural sinuses without pial venous reflux, and correspond to Borden Type I and Merland-Cognard Types I and IIa. Modified Type II fistulas drain into dural sinuses, and are further subdivided as having symptomatic or asymptomatic pial venous reflux. Modified Type II DAVFs correspond to Borden Type II and Merland-Cognard Types IIb and IIa+b. Modified Type III DAVFs drain directly into pial veins, and are also subdivided as having symptomatic or asymptomatic cortical venous reflux. Modified Type III DAVFs correspond to Borden Type II and Merland-Cognard Types III, IV, and V. This new classification scheme is directly linked to treatment recommendations. DAVFs without pial reflux are electively treated to address intractable symptoms. DAVFs with pial venous drainage are treated to prevent the occurrence of intracranial hemorrhage or nonhemorrhagic neurologic deficits, on an elective basis for the nonsymptomatic lesions and immediately for the symptomatic ones.

## Evolutive Potential of DAVFs, or Can Morphologic Features and Classification Grade Change Over Time?

The natural history of DAVFs remains poorly understood, in part because of the limited number

of case studies evaluating their angiographic progression. This lack of data in turn affects management decision making. It is generally accepted that, in view of their well-established association with aggressive clinical behavior, DAVFs with pial reflux require therapy. The management of the so-called benign DAVFs, low-grade lesions with non–life-threatening presentations and without pial venous drainage, remains controversial. The first point of contention is how benign these lesions really are from a patient's standpoint. For example, many patients whose life is rendered miserable by constant tinnitus would argue against being classified as "asymptomatic." Tinnitus can be associated with sleep disturbance, anxiety, depression, irritation, and concentration difficulties.[20] In their practice the authors do treat low-grade DAVFs producing life-altering tinnitus. The second and more controversial question is whether a DAVF should be addressed at an early stage, when treatment is technically simple and the prospect of a cure high (**Fig. 5**A, B), rather than at a later stage when treatment is technically more challenging and a successful therapy less likely (see **Fig. 5**B, C). A better understanding of the evolutive potential of low-grade DAVFs would help to address this point. Only anecdotal evidence is available at present, including case reports showing that DAVFs can either undergo spontaneous regression or evolve into more malignant types with associated pial reflux.[21–31] Although rarely documented, the progression of a DAVF from low grade to high grade is a concern already mentioned by Cognard and colleagues[14] in their initial series. Of importance, the investigators stressed the fact that a change in clinical status, either the

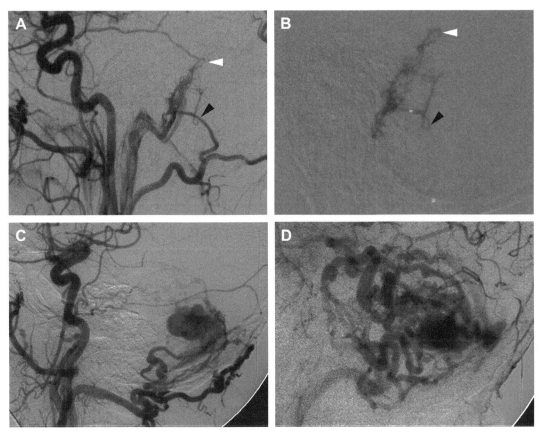

**Fig. 5.** Variation in shunt complexity and drainage pattern of transverse sinus DAVFs. (*A*) Digital subtraction angiography (DSA), common carotid injection, lateral view. Transverse/sigmoid junction DAVF in a 40-year-old woman presenting with headache and tinnitus. The DAVF shows a simple architecture, with a single arteriovenous shunt receiving contributions from the occipital (*black arrowhead*) and middle meningeal (*white arrowhead*) arteries. The venous drainage is dural and antegrade (Merland-Cognard Type I, Borden Ia). The patient elected for treatment because of the tinnitus. (*B*) Same patient as in *A*, lateral fluoroscopic view after embolization of the shunt showing the distribution of liquid embolic agent (NBCA, Trufill, Codman Neurovascular). The meningeal network feeding the lesion was completely cast through a single transarterial injection, including both the occipital (*black arrowhead*) and middle meningeal (*white arrowhead*) contributions. The 2 white artifacts indicate the position of the microcatheter during embolization. (*C*) DSA, common carotid injection, lateral view. Transverse sinus DAVF in a 55-year-old man presenting with headache, dizziness, and tinnitus. Several occipital artery branches are connected to an isolated sinus segment without direct dural outflow. The venous drainage is through a prominent venous ectasia into a dilated network of pial cerebellar veins, with secondary opacification of the sigmoid and straight sinuses (seen in *D*). Multiple other feeders were documented from the opposite external carotid artery and from both vertebral arteries, which were found during treatment to supply several foci of arteriovenous shunting (Merland-Cognard Type IV, Borden IIIb). (Copyright © 2007 Phillipe Gailloud.)

disappearance of an old symptom or the onset of a new symptom, must raise the suspicion of a change in drainage pattern and prompt new investigations. In their practice the authors have observed DAVF progress to higher grade lesions, in some cases with deleterious neurologic manifestations such as visual loss or intracranial hemorrhage, in 3 clinical situations: spontaneously, after an uneventful diagnostic cerebral angiogram, or after partial treatment **Fig. 6** shows an example of spontaneous modification in drainage pattern occurring within a short period of time (1 month). Such changes likely involve multifactorial mechanisms, including changes in the volume of arteriovenous shunt and/or the development of venous flow impairment (venous stenosis or thrombosis).

## SUMMARY

Classification schemes of DAVFs have typically been based on angiographic features, in particular

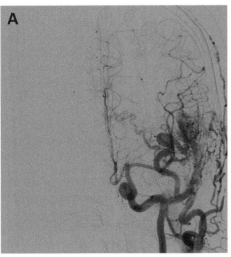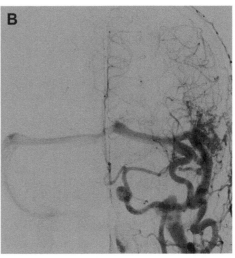

**Fig. 6.** A 51-year-old man with constant left pulsatile tinnitus, noted to progressively worsen over the past 6-month period, and negative noninvasive imaging workup including MRI/MRA and skull base CT. (*A*) DSA, left common carotid injection, anteroposterior view, obtained during diagnostic angiography (June 23, 2011). A left transverse sinus DAVF is documented, principally fed by multiple branches of the left occipital artery, with purely antegrade drainage into the left internal jugular vein (Merland-Cognard Type I). (*B*) DSA, left common carotid injection, anteroposterior view, obtained at the beginning of the therapeutic procedure performed 1 month later (July 25, 2011). Retrograde drainage into the right transverse sinus and right internal jugular vein is now observed (Merland-Cognard Type IIa). (Copyright © 2007 Phillipe Gailloud.)

their pattern of venous drainage. While confirming the link between pial reflux and DAVF aggressiveness, recent studies have also emphasized the importance of the mode of initial presentation as a predicting factor for subsequent significant clinical events. The classification schemes currently in use and their refined versions are important tools for the management of DAVFs, in particular for treatment recommendation and patient counseling. It should be remembered, however, that DAVFs are dynamic lesions that do not fit easily into static classification patterns. The impact of this evolutive potential on DAVF management remains to be determined.

# REFERENCES

1. Yasargil MG. Microneurosurgery. Stuttgart, New York: Georg Thieme - Thieme Stratton; 1987.
2. Perrini P, Nannini T, Di Lorenzo N. Francesco Rizzoli (1809-1880) and the elusive case of giulia: the description of an "arteriovenous aneurysm passing through the wall of the skull". Acta Neurochir (Wien) 2007;149:191–6 [discussion: 196].
3. Sachs E. The diagnosis and treatment of brain tumors. St Louis (MO): Mosby; 1931.
4. Sachs E. Diagnosis and treatment of brain tumors and care of the neurosurgical patient. St Louis (MO): Mosby; 1949.
5. Aminoff MJ. Vascular anomalies in the intracranial dura mater. Brain: a journal of neurology 1973;96: 601–12.
6. Bergstrand H, Olivecrona H, Tönnis W. Gefässmissbildungen und gefässgeschwülste des gehirns. Leipzig (Germany): Georg Thieme Verlag; 1936.
7. Castaigne P, Bories J, Brunet P, et al. Meningeal arterio-venous fistulas with cortical venous drainage. Rev Neurol 1976;132:169–81 [in French].
8. Houser OW, Baker HL Jr, Rhoton AL Jr, et al. Intracranial dural arteriovenous malformations. Radiology 1972;105:55–64.
9. Obrador S, Soto M, Silvela J. Clinical syndromes of arteriovenous malformations of the transverse-sigmoid sinus. J Neurol Neurosurg Psychiatry 1975;38:436–51.
10. Obrador S, Urquiza P. Arteriovenous angioma of the tentorium cerebelli. Rev Esp Otoneurooftalmol Neurocir 1951;10:387–92 [in Undetermined Language].
11. Djindjian R, Merland JJ, Théron J. Super-selective arteriography of the external carotid artery. Berlin, New York: Springer-Verlag; 1978.
12. Borden JA, Wu JK, Shucart WA. A proposed classification for spinal and cranial dural arteriovenous fistulous malformations and implications for treatment. J Neurosurg 1995;82:166–79.
13. Brown RD Jr, Wiebers DO, Nichols DA. Intracranial dural arteriovenous fistulae: angiographic predictors of intracranial hemorrhage and clinical outcome in nonsurgical patients. J Neurosurg 1994;81:531–8.

14. Cognard C, Gobin YP, Pierot L, et al. Cerebral dural arteriovenous fistulas: clinical and angiographic correlation with a revised classification of venous drainage. Radiology 1995;194:671–80.

15. Davies MA, TerBrugge K, Willinsky R, et al. The validity of classification for the clinical presentation of intracranial dural arteriovenous fistulas. J Neurosurg 1996;85:830–7.

16. Soderman M, Pavic L, Edner G, et al. Natural history of dural arteriovenous shunts. Stroke; a journal of cerebral circulation 2008;39:1735–9.

17. Strom RG, Botros JA, Refai D, et al. Cranial dural arteriovenous fistulae: asymptomatic cortical venous drainage portends less aggressive clinical course. Neurosurgery 2009;64:241–7 [discussion: 247–8].

18. Zipfel GJ, Shah MN, Refai D, et al. Cranial dural arteriovenous fistulas: modification of angiographic classification scales based on new natural history data. Neurosurg Focus 2009;26:E14.

19. Gobin YP, Rogopoulos A, Aymard A, et al. Endovascular treatment of intracranial dural arteriovenous fistulas with spinal perimedullary venous drainage. J Neurosurg 1992;77:718–23.

20. Langguth B. A review of tinnitus symptoms beyond 'ringing in the ears': a call to action. Curr Med Res Opin 2011;27:1635–43.

21. Cognard C, Houdart E, Casasco A, et al. Long-term changes in intracranial dural arteriovenous fistulae leading to worsening in the type of venous drainage. Neuroradiology 1997;39:59–66.

22. Endo S, Koshu K, Suzuki J. Spontaneous regression of posterior fossa dural arteriovenous malformation. J Neurosurg 1979;51:715–7.

23. Hansen JH, Sogaard I. Spontaneous regression of an extra- and intracranial arteriovenous malformation. Case report. J Neurosurg 1976;45:338–41.

24. Kim DJ, terBrugge K, Krings T, et al. Spontaneous angiographic conversion of intracranial dural arteriovenous shunt: long-term follow-up in nontreated patients. Stroke; a journal of cerebral circulation 2010;41:1489–94.

25. Landman JA, Braun IF. Spontaneous closure of a dural arteriovenous fistula associated with acute hearing loss. AJNR Am J Neuroradiol 1985;6:448–9.

26. Luciani A, Houdart E, Mounayer C, et al. Spontaneous closure of dural arteriovenous fistulas: report of three cases and review of the literature. AJNR Am J Neuroradiol 2001;22:992–6.

27. Magidson MA, Weinberg PE. Spontaneous closure of a dural arteriovenous malformation. Surg Neurol 1976;6:107–10.

28. Olutola PS, Eliam M, Molot M, et al. Spontaneous regression of a dural arteriovenous malformation. Neurosurgery 1983;12:687–90.

29. Pritz MB, Pribram HF. Spontaneous closure of a high-risk dural arteriovenous malformation of the transverse sinus. Surg Neurol 1991;36:226–8.

30. Satomi J, Satoh K, Matsubara S, et al. Angiographic changes in venous drainage of cavernous sinus dural arteriovenous fistulae after palliative transarterial embolization or observational management: a proposed stage classification. Neurosurgery 2005;56:494–502 [discussion: 494–2].

31. Voigt K, Sauer M, Dichgans J. Spontaneous occlusion of a bilateral caroticocavernous fistula studied by serial angiography. Neuroradiology 1971;2:207–11.

# Selection of Treatment Modalities or Observation of Arteriovenous Malformations

John C. Barr, MD, Christopher S. Ogilvy, MD*

## KEYWORDS

- Arteriovenous malformations • Surgical excision
- Endovascular embolization • Radiosurgery

Cerebral arteriovenous malformations (AVMs) have variable modes of presentation. The hemorrhagic presentation of these lesions, as identified in the prospective trials of the New York Islands AVM Hemorrhage Study and Northern Manhattan Stroke Study groups, is 0.42 per 100,000 and 0.55 per 100,000, respectively.[1] Evidence based on observation of patients with known lesions shows that the natural history of the disease is unchanged without intervention, even in symptomatic patients. Ondra and colleagues[2] showed in a study of 160 patients followed over 24 years without intervention that the combined major morbidity and mortality was 2.7% per year.[3] This per year risk percentage remained unchanged throughout the course of observation. In light of this, intervention risk should be lower than the natural history of the disease. This article elucidates ideal treatment modalities based on patient-specific factors.

## FACTORS INFLUENCING MODALITY OF TREATMENT

Once the decision is made to treat an AVM, the type of treatment is based on lesion-specific factors (size, location, and angiographic anatomy) and patient-specific factors. The first patient-specific factor to consider is age. A younger patient, who is more likely to benefit from long-term cure and symptom relief, is often at lower treatment-related risks compared with older patients. The overall health and neurologic state of the patient must also be considered preoperatively, because those with significant medical comorbidities may have reduced longevity, which is taken into account when considering the natural history of these lesions. Lawton and colleagues[4,5] discuss multiple factors influencing outcome in the setting of hemorrhage, with a positive correlation with younger age, AVMs in noneloquent territory, and Spetzler-Martin Grades 3 or less. AVMs that display diffuse hemispheric or bilateral cerebral involvement may not be amenable to any treatment modality, and thus goals of care may be more palliative or toward symptom relief (**Fig. 1**).

Seizures associated with AVMs can occur as the presenting symptom or de novo posttreatment. Patients who have had prior hemorrhage, particularly in the temporal lobe, are more prone to seizures. Piepgras and colleagues[3] report that in patients with preoperative seizures, 83% were seizure-free on follow-up, and the remaining had interval improvement in regards to occurrence. In patients presenting without seizures, 6% developed de novo seizures postoperatively. These findings show significant improvement compared with previous studies, likely relating to improvements

Neurosurgical Service, Endovascular and Neurovascular Neurosurgery, Massachusetts General Hospital, 55 Fruit Street, Boston, MA 02114, USA
* Corresponding author. Neurosurgical Service, Massachusetts General Hospital, WAC–745, 55 Fruit Street, Boston, MA 02114.
E-mail address: cogilvy@partners.org

Neurosurg Clin N Am 23 (2012) 63–75
doi:10.1016/j.nec.2011.09.010
1042-3680/12/$ – see front matter © 2012 Elsevier Inc. All rights reserved.

**A**        **B**

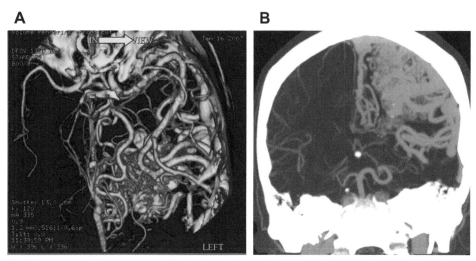

**Fig. 1.** (A, B) A 25-year-old woman with progressive parasthesias and complaints of right hand clumsiness revealing a diffuse, large AVM with arterial supply from anterior cerebral artery (ACA), middle cerebral artery (MCA), posterior cerebral artery (PCA), and external carotid artery (ECA) territories. A 1.7-cm flow-related aneurysm is also noted (*arrow*). (*Courtesy of* Massachusetts General Hospital, Department of Neurosurgery and Neurointerventional Radiology, Boston, MA.)

in surgical techniques.[6] In patients who undergo surgical resection, it is advocated to resect the surrounding gliotic and hemosiderin-stained tissue if possible, which can improve seizure control in patients with this as a presenting symptom. Cao and colleagues[7] used intraopertive electrocorticography to delineate additional surrounding epileptic discharges for bipolar electrocoagulation with significant improvement in seizure control noted on follow-up.

The location of a lesion, in particular with reference to eloquence of cortex, also influences treatment strategies. Historically, lesions in the sensory-motor strip have been less amenable to surgical intervention because of a presumed increase in morbidity. Kato and colleagues[8] demonstrated improvement in 15 of 17 patients treated with surgery. Motor-evoked potentials were used intraoperatively to demonstrate a functional shift in the cortex away from the AVM nidus, thus allowing safe resection.[9,10] Additionally, in multiple other studies patients with occipital lobe vascular malformations treated with surgical resection or stereotactic radiosurgery have been shown to have seizure improvement or resolution posttreatment with minimal risk to worsening visual function. Based on this, all modalities of therapy may currently be considered for lesions in eloquent cortex.

Giant AVMs, which compromise less than 10% of all malformations, present a unique situation in that these lesions are more prone to ischemia secondary to steal phenomenon.[6] This is thought to result from the loss of the autoregulatory

compensation caused by the prolonged dilated state from persistent high flow through these lesions.[11] These lesions often have extensive collateral recruitment from multiple vascular beds, which can be demonstrated with angiography (**Fig. 2**). Treatment goals are based on the location, extent of hemispheric involvement, and overall condition of the patient. Staged endovascular treatments may be used at times, but the goal of treatment needs to be carefully planned. Volume reduction may be possible with subsequent radiosurgery to the remaining nidus, yet conclusive proof of this therapy is not available. At times, it is necessary to target an intranidal aneurysm with endovascular therapy if the lesion is the obvious source of hemorrhage. Angiographic cure may not be possible in such cases where diffuse involvement is noted, and in such cases, no therapy is recommended. In a review of 53 patients with either Spetzler-Martin Grade IV to V AVMs, Chang and colleagues[12] reported good outcomes in patients with symptomatic giant AVMs (hemorrhage [n = 20]; seizure [n = 18]; progressive neurologic decline [n = 7]; and headache [n = 8]) with multimodal treatment strategies (**Table 1**).[13,14] Yet even in this report, there is a bias toward patients with lesions favorable for treatment.

The association of aneurysms in conjunction with cerebral AVMs is an issue in about 20% to 25% of patients with AVMs. These may be incidental aneurysms in a separate vascular bed from the AVM. Aneurysms occurring on expected locations, such as the circle of Willis, that ultimately give supply to the AVM are likely to be

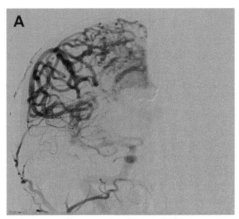 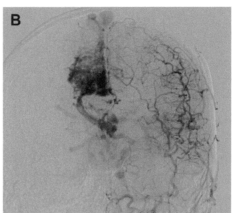

**Fig. 2.** (*A, B*) Giant right parietal AVM in a 25-year-old woman presenting with generalized tonic–clonic seizures. The right common carotid injection displays arterial supply from ACA, MCA, PCA, and ECA territories. The left CCA injections show the AVM parasitizing blood supply from the contralateral ACA and MCA vessels. (*Courtesy of Massachusetts General Hospital, Department of Neurosurgery and Neurointerventional Radiology, Boston, MA.*)

flow-related aneurysms and are thought to arise secondary to a hyperdynamic circulatory state induced by the AVM.[15] Yasargil and coworkers[15] comment on the association, including aneurysms less than 3 mm, as being approximately 10.8%, although no direct relationship between either size or degree of flow through the AVM as determined angiographically was associated with the presence of aneurysms. Cortical AVMs, in particular frontal and occipital, seem to have higher preponderance of associated aneurysms (**Table 2**), and deeper locations, such as basal ganglia and brainstem lesions, were less likely to have flow-related aneurysms (**Fig. 3**).

In one study, the risk of hemorrhage of an AVM associated with an aneurysm was shown to be 7% at 5 years versus a baseline risk of AVM hemorrhage without aneurysm reported at 2% to 4% per year.[16] This remains controversial, because separate studies by Miesal and Thompson and colleagues have not shown any increase in correlation.[17] Although intranidal aneurysms have been associated with increased hemorrhage from an AVM, this has not been shown conclusively. Intranidal aneurysms adjacent to a ventricle may be at increased risks of recurrent hemorrhage (**Table 3**). Batjer and colleagues also noted a higher likelihood of rupture associated with pedicle or feeding artery

aneurysms.[6] In the setting of hemorrhage from a cerebral AVM associated with a nidal, pedicle branch, or flow-related aneurysm, Yasargil and coworkers[15] comment on multiple studies that the AVM is more likely the source of hemorrhage, except in the posterior fossa.[15] Treatment should be focused on the aneurysm if it is the cause of hemorrhage. In the setting of a nonhemorrhagic presentation, aneurysms that are distal or flow-related may regress with AVM treatment of the aneurysm and those arising from the circle of Willis are unlikely to regress with time (**Fig. 4**).[17–20]

## TIMING OF TREATMENT

The reported morbidity associated with the initial hemorrhage from an AVM is relatively low, as

**Table 1**
**37-month follow-up in 53 patients treated with Spetzler-Martin Grade IV or V AVMs**

| Neurologic Status | Excellent | Good | Poor | Deceased |
|---|---|---|---|---|
| Pretreatment | 31 (58%) | 17 (32%) | 5 (9%) | — |
| Posttreatment | 27 (51%) | 15 (28%) | 3 (6%) | 8 (15%) |

**Table 2**
**Site of AVM and frequency of associated aneurysm**

| Site of AVM | Total No. | No. Patients with Aneurysms | % with Aneurysm |
|---|---|---|---|
| Frontal | 48 | 12 | 25 |
| Parietal | 49 | 2 | 4.1 |
| Temporal | 53 | 6 | 11.3 |
| Insular | 23 | 5 | 21.7 |
| Occipital | 30 | 7 | 23.3 |
| Cerebellar | 58 | 6 | 10.3 |
| Hippocampal | 17 | 2 | 11.8 |

*Data from* Yasargil M. Microneurosurgery - AVM of the brain, clinical considerations, general and special operative techniques, surgical results, nonoperative cases, cavernous and venous angiomas. In: Microneurosurgery, IIIB. New York: Thieme; 1988. p. 137.

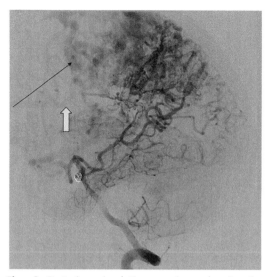

**Fig. 3.** Posterior circulation angiography in the previous patient reveals an additional flow-related SCA aneurysm status post coil embolization (*thick arrow*). Pronounced venous hypertension changes and ectasia noted in superficial and deep venous drainage pathways (*thin arrow*) on this lateral left vertebral angiogram. (*Courtesy of* Massachusetts General Hospital, Department of Neurosurgery and Neurointerventional Radiology, Boston, MA.)

discussed by Hartmann and colleagues[21] in a study of 115 patients with hemorrhage secondary to AVM rupture. Ninety-seven of these patients were found to be independent in their daily activities (Rankin Score 1), with 15 being Rankin Score 2 or 3, and only three patients being severely disabled. Data from the prospective Columbia AVM Databank showed the median Rankin Score to be 2 in a study of 241 AVM patients. Of the AVM hemorrhage subtypes, parenchymal hemorrhage was associated with a higher neurologic morbidity. The reported rerupture risk in the first year was reported at 6% to 18%, and returning to baseline risk after the first

year.[22] It was also noted that in 120 patients who presented with AVM hemorrhage and underwent surgery, there was a mean change in Modified Rankin Score (MRS) score of +0.89 after resection. This can be attributed to the hemorrhage masking the effect of the morbidity of a craniotomy. Hematoma absorption in patients operated weeks to months after rupture also generates cavities and encephalomalacia that improve surgical access to the nidus that might otherwise have necessitated corticectomy.[4] Unless the AVM and hemorrhage have resulted in an expected major neurologic deficit in that territory, it is advisable to allow the patient time for neurologic recovery.[6] In the urgent setting of a hematoma with resulting mass effect and a neurologic deficit, surgical intervention with evacuation of the hematoma is recommended. This should then be followed by appropriate diagnostic imaging and angiography to fully delineate and characterize the arterial supply and venous outflow in lieu of attempted resection in the same setting. Resection of the AVM at the time of hematoma evacuation could result in significant blood loss and a higher risk of ischemic complications secondary to resection of parenchymal branches along with the vasculature recruited by the AVM. In regards to the timing of radiosurgery after hematoma, Maruyama and colleagues[23] noted in a study of patients status posthemorrhage with hematoma that waiting more than 6 months before treatment to allow for hematoma reabsorption put the patient at greater risk of rehemorrhage in the interval preceding treatment. However, the hematoma should be resolved to the point where it does not alter the accurate targeting for radiosurgery.

## SURGICAL INTERVENTION

The history of surgical resection of AVMs dates back to the 1920s, where outcomes were typically poor. The development of cerebral angiography by Moniz in 1927 provided an essential understanding of the vascular anatomy and hemodynamics of these lesions.[24] The acceptance of en bloc resection of these lesions did not become part of standard surgical technique until 1957 after the publication of Olivecrona's and Landenheim's paper.[25] Technologic advances, such as the introduction of microneurosurgery by Yasargil in 1969 and bipolar cauterization by Malis, have resulted in a significant reduction in morbidity and mortality compared to the initial documented operative resections.[24]

The principal benefit of surgical resection is the immediate cure (**Fig. 5**). Additionally, in a study of 54 patients with epilepsy and without a history of

| Table 3 | |
|---------|---|
| **AVM-associated aneurysm classification** | |
| **Aneurysm Classification** | **Location** |
| I | Anatomically unrelated |
| II | Proximal portion of major feeding vessel |
| III | Pedicle branch of major feeding vessel |
| IV | Intranidal |

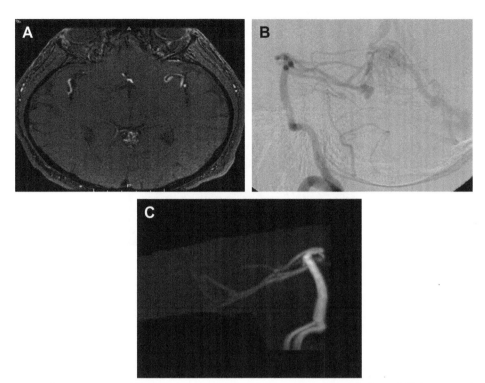

**Fig. 4.** Imaging from a 70-year-old man who had a 15-year history of vertigo. (*A*) Time-of-flight MR angiography depicting a superior vermian AVM. (*B*) Angiography displays arterial supply from the right superior cerebellar artery and venous drainage by the superior vermian vein to the torcular of Herophili. A right cerebellomesence-phalic segment 7-mm aneurysm of the right SCA is noted. (*C*) New resolution on follow-up magnetic resonance angiography 2 years after proton therapy. Interval reduction in the aneurysm is also noted.

hemorrhage who underwent total surgical resection of the AVM, excellent (70%) and good (18.5%) results in terms of seizure control were noted.[26] Treatment of AVMs even in eloquent areas, such as in the occipital lobe and dominant superior temporal gyrus, has had promising results when surgery has been used as the primary modality of therapy. This series had only 1 of 22 total patients with occipital AVMs who developed worsening of a homonymous hemianopsia.[24] However, this and other reports are subject to selection bias.

The process of excision of the AVM after dural opening includes identification of the malformation, elimination of superficial feeding arteries, circumferential dissection of the nidus with control of deep arterial pedicles, and transection of the venous system.[27] To proceed with surgical resection, a preoperative angiogram and magnetic resonance imaging for stereotactic localization intraoperatively are essential. Careful planning of the surgical attack must be done to include potential avenues of dissection and areas to avoid. Lesions, particularly in the sylvian fissure and ones involving pericallosal vessels, are prone to have vessels *en passage* that must be skeletonized

and with only resection of the small side branches supplying the nidus, while maintaining supply to the main trunk.[27] It is also critically important to identify arterialized veins before resection, because early venous coagulation can result in significant intraoperative hemorrhage. If there is any question regarding a specific vessel, a temporary clip may be used. Once the superficial arterial supply is controlled, dissection of the nidus can ensue. A hemosiderin or gliotic rim may be present and provide a plane of dissection around the nidus. The apex of deeper lesions tends to be periventricular and thus identification and bipolar coagulation of these vessels are critically important to prevent vessel retraction and delayed hematoma formation.[6,27] Maintenance of the major draining veins is essential and if hemorrhage is encountered from these sources, it is preferable to use hemostatic agents as a primary method of control instead of cauterization and ligation of the vein to preserve venous outflow from the AVM. Once all arterial feeders to the nidus have been identified and coagulated, then the direct venous outflow can be occluded and the nidus resected. The resection bed should be carefully inspected

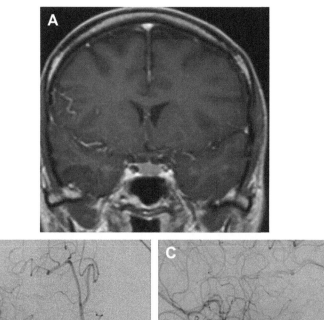

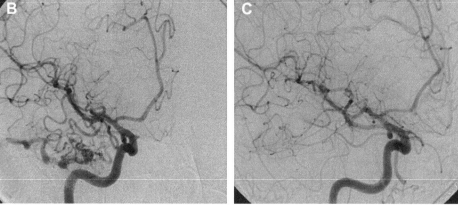

**Fig. 5.** (*A–C, clockwise*) Imaging of a 57-year-old right-handed woman with new-onset seizures depicting a Spetzler-Martin I right temporal AVM. Angiography confirmed feeders from right anterior temporal artery, right inferior division M3 branches, and right PCA inferior temporal branches. Postoperative angiogram reveals a complete resection. (*Courtesy of* Massachusetts General Hospital, Department of Neurosurgery and Neurointerventional Radiology, Boston, MA.)

microscopically to obtain hemostasis, during which the blood pressure is maintained 15 to 20 mm Hg above the baseline for the patient.[27] Once this is complete, oxidized cellulose (Surgicel) can be used to line the nidus bed, and the patient's goal blood pressure should not be allowed to be higher than the normal mean for the first 24 hours postoperatively.

In addition to the general resection principles discussed previously, the location of the AVM carries significant weight in regards to surgical planning. For example, traditionally the convexity AVM is approached perpendicularly, but the parafalcine AVM should be approached tangentially,[28] which allows for the use of gravity retraction. As further detailed by Kim,[29] the parafalcine lesions are divided into zones, and proper surgical positioning is determined based on the zone of the lesion. Lesions of the posterior fossa account for approximately 10% of all intracranial AVMs.[30]

Based on the location within the posterior fossa, the positioning must allow for maximal exposure and cerebrospinal fluid diversion by opening of an adjacent cistern. For lesions of the cerebellar tonsils, fourth ventricle, and vermis, patients are positioned prone with the head in a flexed position. This allows for maximal exposure for dissection of the posterior inferior cerebellar artery and superior cerebellar artery vessels in the case of vermian lesions. Alternatively, a lateral position with the head turned and flexed may be used. Superficial brainstem AVMs are most commonly situated in the anterolateral aspect of the brainstem surface and are associated with the cerebellopontine angle.[6] Typical arterial feeders to an AVM in this territory are likely to be anterior–inferior cerebellar artery and superior cerebellar artery and a lateral position is recommended to enhance exposure.

To determine the risks of AVM surgery, the Spetzler-Martin Grading Scale was developed in

1986. This grading system (see **Fig. 5**) allowed for risk stratification to surgical resection based on the size of the AVM, pattern of venous drainage, and whether it resided in an eloquent location of the brain. The results as seen in **Table 4** from a study of 100 consecutive patients show there is a significant increase in surgical morbidity and mortality as the grade increases. A supplementary grading system has also been devised to further consider the diffuseness of the lesion, hemorrhagic presentation, patient age, and deep perforating arterial supply in conjunction with the previous grading system. When used with the Spetzler-Martin Grading Scale, the predictive value based on the MRS was more significantly correlated with patient outcomes.[5,31] Recently, a three-tier system, combining Spetzler-Martin Grades I to II (group A) and IV to V (group C) is now used with similar predictive outcome values and simplifies treatment strategies. Based on these studies, surgical resection is reserved for group A.[32]

## EMBOLIZATION

The first report of embolization of a brain AVM appeared in 1960, with a documented cure of a left sylvian fissure AVM embolized with four spheres of methyl methacrylate.[33] Endovascular techniques have advanced greatly and reported cure rate for AVMs by embolization alone varies between 10% and 40%.[34] A higher yield of total obliteration is expected in a single-pedicle feeder that is small in size. Total obliteration seems related to the anatomic arrangement of the feeding vessels, such as in the case of an AVM with indirect leptomeningeal collaterals or feeders *en passage* influence the capability to safely embolize the lesion entirely.[27] Although achieving angiographic cure as a unimodal treatment strategy is not always possible, embolization can be used

for achieving significant AVM volume reduction. As an adjunct to surgery or radiosurgery, this is an essential treatment modality in the larger AVMs that are located in eloquent regions of the parenchyma and is typically performed over multiple staged treatments. Multiple methods of endovascular embolization of an AVM nidus include using such materials as Onyx, Gelfoam, platinum coils, polyvinyl alcohol (PVA), and *N*-butyl cyanoacrylate (NBCA).

The Onyx liquid embolic system was first approved in Europe in 1999 for embolization of intracranial and peripheral vasculature lesions, including cerebral AVMs and vascular tumors.[35,36] In a study of 117 patients treated with Onyx (54) or NBCA (63), in which success was determined by more than 50% reduction in AVM volume, Onyx use was found to be successful in 96% of the cases versus 85% for NBCA.[35] Increased penetration throughout the AVM nidus is likely because of the precipitating reaction and cohesive nature of Onyx. This along with the slower and longer injection rate results in much more effective intranidal penetration, and higher likelihood of anatomic cures and higher volume reductions in large AVMs allowing them to be amenable to adjunctive radiosurgical treatment (**Fig. 6**).[35] Because of the increased ability of nidal penetration by Onyx, one must be careful not to occlude the venous outflow, which can result in an increased chance of posttreatment hemorrhage. In comparing Onyx with NBCA, there was not a detectable difference in the rate of posttreatment hemorrhage, although the author stated this could be confounded by a small sample size.[35] A potential deterrent to the use of Onyx, which consists of ethylene vinyl alcohol and dimethyl sulfoxide, is the known toxicity of dimethyl sulfoxide. However, dimethyl sulfoxide in treatment doses has not been noted to carry additional toxicity in multiple animal and preclinical studies.[35,37,38] Reports of posttreatment headaches, nuchal rigidity, and rash have been reported. The risk of permanent neurologic deficit or morbidity ranged from 2% to 7% in a review of multiple large trials. In using liquid embolic agents, it is critically important to observe for reflux of the agent, because hardening of the cast can adhere to the microcatheter making catheter removal difficult.

Alternative embolization material that has been used includes PVA. Proponents of the use of this and other dehydrated alcohol state that the efficacy lies behind its immediate cytotoxic effects on the endothelium of vessels, inducing thrombosis of the vessel.[39] Although these modalities have been effective for treatment of cerebral AVMs, sequential follow-up revealed as high as

**Table 4**
**Surgical outcome data based on Spetzler-Martin grading**

| Grade | #Cases | % No Deficit | % Minor Deficit | % Major Deficit |
|---|---|---|---|---|
| I | 23 | 100 | 0 | 0 |
| II | 21 | 95 | 5 | 0 |
| III | 25 | 84 | 12 | 4 |
| IV | 15 | 74 | 20 | 7 |
| V | 16 | 69 | 19 | 12 |

*Data from* Spetzler R, Martin N. A proposed grading system for arteriovenous malformations. J Neurosurg 1986;65(4): 476–83.

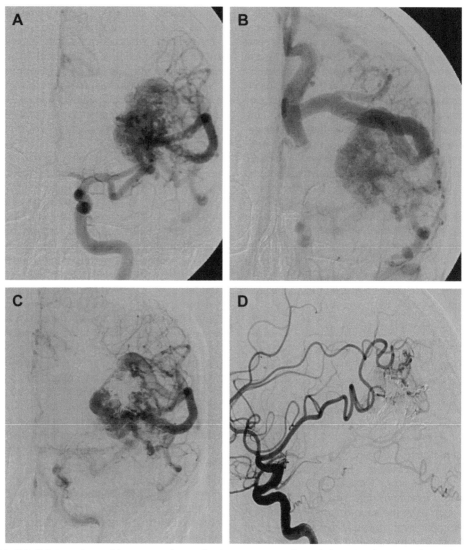

**Fig. 6.** (*A, B*) Left internal carotid artery angiography demonstrates a large left parietal AVM with a nidus approximately 4 cm. Supply is from the right MCA territory with venous drainage to the superior sagittal and transverse sinuses. (*C*) An approximately 40% reduction with stage I Onyx embolization through the left angular artery. (*D*) Near complete obliteration after stage II Onyx embolization by a left parietal inferior division MCA branch. (*Courtesy of* Massachusetts General Hospital, Department of Neurosurgery and Neurointerventional Radiology, Boston, MA.)

43% recanalization rates within 13 months of follow-up.[40,41] A comparison of postoperative hemorrhagic rates were higher in the PVA versus the NBCA group.[40] Additional documented risks include the cytotoxic effect to brain parenchyma when administered at high concentrations along with the risk of developing pulmonary hypertension. Although the overall procedural complication rates were similar between NBCA and PVA, the rate of postresection hemorrhage was significantly higher in the PVA group.[33] Therefore, volume infusions for treatment should not exceed 1 mL/kg.[39]

Coil embolization by itself is limited to adjunctive therapy, unless in the setting of a single arterial feeder because of the limited ability to have coil penetration within the nidus itself. Preoperative superselective angiography of pedicle branch feeders for coil embolization can greatly reduce the AVM volume and assist with resection. Additionally, cerebral AVMs associated with high-flow AVFs present a therapeutic challenge to surgical and radiosurgical techniques, resulting in higher rates of incomplete AVM obliteration. These high-flow shunts are more amenable to endovascular coil placement instead of liquid embolic agent to prevent early venous flow occlusion and thus aid with additional treatment modalities.[42]

Similar general principles for embolization treatment exist as with surgical resection, in that strict blood pressure parameters must be set, and one must not occlude the venous outflow before all arterial supply is identified and obliterated. Additionally, careful manipulation of the microcatheter must be maintained through the pedicle branches, which typically have a more delicate and friable vascular architecture. Cortical branches that are in question of supplying eloquent cortex and the nidus can have a preembolization functional evaluation with a sodium amytal test.[43]

## RADIOSURGERY

Radiosurgery is typically reserved for compact lesions, usually less than 3 cm. It is also a preferred treatment strategy for patients who are not favorable surgical candidates either radiographically (Spetzler-Martin Grades >3) or based on other existing comorbidities. Several different techniques are available to deliver a high dose of radiation to the AVM nidus while minimizing dose to surrounding brain. With stereotactic imaging, a focal high dose is delivered to the nidus, with the goal of minimizing radiation to the surrounding normal brain tissue. This mode of treatment is highly beneficial to lesions located in central structures, such as the brainstem, thalamus, and basal ganglia. The outcome data on central AVMs (mean volume of 4 cm$^3$ with a mean dose of 23 Gy) versus peripheral AVMs demonstrate lower obliteration rates along with the increased propensity of developing sequelae from radiation edema in follow-up studies. These data suggest that Gamma Knife surgery is an effective treatment modality for central lesions.[8] Treatment strategies are performed by a team composed of a neurosurgeon, radiation oncologist, and medical physicist.[44] In a study of 41 patients who had a previous AVM rupture, postradiosurgery decline in their MRS score was noted in 17%. Notably, in this same study, it was concluded that patients with ruptured and unruptured AVMs had a similar chance of neurologic deterioration.[45] Neurologic outcome with radiosurgery has had a better predictive value by use of the Pollock-Flickinger grading system, which evaluates outcome based on preoperative data that include patient age, AVM volume, previous embolization, number of draining veins, and AVM location.[46]

Recommended follow-up includes annual evaluations to assess for neurologic function with magnetic resonance imaging and magnetic resonance angiography to evaluate for AVM volume and affect, if any, on surrounding tissue. With timing for successful treatment spanning from 12 to 36 months, angiography should be completed at the latter to evaluate for residual AVM nidus and subsequent need for radiosurgery retreatment or alternative treatment strategies (see **Fig. 4**).[46] It is essential to inform the patient that although undergoing treatment for the AVM via radiosurgery, the risk of hemorrhage is not eliminated because of the delayed timing for obliteration with this technique. The exact risk of hemorrhage after radiation is not definite based on current literature. In one retrospective evaluation of 500 patients after Gamma Knife therapy there was a risk of reduction of hemorrhage of 54%.[47] Larger AVMs and the older patient population may be risk factors with this interval increase during treatment.[48] The pathophysiology of the hemorrhage during this window may be caused by an acute inflammatory response after tissue irradiation, resulting in structural and functional vascular changes that can lead to vessel thrombosis.[49] In the subset of patients presenting with seizures, improvement in seizure control seems altered related to AVM obliteration. In a study of patients with known rolandic area AVMs and seizure presentation, 40.7% had improved seizure control during the latency period and 51.8% had complete resolution with obliteration of the nidus.[50] Lim and colleagues[51] reported even better results with cerebral AVMs in multiple different areas, and in patients presenting with medically intractable seizures secondary to the AVM. The rates of complete obliteration after radiosurgery are found to be significantly greater in AVMs less than 3 cm and in lower Spetzler-Martin grades.

Multiple series have been published regarding proton radiosurgery, Gamma Knife therapy, linear particle accelerator (LINAC), and more recently cyberknife treatment results. Proton-beam therapy uses a Bragg peak at the point of deceleration of a particle beam of accelerated protons. Photon energy follows the law of exponential decay, consequently resulting in its energy being deposited over the path to the target. Considering this, proton therapy has the distinct advantage of not losing energy before or after the target.

In a study of 300 AVM patients treated solely with helium ion radiosurgery, complete angiographic cure was noted in 80% to 85% of patients with at least 3-year follow-up. In this study, AVMs greater than 14 cm$^3$ were found to have 60% to 70% angiographic obliteration in this same timeline. Dosing used was approximately 20 to 25 Gy. The advantage of heavy charged particle radiation, such as helium ion radiosurgery, is that the physical properties of these particles allows for the shaping of individual beams to encompass the contours and complex shape of the AVM.[52]

LINAC therapy uses x-rays derived from electron-photon administration and has been demonstrated by Blamek and colleagues[53] to have successful complete obliteration in 77% of patients with an average of 28-month follow-up. It was noted that dosing less than 15 Gy significantly reduced the probability of obliteration.[53] In regards to the larger lesions that spanned greater than 25 mm in diameter, obliteration at 1 year was noted to be 40% in these lesions.[44] In contrast to this, the Leksell Gamma Knife uses a cobalt source for the administration of gamma rays to the AVM target. In addition to the outcome results of the Gamma Knife trials in **Table 5**, Lunsford and colleagues[54] document 80% complete obliteration at 2 years.

In regards to the patient population without obliteration after radiosurgery treatment, retreatment can be performed. The Stockholm radiosurgery group comments on achieving angiographic cure with second or salvage therapy, although with a higher complication rate of 14%.[44]

Radiation-induced sequelae include subjective complaints of headache, nausea, and vomiting in the acute posttreatment stage. The delayed complications include neurologic deterioration secondary to radiation-induced necrosis. Lunsford and colleagues[54] reported a 4.4% of neurologic deficits likely secondary to radiation injury that occurred between 4 and 18 months after treatments. Improved neurologic recovery was noted in this study with steroid administration. The documented risk for developing a permanent radiation-induced neurologic deficit was 3.8%.[44] Actual risks with proton therapy were best predicted using a model

that accounted for treatment dose and volume, lesion location, and patient age.[55] Doses greater than 34.6 Gy have been known to lead to a relatively high complication rate in contrast to results from the study by Levegrun and colleagues[31] with stereotactic linear accelerator treatment and a median dose of 19 Gy and 80% isodose administered with no resulting radiation necrosis.[56–58] Although rare, additional documented findings postradiosurgery treatments include the development of intracerebral vascular stenosis and dural arteriovenous fistula development.

## MULTIMODAL TREATMENT

The outcome for AVM treatment of immediate elimination of hemorrhagic risk and cure is only offered by open surgery. Microsurgical resection is not always an option because of the risks that invariably increase with larger, deeper lesions, and those in eloquent areas. Because of this, combining therapies to either make lesions more safely approached by surgery or for overall volume reduction has become more and more prevalent compared with one-dimensional treatment strategies, in particular for Spetzler-Martin Grade 3 or higher lesions. Radiosurgery has been noted to facilitate AVM surgical resection along with decreasing operative morbidity by reduction in AVM volume and subsequent Spetzler-Martin grades compared with patients with similar AVMs who were not radiated.[59,60] In a study of lesions greater than 3 cm, staged embolization performed with subsequent stereotactic radiosurgery was found to be an effective means of treatment for Spetzler-Martin grades greater than 4 (**Fig. 7**). Of the 19 patients with angiography follow-up, complete obliteration was noted in 13 of the patients.[56] In a larger study of patients

## Table 5
### Major AVM outcome series comparing different radiosurgery modalities

| Reference | Colombo et al | Pollock et al | Karlsson et al | Steinberg et al | Colombo et al | Friedman et al |
|---|---|---|---|---|---|---|
| Device | Cyberknife | Gamma knife | Gamma knife | Proton | LINAC | LINAC |
| # Patients | 279 | 313 | 945 | 86 | 180 | 388 |
| Angiographic cure rate % | 81 | 61 | 56 | 92 | 80 | 67 |
| Permanent neurologic deficit % | 0 | 9 | 5 | 11 | 2 | 2 |
| Hemorrhage | 8 | 8 fatal | 55 | 10 | 15 (5 fatal) | 25 (5 fatal) |

*Data from* Youmans neurological surgery. 5th edition. New York: WB Saunders; 2004. p. 4079; and Colombo Cyberknife results.

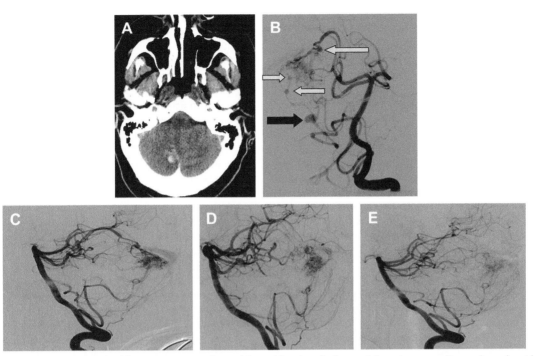

**Fig. 7.** (A–E) A 54-year-old woman presenting with sudden headache and imaging revealing subarachnoid hemorrhage (A). She was taken for diagnostic angiography, where a 2-cm AVM nidus supplied by the right SCA and right anterior inferior cerebellar artery-posterior inferior cerebellar artery complex is noted. An associated 7-mm pseudoaneurysm (*black arrow*) along with three smaller aneurysms less than 3 mm are also present (*blue arrows*). (C, D) Results status post–staged Onyx embolization of the aneurysm and AVM. Angiography 1 year after proton-beam radiosurgery reveals significant flow reduction through the nidus. (*Courtesy of* Massachusetts General Hospital, Department of Neurosurgery and Neurointerventional Radiology, Boston, MA.)

treated with embolization and LINAC radiosurgery, 77% of AVMs were reduced in size for LINAC radiosurgery, with 65% of those resulting in eventual complete occlusion.[61] Even though both of these studies display significant reduction and obliteration rates in complex AVMs, both studies have documented greater than 10% morbidity rates.

## SUMMARY

The understanding of AVMs has undergone significant changes and improvements regarding diagnosis and management. This coincides with the development of technologic advances in imaging modalities, microsurgical techniques, and follow-up outcome data of adjuvant treatment modalities, such as endovascular and radiosurgery techniques, which can be used separately or in conjunction. Determining the treatment modality ultimately depends on understanding the pathophysiology of AVMs. Multiple factors including age of presentation, constellation of symptoms, size and location of the lesion, and the timing of therapy along with clinical presentation influences the decision of the treating clinician. Based on these factors, the proper treatment arm or

combination thereof can be determined versus observation. The latter is an option as long as a firm understanding of the natural history of the lesion is considered in relation to the risk of treatment and neurologic sequela from such intervention. The results of ongoing and future randomized trials will provide further insight into the pathophysiology and indications for treatment, which can be further stratified to individualize treatment based on patient and lesional characteristics.

## REFERENCES

1. Stapf C, Mohr J, Pile-Spellman J, et al. Epidemiology and natural history of arteriovenous malformations. Neurosurg Focus 2001;11(5):1–6.
2. Ondra S, Troup H, George E, et al. The natural history of symptomatic arteriovenous malformations of the brain: a 24 year follow up assessment. J Neurosurg 1990;73(3):387–91.
3. Piepgras D, Sundt T, Ragoowansi A, et al. Seizure outcome in patients with surgically treated cerebral arteriovenous malformations. J Neurosurg 1993;78:5–11.
4. Lawton M, Du R, Tran M, et al. Effect of presenting hemorrhage on outcome after microsurgical

resection of brain arteriovenous malformations. Neurosurgery 2005;56(3):485–93.

5. Lawton M, Kim H, Mculloch C, et al. A supplementary grading scale for selecting patients with brain arteriovenous malformations for surgery. Neurosurgery 2010;66(4):702–13.

6. Atlas S, Do H. Intracranial vascular malformations and aneurysms. In: Magnetic resonance imaging of the brain and spine. Philadelphia: Lippincott Williams & Wilkins; 2009. p. 695–771.

7. Cao Y, Wang R, Yang L, et al. Bipolar electrocoagulation on cortex after AVMs lesionectomy for seizure control. Can J Neurol Sci 2011;38(1):48–53.

8. Kato Y, Sano H, Kanaoka N, et al. Successful resection of arteriovenous malformations in eloquent areas diagnosed by surface anatomy scanning and motor evoked potential. Neurol Med Chir (Tokyo) 1998;38: 217–21.

9. Kiran N, Kale S, Kasliwal M, et al. Gamma knife radiosurgery for arteriovenous malformations of basal ganglia, thalamus and brainstem–a retrospective study comparing the results with that for AVMs at other intracranial locations. Acta Neurochir 2009; 151(12):1575–82.

10. Kondziolka D, Nixon B, Lasjaunias P, et al. Cerebral arteriovenous malformations and associated arterial aneurysms: hemodynamic and therapeutic considerations. Can J Neurol Sci 1988;15:130–4.

11. Marks M, Lane B, Steinberg GK, et al. Vascular characteristics of intracerebral arteriovenous malformations in patients with clinical steal. AJNR Am J Neuroradiol 1991;12:489–96.

12. Chang S, Marcellus M, Marks M, et al. Multimodality treatment of giant intracranial AVMs. Neurosurgery 2007;61(1):432–42.

13. Chen C, Chapman P, Petit J, et al. Proton radiosurgery in neurosurgery. Neurosurg Focus 2007;23(6):52.

14. Choi J, Henning M, Sciacca R. Clinical outcome after first and recurrent hemorrhage in patients with untreated brain AVM. Stroke 2006;37:1243–7.

15. Yasargil MG, Teddy P, Valavanis A. Location of AVMs. In: Microneurosurgery, IIIA. New York: Theime; 1987. p. 183–5.

16. Brown R, Wiebers D, Forbes G. Unruptured intracranial aneurysms and vascular malformations: frequency of intracranial hemorrhage and relationship with lesions. J Neurosurg 1990;73:859–63.

17. Thompson R, Steinberg G, Levy R, et al. The management of patients with arteriovenous malformations and associated intracranial aneurysms. Neurosurgery 1998;43(2):202–11.

18. Weigele J, Riyadh N, Al-Okaili R, et al. Endovascular management of brain arteriovenous malformations. In: Interventional neuroroadiology. New York: Informa Healthcare; 2008. p. 283–6.

19. Redekop G, TerBrugge K, Montanera W, et al. Arterial aneurysms associated with cerebral arteriovenous malformations: classification, incidence, and risks of hemorrhage. J Neurosurg 1998;89:539–46.

20. Saatci I, Geyik S, Yavuz K, et al. Endovascular treatment of brain arteriovenous malformations with prolonged intranidal Onyx injection technique: long-term results in 350 consecutive patients with completed endovascular treatment course. J Neurosurg 2011; 115(1):78–88.

21. Hartmann A, Mast H, Mohr J, et al. Morbidity of intracranial hemorrhage in patients with cerebral arteriovenous malformation. Stroke 1998;29(5):931–4.

22. Du R, McDermott M, Dowd C, et al. Neurosurgery at the crossroads: integrated multidisciplinary management of 449 patients with brain arteriovenous malformation. In: Clinical neurosurgery. Congress of Neurosurgery. 2004. p. 100.

23. Maruyama K, Koga T, Shin M, et al. Optimal timing for Gamma Knife surgery after hemorrhage from brain arteriovenous malformations. J Neurosurg 2008;109:73–6.

24. Yamada S. Surgical approaches to AVMs in functional areas of the brain. In: Arteriovenous malformations in functional areas of the brain. New York: Futura; 1999. p. 1–123.

25. Olivecrona H, Ladenheim J. Congenital arteriovenous aneurysms of the carotid and vertebral arterial systems. Berlin: Springer; 1957.

26. Yeh HS, Tew JM, Gartner M. Seizure control after surgery on cerebral arteriovenous malformations. J Neurosurg 1993;78(1):12–8.

27. Fritsch M, Heros R. Surgical management of supratentorial arteriovenous malformations. In: Youmans neurological surgery. 5th edition. New York: WB Saunders; 2004. p. 2231–48.

28. Yong B, Young W, Lawton M. Parafalcine and midline arteriovenous malformations: surgical strategy, techniques, and outcomes. J Neurosurg 2011;114: 984–93.

29. Kim Y, Young W, Lawton L. Parafalcine and midline arteriovenous malformations: surgical strategy, techniques, and outcomes. J Neurosurg 2011;114(4): 984–93.

30. Batjer H, Samson D. Arteriovenous malformations of the posterior fossa. J Neurosurg 1986;64:849–56.

31. Levegrun S, Holger H, Essiq M, et al. Radiation induced changes of brain tissue after radiosurgery in patients with arteriovenous malformations: correlation with dose distribution parameters. Int J Radiat Oncol Biol Phys 2004;59(3):796–808.

32. Spetzler R, Ponce FA. A 3-tier classification of cerebral arteriovenous malformations. Clinical article. J Neurosurg 2011;114(3):842–89.

33. Harrigan M, Deveikis J. Arteriovenous malformations. In: Handbook of cerebrovascular disease and neurointerventional techniques. New York: Humana Press; 2009. p. 522.

34. Berenstein A, Lasjaunias P. Surgical neuroangiography: endovascular treatment of cerebral lesions, vol. 4. Berlin: Springer Verlag; 1992. p. 317.

35. Loh Y, Duckwiler G. Clinical article: a prospective multicenter, randomized trial of the Onyx liquid embolic system and N-butyl cyanoacrylate embolization of cerebral arteriovenous malformations. J Neurosurg 2010;113:733–41.

36. Luessenhop AJ, Rosa L. Cerebral arteriovenous malformations. Indications for and results of surgery, and the role of intravascular techniques. J Neurosurg 1984;60:14–22.

37. US Food and Drug Administration. Summary of safety and effectiveness data. Washington, DC: US Department of Health and Human Services; 2005.

38. Valvanis A, Yasargil MG. The endovascular treatment of brain arteriovenous malformations. Adv Tech Stand Neurosurg 1998;24:131–214.

39. Morris P. Embolization of pial arteriovenous malformations. In: Practical neuroangiography. Philadelphia: Lippincott Williams & Wilkins; 2007. p. 456–63.

40. Sorimachi T, Koike T, Takeuchi S, et al. Embolization of cerebral arteriovenous malformations achieved with polyvinyl alcohol particles: angiographic reappearance and complications. AJNR Am J Neuroradiol 1999;20(7):1323–8.

41. Spetzler R, Martin N. A proposed grading system for arteriovenous malformations. J Neurosurg 1986; 65(4):476–83.

42. Yuki I, Kim R, Duckwiler G, et al. Treatment of brain arteriovenous malformations with high-flow arteriovenous fistulas: risks and complications associated with endovascular embolization in multimodality treatment. J Neurosurg 2010;113(4):715–22.

43. Rauch R, Vinuela F, Dion J, et al. Preembolization functional evaluation in brain arteriovenous malformations: the ability of superselective Amytal test to predict neurological dysfunction before embolization. AJNR Am J Neuroradiol 1992;13:309–14.

44. Friedman W, Foote K. Radiosurgery for arteriovenous malformations. In: Youmans neurological surgery. 5th edition. New York: WB Saunders; 2004. p. 4073–85.

45. Pollock B, Brown R. Use of the Modified Rankin Scale to assess outcome after arteriovenous malformation radiosurgery. Neurology 2006;67(9):1630–4.

46. Pollock B, Flickinger J. A proposed radiosurgery-based grading system for arteriovenous malformations. J Neurosurg 2002;96(1):79–85.

47. Maruyama K, Kawahara N, Shin M, et al. The risk of hemorrhage after radiosurgery for cerebral arteriovenous malformations. N Engl J Med 2005;252(2):146–53.

48. Karlsson B, Lax I, Soderman M. Risk for hemorrhage during the 2-year latency period following Gamma Knife radiosurgery for arteriovenous malformations. Int J Radiat Oncol Biol Phys 2001;49(4):1045–51.

49. Celix J, Douglas J, Haynor D, et al. Thrombosis and hemorrhage in the acute period following Gamma Knife surgery for arteriovenous malformations. Case report. J Neurosurg 2009;111(1):124–31.

50. Andrade-Souza Y, Ramani M, Scora D, et al. Radiosurgical treatment for rolandic arteriovenous malformations. J Neurosurg 2006;105(5):689–97.

51. Lim Y, Lee C, Koh J, et al. Seizure control of Gamma Knife radiosurgery for non-hemorrhagic arteriovenous malformations. Acta Neurochir Suppl 2006; 99:97–101.

52. Fabrikant J, Levy R, Steinberg G. Charged-particle radiosurgery for intracranial vascular malformations. Neurosurg Clin N Am 1992;3(1):99–139.

53. Blamek S, Tarnawski R, Miszczyk L. LINAC-based stereotactic radiosurgery for brain arteriovenous malformations. Clin Oncol (R Coll Radiol) 2011; 23(8):525–31.

54. Lunsford L, Kondziolka D, Flickinger J, et al. Stereotactic radiosurgery for arteriovenous malformations of the brain. J Neurosurg 1991;75(4):512–24.

55. Barker F, Butler W, Lyons S, et al. Dose-volume prediction of radiation-related complications after proton beam radiosurgery for cerebral arteriovenous malformations. J Neurosurg 2003;99:254–63.

56. Blackburn S, Ashley W, Rich K, et al. Combined endovascular embolization and stereotactic radiosurgery in the treatment of large arteriovenous malformations. J Neurosurg 2011;114(6):1758–67.

57. Steinberg G, Fabrikant J, Marks M, et al. Stereotactic heavy charged particle Bragg peak radiation for intracranial arteriovenous malformations. N Engl J Med 1990;323:96–101.

58. Steinberg G, Marks M, Levy R, et al. Multimodality treatment of vascular malformations in functional brain areas, using stereotactic radiosurgery, embolization, and microsurgery. In: Arteriovenous malformations in functional areas of the brain. New York: Futura; 1999. p. 181–95.

59. Sanchez-Mejia R, McDermott M, Tan J, et al. Radiosurgery facilitates resection of brain arteriovenous malformations and reduces surgical morbidity. Neurosurgery 2009;64(2):231–8.

60. Silander H, Pellettieri L, Enblad P, et al. Fractionated stereotactic proton beam treatment of cerebral arteriovenous malformations. Acta Neurol Scand 2004; 109(2):85–90.

61. Gobin Y, Laurent A, Merienne L, et al. Treatment of brain arteriovenous malformations by embolization and radiosurgery. J Neurosurg 1996;85: 19–28.

# Selection of Treatment Modalities or Observation of Dural Arteriovenous Fistulas

Alexandra R. Paul, MD[a], Geoffrey P. Colby, MD, PhD[b],
Judy Huang, MD[b], Rafael J. Tamargo, MD[b],
Alexander L. Coon, MD[b],*

## KEYWORDS

- Dural arteriovenous malformation
- Dural arteriovenous fistula • Endovascular

Cranial dural arteriovenous malformations, commonly referred to as dural arteriovenous fistulas (DAVFs), are abnormal shunts between dural arteries and a dural venous sinus or a cortical vein. DAVFs occur throughout the intracranial space, but are most often located near and involve 1 or more dural venous sinuses. Depending on the extent of the lesion and its associated venous drainage, DAVFs are either managed conservatively by observation or treatment is recommended. Various treatment options for DAVFs are available, including endovascular embolization, open surgery, and radiosurgery.[1–4] The clinical decision pathways for managing patients with DAVFs are discussed in this article.

## REVIEW OF DAVF CLASSIFICATION SCHEMES

To appropriately triage a patient with a DAVF, it is essential to first understand the anatomy of the fistula and the involved venous pathways. Various classifications schemes have been devised to describe these lesions, and the Borden and the Cognard schemes are the most widely used.[5,6] The key feature for both of these grading systems is the direction and severity of venous drainage, and these features ultimately determine the clinical significance of the lesion and influence the decision to treat.

The Borden classification system groups DAVFs into 3 main types based on the location of venous drainage (dural sinus and/or cortical vein) and on whether cortical venous reflux (CVR) is present or absent. Borden type 1 DAVFs have anterograde venous drainage into a dural sinus and no CVR. Type 2 lesions drain retrogradely into dural sinuses and also into cortical veins, with associated CVR. Type 3 lesions drain directly into a cortical veins, causing significant CVR.[5]

The Cognard system groups DAVFs into 5 main types based on the direction of venous sinus drainage (anterograde or retrograde), the presence or absence of CVR, and the type of venous outflow (eg, nonectatic vs ectatic cortical veins). A Cognard type 1 DAVF has anterograde flow with no CVR. A type II DAVF drains into a sinus with retrograde flow in the sinus (type IIA), retrograde flow in a cortical vein (type IIb), or retrograde flow in the sinus and cortical veins (type II A+B). Type III DAVF drains retrogradely into a nonectatic

The authors have no financial disclosures or conflicts of interest.
[a] Division of Neurosurgery, Albany Medical Center Hospital, 47 New Scotland Avenue, MC 10, Albany, NY 12208, USA
[b] Department of Neurosurgery, Johns Hopkins University School of Medicine, The Johns Hopkins Hospital, 600 North Wolfe Street, Meyer 8-181, Baltimore, MD 21287, USA
* Corresponding author.
*E-mail address:* Acoon2@jhmi.edu

Neurosurg Clin N Am 23 (2012) 77–85
doi:10.1016/j.nec.2011.09.004
1042-3680/12/$ – see front matter Published by Elsevier Inc.

cortical vein, and type IV drains into an ectatic cortical vein. Lastly, Cognard type V DAVFs drain into a spinal perimedullary vein.[6]

Both of these classification systems highlight the importance of CVR; however, Zipfel and colleagues[7] proposed modification of these classic schemes to include clinical information about whether or not the CVR is symptomatic. This modification is based on studies by Soderman and colleagues[8] and Strom and colleagues[9] that show that patients presenting with intracranial hemorrhage (ICH) or nonhemorrhagic neurologic deficit (defined as symptomatic CVR) have a greater neurologic risk and death than patients who present incidentally or solely with symptoms of increased dural sinus drainage (defined as asymptomatic CVR).[8,9] The new scale proposed by Zipfel and colleagues[7] is as follows: 1) type 1 DAVFs drain only into a dural sinus and have no CVR; 2) type 2 DAVFs drain into a dural sinus and have either asymptomatic or symptomatic CVR; and 3) type 3 DAVFs drain directly into cortical veins and have either asymptomatic or symptomatic CVR. Neurologic risk increases from type 1 lesions to type 2 or 3 lesions with asymptomatic CVR (1.4–1.5% annual risk of ICH) to type 2 or 3 lesions with symptomatic CVR (7.4%–7.6% annual risk of ICH). Zipfel and colleagues[7] recommend that patients with symptomatic CVR (type 2 or 3 DAVF) undergo immediate, definitive treatment of the fistula by an endovascular or open surgical approach. Stereotactic radiosurgery is not recommended in these patients because of the time delay required for occlusion of the fistula.

Carotid cavernous fistulas (CCFs) are another important group of DAVFs. The most widely used classification system for these fistulas is the Barrow system. CCFs are categorized into direct (Barrow type A) and indirect (Barrow types B–D). Indirect CCFs are DAVFs with arterial feeders from the internal carotid artery (Barrow type B), external carotid artery (Barrow type C), or both (Barrow type D).[10]

## THE NATURAL HISTORY OF DAVFs

Insight into the natural history of DAVFs has been instrumental in the development of clinical decision pathways for managing patients with DAVFs. The natural history of DAVFs is known to be highly variable, and the potential of the lesion to cause morbidity and mortality needs to be weighed against the risks of the intervention used for treatment.[11] Many studies have tried to identify independent factors predictive of the natural history of DAVFs to develop informed treatment plans and decrease mortality and morbidity. Many patients with DAVFs have a benign course,

but 7% to 20% present with ICH.[12] Mortality and morbidity of a hemorrhagic presentation of a DAVF has been estimated to be 20% to 30% with poor long-term prognosis.[11] Individual factors related to the natural history of DAVFs should be carefully considered when making clinical decisions regarding treatment versus observation.

### Location

Awad and colleagues[11] analyzed 377 cases of DAVFs in a meta-analysis. They defined aggressive neurologic behavior as hemorrhage or progressive focal neurologic deficit other than ophthalmoplegia. The investigators found that DAVFs located at the tentorial incisura (8.4% of cases) were most often associated with aggressive neurologic behavior, and 96.9% of these tentorial lesions (31 out of 32) were associated with a hemorrhagic or nonhemorrhagic stroke. Conversely, DAVFs located at the transverse-sigmoid sinuses (62.6% of cases) and at the cavernous sinus (11.9% of cases) were least likely to be associated with aggressive neurologic behavior. Only about 10% of these lesions were associated with aggressive behavior. However, the investigators found that there was no location of DAVFs that completely precluded aggressive neurologic behavior.

In an analysis of 402 patients, Singh and colleagues[12] found that patients were more likely to present with ICH if they had a DAVF in ethmoidal or posterior fossa locations. Twelve patients in their series had ethmoid DAVFs, and 9 of these patients (75%) presented with ICH. Thirty-two patients had DAVFs in the posterior fossa, and 17 (53%) of these patients presented with ICH. The odds ratio (OR) for a hemorrhagic presentation of a DAVF in the posterior fossa is 4. Patients harboring DAVFs in cavernous, marginal, and transverse-sigmoid sinus locations were least likely to present with ICH. Hemorrhage rates were 6.1% (10 of 163 patients) for cavernous sinus lesions, 5.9% (1 of 17 patients) for fistulas in the marginal sinus, and 15.3% (19 of 124 patients) for DAVFs of the transverse-sigmoid sinus.

The anatomic location of a DAVF likely has no direct correlation with aggressive clinical course.[13] The more reasonable explanation for the findings mentioned earlier is that certain cranial locations, secondary to local venous anatomy, have a higher likelihood of developing CVR. The severity of the CVR then dictates the clinical course.

### Venous Drainage

It is generally accepted that the presentation of a DAVF is dictated by its venous drainage pattern.

The pattern of venous drainage is used to classify DAVFs into high-risk and low-risk groups.[12] In the meta-analysis of 377 cases of DAVFs, Awad and colleagues[11] analyzed the relationship between angiographic features of DAVFs and aggressive neurologic behavior. Aggressive neurologic behavior was correlated with leptomeningeal retrograde venous drainage, variceal or aneurysmal venous dilatations, and galenic venous drainage. Less than 1% of nonaggressive DAVFs were found to exhibit these 3 features simultaneously. However, every aggressive DAVF exhibited 1 or more of the 3 angiographic features. The presence of high-flow shunting or contralateral arterial contribution did not correlate with aggressive neurologic behavior.

In a series of 402 patients with DAVFs, Singh and colleagues[12] found that patients presenting with ICH were more likely to have angiographic evidence of venous sinus thrombosis and CVR. Eighty-five percent of patients with DAVFs presenting with ICH had angiographic evidence of CVR, compared with 22% of patients with nonhemorrhagic DAVFs ($P<.001$, OR 10.5). Venous sinus thrombosis was found in 33% of patients with DAVFs presenting with ICH and only 18% of patients with a nonhemorrhagic presentation ($P = .004$). Ninety-five percent of DAVFs were classified as Borden type II and III compared with 45% in the nonhemorrhagic group ($P<.001$).

Strom and colleagues[9] sought to differentiate between symptomatic CVR and asymptomatic CVR to further risk stratify patients diagnosed with type 2 and 3 DAVFs. Patients with symptomatic CVR were defined as presenting with symptoms of cortical venous hypertension, namely ICH or nonhemorrhagic neurologic deficits (progressive dementia, seizures, parkinsonism, cerebellar symptoms, or other focal deficits). Patients with asymptomatic CVR presented incidentally or with isolated symptoms of increased dural sinus drainage (ie, pulsatile tinnitus for lesions of the transverse-sigmoid sinus). The investigators followed 28 patients with persistent cortical venous drainage (Borden type 2 and 3), and they found that the frequency of ICH or nonhemorrhagic neurologic deficit was significantly lower in patients with asymptomatic CVR (5.9%) versus symptomatic CVR (45.5%, $P = .022$). The annual event rate for either ICH or nonhemorrhagic neurologic deficit in patients with symptomatic cortical venous drainage was 19.0% compared with 1.4% in patients with asymptomatic cortical venous drainage. These data suggest that DAVFs with asymptomatic CVR are less aggressive than those with symptomatic CVR.[9]

## Demographics and Symptoms

Singh and colleagues[12] found DAVFs to be more prevalent in women compared with men but found that men were more likely to present with ICH (74% vs 36%, $P<.01$, OR 3.4). A history of smoking was more common in patients presenting with ICH (23% vs 12%, $P = .008$), and Hispanic patients were more likely to present with ICH than a nonhemorrhagic presentation (15% vs 8%, $P = .05$).

Singh and colleagues[12] also analyzed specific symptoms and their association with ICH. Headache, pulsatile tinnitus, and visual changes were the most common symptoms on presentation; however, headache, focal neurologic deficit, and seizure were significantly associated with ICH at presentation. Focal neurologic deficit was found to have an OR of 4.7 for hemorrhagic presentation in patients with DAVFs.

## MANAGEMENT OF BENIGN DAVFs

The decision to treat an intracranial DAVF or to manage it conservatively with observation is based on both lesion-specific factors and patient-specific factors. Lesion-specific factors include the flow velocity (high flow vs slow flow), location, and venous drainage direction and anatomy, including presence of CVR or venous ectasia. Patient-specific factors include the primary presentation, severity of symptoms, and associated patient comorbidities. Various treatment modalities are available for DAVFs, and these include endovascular embolization (transarterial, transvenous, or both), open surgery, radiosurgery, or a combination of these strategies.

Borden type 1 DAVFs and Cognard type I and type IIa fistulas without cortical venous drainage are generally considered benign secondary to absence of CVR. In some institutions, these fistulas are treated with conservative management by observation unless the associated symptoms are severe.[14] Although the primary goal of DAVF treatment is cure, in some cases therapy should be directed primarily at palliation of symptoms by reduction of flow[15,16] and not necessary at cure. Attempted complete angiographic cure of a benign fistula might be associated with increased risk of procedural complications, and therefore might not be warranted. Endovascular treatment is often the best option for palliative therapy, and the risks of endovascular treatment include arterial dissection, stroke, pulmonary embolism, infarction of cranial nerves, and redirection of venous drainage toward cortical veins.[17]

However, fistulas that are classically labeled benign must still be monitored if cure is not achieved because these lesions have the propensity to transform into higher grade, aggressive lesions. Cognard and colleagues[14] reported a series of 7 patients with DAVFs on the transverse or sigmoid sinuses that were initially benign (5 patients with Cognard type I lesions and 2 patients with type IIa lesions) but were later found to have changes in venous drainage patterns on follow-up angiography (from 1 month to 20 years). Five of the patients developed CVR secondary to either stenosis or thrombosis of the draining veins, increased arterial flow, the appearance of a new fistula, or extension of the initial fistula shunt. Based on these results, Cognard and colleagues[14] recommended close clinical observation of type I and IIa fistulas that are treated conservatively with observation or with an incomplete intervention. Repeat angiography should be performed for any change in clinical condition. If stenosis of the venous drainage pathway is present, increased vigilance is necessary because these lesions are likely at greater risk for progression.

Satomi and colleagues[9] reported a series of 117 patients with benign cranial DAVFs, only 3 of which were asymptomatic at the time of presentation. Of these 117 patients, 73 (62%) underwent conservative management with observation, 43 (37%) underwent palliative embolization for treatment of symptoms, and 1 (1%) patient had surgical treatment. Follow-up was available for 112 patients (95.7%), with a median follow-up period of 27.9 months, and repeat angiography was performed in 50 patients because of a change in symptoms. The investigators reported that tolerable, stable disease was achieved in 98.5% of the patients with observational management. Of the 50 patients with follow-up angiography, changes in venous drainage occurred in 5 cases, and each of these cases was associated with progressive thrombosis in the affected sinus. Two patients who were managed with observation had new development of CVR. The investigators therefore concluded that most patients with benign DAVFs can be managed satisfactorily with either observation or palliative intervention. However, patients with benign DAVFs have a 2% risk of developing CVR and therefore require close clinical follow-up and repeat angiography for changes in symptoms.

## MANAGEMENT OF AGGRESSIVE DAVFs

As described in detail earlier, Borden type 2 and 3 DAVFs and Cognard type IIb to V DAVFs are considered aggressive lesions secondary to the presence of CVR and the propensity for hemorrhage and nonhemorrhagic neurologic deficits.[18,19]

Aggressive fistulas have also been divided into 2 main types: (1) sinus fistulas, which have retrograde drainage into a sinus and into leptomeningeal veins (also called red veins because they are arterialized), and (2) nonsinus fistulas, which have pure leptomeningeal drainage.[20] Even though recent reports suggest that not all patients with leptomeningeal drainage are identical and that groups of patients with asymptomatic CVR have a more favorable course than those with symptomatic CVR,[7–9] treatment is still justified because of the significant long-term risk. For fistulas with symptomatic CVR, Zipfel and colleagues[7] recommend prompt evaluation and immediate, definitive treatment.

Accurate definition of the type of lesion should be the initial management step for all aggressive DAVFs. Treatment options for aggressive fistulas include both endovascular and open surgical approaches. Radiosurgery is generally not used for these cases as a first-line therapy, unless the patient is unable to tolerate an endovascular or open surgical procedure. However, radiosurgery can be used as a salvage therapy for aggressive fistulas that have been refractory to other treatment options. Most patients benefit from a combination of treatments. Several factors influence the selection of a treatment modality.

### Transarterial Embolization

Transarterial embolization is ideally used for high-grade DAVFs, such as those with direct cortical venous drainage, or situations in which venous access is limited. Nelson and colleagues[1] listed the following advantages of transarterial procedures for DAVFs: the arteriovenous fistula transition can definitely be occluded through a transarterial approach, decreasing the possibility of flow diversion into an alternate venous pathway[2]; treatment is not limited by venous access (eg, stenotic or thrombosed venous sinuses)[3]; fistula treatment does not require sacrificing a functional venous pathway[4]; de novo DAVFs can develop at secondary site following transvenous embolization, possibly as a result of venous hypertension; and[5] complications specific to transvenous routes can be avoided (eg, abducens nerve palsy from catheterization of the superior petrosal sinus).[21]

Transarterial embolization with n-butyl cyanoacrylate (NBCA) for DAVFs has a high cure rate, ranging from 64% to 100%, with some documented transient palsies but no permanent complications.[22–24] Geudin and colleagues[22] treated 38 patients with DAVFs with CVR with solely transarterial cyanoacrylate glue (Histoacryl, B. Braun, Melsungen, Germany) or Glubran 2

(GEM S.r.l., Viareggio, Italy) embolization. A complete cure was achieved after a single session in 76% (29/38) of patients. A cure rate of 89.5% (34/38) was reported, with 29 patients achieving immediate cure and 5 patients showing postembolization secondary thrombosis. Two transient cases of cerebellar syndrome were reported but both patients recovered rapidly. They noted no permanent complications as well as no endovascular therapy-related mortality. Acrylic glue has been proved to be effective and stable for use in endovascular procedures for more than 30 years. Some investigators argue that glue is advantageous in terms of cost and long-term stability compared with newer liquid agents such as Onyx (ev3, Irvine, CA, USA).

In the past several years, Onyx has been increasingly used in the endovascular treatment of DAVFs. Onyx is a favorable agent because of its properties and predictability during injection. Prolonged injections can be performed through a single feeding vessel with excellent nidus penetration and retrograde embolization of additional feeders. Onyx can also be used for venous sinus occlusion from an arterial injection.

Several large series have now been published, reporting cure rates between 61% and 91%, with complication rates between 0% and 16%. Some investigators have reported cure rates of transarterial Onyx of 100% in small series with no complications reported.[25–27] In 1 series, the treatment of DAVFs with cortical venous drainage with transarterial Onyx in 30 patients were prospectively analyzed. Complete angiographic cure was observed in 80% (24/30) of cases, with 83% (20/24) of these cures achieved after a single procedure. Two complications were reported: a postprocedure hemorrhage secondary to venous outlet thrombosis and 1 temporary cranial nerve palsy.[28]

The role of transarterial Onyx in patients with grade I and grade II DAVFs has also been studied. Anatomic cure was achieved in 50% (13/26) of patients and clinical cure was achieved in 65.4 % (17/26) of patients. All anatomic cures were achieved in a single procedure and follow-up angiography showed no recurrence.[29]

## Transvenous Embolization

Transvenous approaches are also commonly used for treatment of certain DAVFs. Transvenous embolization is generally preferred when the primary arterial feeders to a fistula arise from the internal carotid artery or the vertebral artery, because these arterial pedicles can be small, and reflux of an embolic agent during a transarterial approach is not tolerated. Other situations in

which a transvenous approach is useful are when potential extracranial-intracranial collaterals exist and when the arterial supply to cranial nerves is at risk. In addition, fistulas involving the cavernous sinus, such as CCFs, are typically approached transvenously.[28,30,31]

Selection of a transvenous route depends on the specific venous anatomy of the patient and the dominant venous outflow of the fistula. A transvenous approach is not ideal when the affected sinus is stenotic, compartamentalized, or occluded upstream or downstream of the fistula point. Care must be taken during a transvenous procedure not to inadvertently occlude a critical normal vein, which can cause a venous stroke, or to partially occlude the venous outlet without complete obliteration of the fistula, which can promote CVR and worsen the grade of the fistula.[32–34] In certain circumstances, a combined surgical-transvenous approach, such as the combined surgical-endovascular approach to the cavernous sinus via the superior ophthalmic vein, is warranted.[35]

Since first being pioneered in the late 1970s by Mullan[30] and Hosobuchi,[31] a transvenous approach has become the preferred method of treatment of indirect CCFs.[28] The 2 largest series to date showed complete obliteration in 87% to 91% of patients with indirect CCFs treated with transvenous coils with a procedure-related permanent morbidity of 0% to 2.3%.[36,37] Studies analyzing the long-term outcome in patients who underwent coil embolization of CCFs found a 44% rate of persistent cranial nerve deficits with disturbance of oculomotor and visual functions and a significant correlation between coil volume and persistent diplopia and persistent cranial nerve VI paresis.[38]

Liquid embolics can also be used for treatment of indirect CCFs, either as a primary agent or as an adjunct to coil embolization. Wakhloo and colleagues[39] evaluated the efficacy and safety of transvenous NBCA alone or in combination with coils in a series of 14 patients with indirect CCFs. Eighty-eight percent (7/8) of the patients treated with a combination of NBCA and coils had complete angiographic obliteration of the CCF. Eighty-three percent of patients (5/6) treated with NBCA alone achieved immediate obliteration of the CCF. Onyx has also been used as an adjuvant to coils in transvenous embolization of indirect CCFs. Complete angiographic cure rates ranged from 67% to 100%, with complications between 0% and 33%.[40–43]

## Surgery

Open surgical treatment of DAVFs remains a versatile and effective option for management of various aggressive intracranial DAVFs.[20] The type of surgical procedure required to treat a fistula depends on whether it is a sinus fistula or a nonsinus fistula. In the case of a sinus fistula, the arterialized sinus is not draining normal brain and can be skeletonized and even excised. For skeletonization, the dura along both sides of the involved sinus is incised and extensively coagulated to disconnect the arterial supply. Hemostatic clips can be placed along the cut edges to further prevent future regrowth of bridging vessels. Sundt and colleagues[44,45] were the first to advocate resection of an involved sinus. Certain groups think that the arterialized, pathologic segment of a sinus fistula can be safely resected without any risk of venous hypertension or infarct regardless of the location of the sinus segment or its depth.[20] However, it can be difficult to predict whether adequate collateral venous pathways have developed, and resection of an arterialized sinus is often a serious undertaking with significant risk of substantial blood loss and morbidity.[44] An alternative procedure for open surgical obliteration of the involved sinus is packing the sinus with thrombogenic materials such as Gelfoam (Pfizer, New York, NY, USA), Surgicel (Johnson & Johnson, New Brunswick, NJ, USA), or muscle. Preoperative transarterial embolization, often performed in multiple stages, is commonly used before surgical intervention. Presurgical embolization is particularly important for complex, high-flow lesions to reduce intraoperative blood loss. Collice and colleagues[21] reported a series of 12 patients with sinus fistulas who underwent transarterial embolization followed by surgical excision of the involved sinus. Definitive cure without mortality or major morbidity was obtained in all 12 cases.

Sinus excision is not recommended for a nonsinus fistula because the parent sinus may drain normal cerebral tissue. For nonsinus fistulas, the preferred surgical intervention is the simple interruption of the arterialized draining veins at their dural origin.[20,46,47] A small surgical exposure can be used if precise localization of the fistula is performed. Collice and colleagues[20] reported a series of 22 patients with nonsinus fistulas, 4 of whom had preoperative transarterial embolization. Definitive cure without major complication was achieved in all cases.

Lucas and colleagues[17] performed a meta-analysis of treatments for DAVFs. One of the recommendations of this study is that surgical ligation of arterial feeding vessels is not advised in the modern management of DAVFs. If occlusion of feeding vessels is the goal of treatment, then transarterial embolization is the procedure of choice. This meta-analysis also recommended surgical obliteration as the treatment of choice for anterior fossa DAVFs, finding that 95.5% of anterior fossa DAVFs reviewed were treated successfully by surgery alone. The rationale for this selection is that the ethmoidal feeding vessels for anterior fossa DAVFs arise from branches of the ophthalmic artery, and there is significant risk to the visual system with embolization procedures. However, the risks of surgery are significant, including significant blood loss, direct damage to structures of the central nervous system, stroke, neurologic deficits, infection, and death. Continual advances in endovascular technology have led to safe treatment of these lesions via endovascular approaches as well.[23,48]

Intraoperative angiography (IA) is an important tool during surgery for DAVFs. Pandey and colleagues[49] reported a series of 29 patients who had surgical treatment of DAVFs. Thirty-eight surgeries were performed for DAVF in these 29 patients, and IA was performed in 34 of the surgeries for a total of 44 angiographic procedures. The investigators reported that IA revealed residual fistula in 11 patients (37.9%) after the surgeon determined that the fistula was obliterated. This finding resulted in additional exploration in 10 patients during the same surgery and 1 patient at a later date. However, IA led to false-negative findings in 3 patients (10.7%), thereby justifying the need for additional higher resolution postoperative angiography.

## Radiosurgery

Radiosurgery is available as a sole treatment option for DAVFs or in combination with other treatment modalities. Although there are no established criteria for the use of radiosurgery for DAVF treatment, it is considered an option for benign DAVFs, those with a small fistula nidus, and patients who are either not candidates for either open surgery or endovascular procedures or who have already failed these treatments.[50] Radiosurgery is a noninvasive procedure that is also good for patients with significant medical comorbidities that make them unable tolerate the risks of general anesthesia, open surgery, or endovascular embolization. One main disadvantage of radiosurgery is the latency period between the time of treatment and the effects of treatment, usually a delay of at least 6 months.[51] Radiosurgery is therefore not selected as the primary treatment modality in urgent cases of symptomatic CVR.

Since the introduction of radiosurgery for DAVFs in the 1980s, a variety of reports have been published regarding the use of this technique for both CCFs and non-CCF DAVFs. Obliteration rates for indirect CCFs treated solely with radio-surgery range from 50% to 100%, with 77% of patients having angiographic obliteration. Obliteration rates for non-CCF DAVFs treated by radio-surgery range from 20% to 100%, with 64.3% of patients having angiographic occlusion on follow-up.[50]

Combination therapy for endovascular embolization and radiosurgery has also been widely used for DAVF treatment of both CCFs and non-CCF DAVFs.[52,53] Meta-analysis of combined treatment series by Loumiotis and colleagues[50] showed that combination therapy resulted in complete fistula obliteration in 62.5% of patients with CCFs and 50% of patients with non-CCF lesions. These techniques are thought to be complimentary.[53,54] The embolization procedure provides immediate symptom relief, but might not cure the lesion. The radiosurgery offers no immediate benefit, but has a good chance of longer term permanent occlusion. If combination therapy is chosen to treat an aggressive fistula, embolization should be used first for rapid stabilization of the lesion, followed by radiosurgery for delayed fistula closure.

## SUMMARY

Cranial DAVFs represent an important class of cranial vascular lesions. The clinical significance of these lesions is highly dependent on the pattern of venous drainage, with CVR being an important marker of an aggressive, high-risk fistula. For cases of asymptomatic benign fistulas, conservative management, consisting of observation with follow-up, is a reasonable option. For symptomatic benign fistulas or aggressive fistulas, treatment is recommended. A variety of treatment modalities are available for DAVF management, including endovascular techniques, open surgery, and radiosurgery. A multimodality approach is often warranted and can offer improved chances of achieving a cure.

## REFERENCES

1. Watanabe A, Takahara Y, Ibuchi Y, et al. Two cases of dural arteriovenous malformation occurring after intracranial surgery. Neuroradiology 1984;26:375–80.
2. Nabors MW, Azzam CJ, Albanna FJ, et al. Delayed postoperative dural arteriovenous malformations. Report of two cases. J Neurosurg 1987;66:768–72.
3. Sakaki T, Morimoto T, Nakase H, et al. Dural arteriovenous fistula of the posterior fossa developing after surgical occlusion of the sigmoid sinus. Report of five cases. J Neurosurg 1996;84:113–8.
4. McConnell KA, Tjoumakaris SI, Allen J, et al. Neuroendovascular management of dural arteriovenous malformations. Neurosurg Clin N Am 2009; 20:431–9.
5. Borden JA, Wu JK, Shucart WA. A proposed classification for spinal and cranial dural arteriovenous fistulous malformations and implications for treatment. J Neurosurg 1995;82(2):166–79.
6. Cognard C, Gobin YP, Pierot L, et al. Cerebral dural arteriovenous fistulas: clinical and angiographic correlation with a revised classification of venous drainage. Radiology 1995;194(3):671–80.
7. Zipfel GJ, Shah MN, Refai D, et al. Cranial dural arteriovenous fistulas: modification of angiographic classification scales based on new natural history data. Neurosurg Focus 2009 May;26(5):E14.
8. Soderman M, Pavic L, Edner G, et al. Natural history of dural arteriovenous shunts. Stroke 2008;39(6): 1735–9.
9. Strom RG, Botros JA, Refai D, et al. Cranial dural arteriovenous fistulae: asymptomatic cortical venous drainage portends less aggressive clinical course. Neurosurgery 2009;64(2):241–7.
10. Barrow DL, Spector RH, Braun IF, et al. Classification and treatment of spontaneous carotid-cavernous sinus fistulas. J Neurosurg 1985;62(2):248–56.
11. Awad IA, Little JR, Akrawi WP, et al. Intracranial dural arteriovenous malformations: factors predisposing to an aggressive neurological course. J Neurosurg 1990;72:839–50.
12. Singh V, Smith WS, Lawton MT, et al. Risk factors for hemorrhagic presentation in patients with dural arteriovenous fistulae. Neurosurgery 2008;62:628–35.
13. Satomi J, van Dijk JM, Terbrugge KG, et al. Benign cranial dural arteriovenous fistulas: outcome of conservative management based on the natural history of the lesion. J Neurosurg 2002; 97(4):767–70.
14. Cognard C, Houdart E, Casaco A, et al. Long-term changes in intracranial dural arteriovenous fistulae leading to worsening in the type of venous drainage. Neuroradiology 1997;39(1):59–66.
15. Davies MA, Saleh J, Ter BK, et al. The natural history and management of intracranial dural arteriovenous fistulae. Part 1: Benign lesions. Interv Neuroradiol 1997;3(4):295–302.
16. Fermand M, Reizine D, Melki JP, et al. Long term follow-up of 43 pure dural arteriovenous fistulae. Neuroradiology 1987;29(4):348–53.
17. Lucas CP, Zabramski JM, Spetzler RF, et al. Treatment for intracranial dural arteriovenous malformations: a meta-analysis from the English language literature. Neurosurgery 1997;40(6):1119–32.
18. Duffau H, Lopes M, Janosevic V, et al. Early rebleeding from intracranial dural arteriovenous fistulas: report of 20 cases and review of the literature. J Neurosurg 1999;90(1):78–84.

19. van Dijk JK, TerBrugge KG, Willinsky RA, et al. Selective disconnection of cortical venous reflux as treatment for cranial dural arteriovenous fistulas. J Neurosurg 2004;101(1):31–5.
20. Collice M, D'Aliberti G, Arena O, et al. Surgical treatment of intracranial dural arteriovenous fistulae: role of venous drainage. Neurosurgery 2000;47(1): 56–67.
21. Nelson PK, Russell SM, Woo HH, et al. Use of a wedged microcatheter for curative transarterial embolization of complex intracranial dural arteriovenous fistulas: indications, endovascular technique and outcome in 21 patients. J Neurosurg 2003; 98(3):498–506.
22. Guedin P, Gaillard S, Boulin A, et al. Therapeutic management of intracranial dural arteriovenous shunts with leptomeningeal venous drainage: report of 53 consecutive patients with emphasis on transarterial embolization with acrylic glue. J Neurosurg 2010;112:603–10.
23. Agid R, Terbrugge K, Rodesch G, et al. Management strategies for anterior cranial fossa (ethmoidal) dural arteriovenous fistulas with an emphasis on endovascular treatment. J Neurosurg 2009;110(1):79–84.
24. Shi ZS, Ziegler J, Gonzalez NR, et al. Transarterial embolization of clival dural arteriovenous fistulae using liquid embolic agents. Neurosurgery 2008; 62(2):408–15.
25. Debrun G, Vinuela F, Fox A, et al. Embolization of cerebral arteriovenous malformations with bucrylate. J Neurosurg 1982;56:615–27.
26. Merland JJ, Rufenacht D, Laurent A, et al. Endovascular treatment with isobutyl cyano acrylate in patients with arteriovenous malformation of the brain. Indications, results and complications. Acta Radiol Suppl 1986;369:621–2.
27. Cognard C, Januel AC, Silva NA Jr, et al. Endovascular treatment of intracranial dural arteriovenous fistulas with cortical venous drainage: new management using Onyx. AJNR Am J Neuroradiol 2008;29: 235–41.
28. Gemmete JJ, Ansari SA, Gandhi DM. Endovascular techniques for treatment of carotid-cavernous fistula. J Neuroophthalmol 2009;29(1):62–71.
29. Lv X, Jiang C, Li Y, et al. The limitations and risks of transarterial Onyx injections in the treatment of grade I and II DAVFs. Eur J Radiol 2010. [Epub ahead of print].
30. Mullan S. Treatment of carotid-cavernous fistulas by cavernous sinus occlusion. J Neurosurg 1979;50(2): 131–44.
31. Hosobuchi Y. Electrothrombosis of carotid-cavernous fistula. J Neurosurg 1975;42(1):76–85.
32. Lewis AI, Tomsick TA, Tew JM Jr. Management of tentorial dural arteriovenous malformations: transarterial embolization combined with stereotactic radiation or surgery. J Neurosurg 1994;81(6):851–9.
33. Lownie SP. Intracranial dural arteriovenous fistulas endovascular therapy. Neurosurg Clin N Am 1994 5(3):449–58.
34. Brown RD Jr, Flemming KD, Meyer FB, et al. Natural history, evaluation, and management of intracranial vascular malformations. Mayo Clin Proc 2005 80(2):269–81.
35. Miller NR, Monsein LH, Debrun GM, et al. Treatment of carotid-cavernous sinus fistulas using a superior ophthalmic vein approach. J Neurosurg 1995 84(5):838–42.
36. Kirsch M, Henkes H, Liebig T, et al. Endovascular management of dural carotid-cavernous sinus fistulas in 141 patients. Neuroradiology 2006;48(7) 486–90.
37. Meyers PM, Halbach VV, Dowd CF, et al. Dural carotid cavernous fistula: definitive endovascular management and long-term follow-up. Am J Ophthalmol 2002;134(1):85–92.
38. Bink A, Goller K, Luchtenberg M, et al. Long-term outcome after coil embolization of cavernous sinus arteriovenous fistulas. AJNR Am J Neuroradiol 2010;31(7):1216–21.
39. Wakhloo AK, Perlow A, Linfante I, et al. Transvenous *n*-butyl-cyanoacrylate infusion for complex dural carotid cavernous fistulas: technical considerations and clinical outcome. AJNR Am J Neuroradiol 2005;26(8):1888–97.
40. Elhammady MS, Peterson EC, Aziz-Sultan MA. Onyx embolization of a carotid cavernous fistula via direct transorbital puncture. J Neurosurg 2011;114(1) 129–32.
41. He HW, Jiang CH, Wu ZX, et al. Transvenous embolization with a combination of detachable coils and Onyx for a complicated cavernous dural arteriovenous fistula. Chin Med J (Engl) 2008;121(17):1651–5
42. Suzuki S, Lee DW, Jahan R, et al. Transvenous treatment of spontaneous dural carotid-cavernous fistulas using a combination of detachable coils and Onyx. AJNR Am J Neuroradiol 2006;27(6):1346–9.
43. Lv X, Jiang C, Li Y, et al. A promising adjuvant to detachable coils for cavernous packing: onyx. Interv Neuroradiol 2009;15(2):145–52. [Epub 2009 Sep 1].
44. Sundt TM, Piepgras DG. The surgical approach to arteriovenous malformations of the lateral and sigmoid dural sinuses. J Neurosurg 1983;59(1):32–9.
45. Sundt TM Jr, Nichols DA, Piepgras DG, et al. Strategies, techniques and approaches for dural arteriovenous malformations of the posterior dural sinuses. Clin Neurosurg 1991;37:155–70.
46. Thompson BG, Doppman JL, Oldfield EH. Treatment of cranial dural arteriovenous fistulae by interruption of leptomeningeal venous drainage. J Neurosurg 1994;80(4):617–23.
47. Collice M, D'Albierti G, Talamonti G, et al. Surgical interruption of leptomeningeal drainage as treatment for intracranial dural arteriovenous fistulas

without dural sinus drainage. J Neurosurg 1996; 84(5):810–7.

48. Mack WJ, Gonzalex NR, Jahan R, et al. Endovascular management of anterior cranial fossa dural arteriovenous malformations. A technical report and anatomical discussion. Inter Neuroradiol 2001; 17(1):93–103.

49. Pandey P, Steinberg GK, Westbroek EM, et al. Intraoperative angiography for cranial dural arteriovenous fistula. AJNR Am J Neuroradiol 2011;32(6):1091–5.

50. Loumiotis I, Lanzino G, Daniels D, et al. Radiosurgery for intracranial dural arteriovenous fistulas (DAVFs): a review. Neurosurg Rev 2001;34(3):305–15.

51. Soderman M, Edner G, Ericson K, et al. Gamma knife surgery for dural arteriovenous shunts: 25 years of experience. J Neurosurg 2006;104(6): 867–75.

52. Pollock BE, Nichols DA, Garrity JA, et al. Stereotactic radiosurgery and particulate embolization for cavernous sinus dural arteriovenous fistulae. Neurosurgery 1999;45(3):459–67.

53. Friedman JA, Pollock BE, Nichols DA, et al. Results of combined stereotactic radiosurgery and transarterial embolization for dural arteriovenous fistulas of the transverse and sigmoid sinuses. J Neurosurg 2001; 94(6):886–91.

54. Bavinzski G, Richling B, Killer M, et al. Evolution of different therapeutic strategies in the treatment of cranial dural arteriovenous fistulas-report of 30 cases. Acta Neurochir (Wien) 1996;138(2):132–8.

# Acute Management of Ruptured Arteriovenous Malformations and Dural Arteriovenous Fistulas

Salah G. Aoun, MD, Bernard R. Bendok, MD*,
H. Hunt Batjer, MD

**KEYWORDS**

- Arteriovenous malformations • Acute management
- Rupture • Dural arteriovenous fistulas • Hemorrhagic stroke

## ARTERIOVENOUS MALFORMATIONS

Arteriovenous malformations of the brain (AVMs) are a major cause of stroke in young healthy individuals and present multiple diagnostic and therapeutic challenges, particularly in the acute setting.[1,2] They present as complex tangles of blood vessels with arterial blood flowing directly into the veins without interposed capillary networks and can be associated with other vascular lesions, such as aneurysms or arteriovenous fistulae,[3,4] thus adding to the complexity of patient management. At least 50% of patients with AVM present with hemorrhage[5–8] with the resulting significant morbidity and mortality. Although the flow hemodynamics, biology, epidemiology, and natural history of these lesions have been extensively studied, little data have been published on AVM surgery in the acute setting,[8] and acute surgery has been claimed to possibly increase the risk of persistent neurological deficits.[8] Although it is usually preferable to defer AVM surgery for a few weeks or even months to allow brain swelling to decrease and gliosis to better delineate the lesion to be excised, acute surgical (open and endovascular) management is,

nevertheless, essential in specific clinical and radiological settings. Large life-threatening hematomas, hydrocephalus, and the presence of an accessible and clear rupture site are all potential indications for acute procedural intervention. For a life-threatening hematoma related to AVM hemorrhage, it is generally advised to remove sufficient hematoma to achieve a slack brain without resecting the AVM. Given the differing acute natural history risk related to rehemorrhage, distinguishing between AVM hemorrhage and hemorrhage from an associated pedicle or circle of Willis aneurysm is paramount. Clearly identifying an interventionally accessible intranidal aneurysm may also be an indication for early embolization. Although experience with early intervention for ruptured AVMs is increasingly discussed in the literature, no guidelines have yet been published, and available data are mostly derived from anecdotal case series and limited to level V evidence.

### Epidemiology of AVM Hemorrhage

AVMs are the most common cause of nontraumatic cerebral hemorrhage in patients aged younger than 45 years.[9,10] Patients with AVM not

Department of Neurological Surgery, Northwestern University Feinberg School of Medicine and McGaw Medical Center, 676 North Saint Clair Street, Suite 2210, Chicago, IL 60611, USA
* Corresponding author.
E-mail address: bbendok@nmff.org

Neurosurg Clin N Am 23 (2012) 87–103
doi:10.1016/j.nec.2011.09.013
1042-3680/12/$ – see front matter © 2012 Elsevier Inc. All rights reserved.

only tend to be younger than the rest of the population suffering from cerebral vascular disorders but also seem to have fewer or no medical comorbidities.[11] Hemorrhage in this population can lead to catastrophic outcomes and claim a heavy functional toll on previously healthy young individuals. Thorough knowledge of the natural history, predictors, and presentation of AVM hemorrhage is essential for prudent clinical decision making.

### Initial hemorrhagic presentation
Approximately 50% of AVMs present with hemorrhage,[5,11–14] with reported rates ranging between 32% and 82%, depending on the series.[5] In stroke registries, around 1% of all strokes are attributed to AVM hemorrhage.[12] Intraparenchymal hemorrhage is most commonly observed, but intraventricular and subarachnoid hemorrhage can also occur.[1,10] Annual rupture rates among individuals presenting with symptoms other than hemorrhage range between 2% and 4%,[5,10–12,15,16] with an estimated lifetime risk of hemorrhage of 17% to 90%.[11] It should be noted that most available natural history data are derived from anecdotal case series (level of evidence V). Initial results from The New York Islands AVM study,[17] a prospective population-based database, have been released, but these data are notable for a lack of long-term follow-up. The examination of 284 prospective AVM cases recruited in this database estimated the incidence of first AVM hemorrhage to be approximately 0.51 per 100,000 person-years (95% CI, 0.41 to 0.61) and the prevalence of hemorrhage among diagnosed cases to 0.68 per 100,000 person-years (95% CI, 0.57–0.79). Kondziolka and colleagues[18] suggested a simple model based on life expectancy and the multiplicative law of probability to predict the lifetime risk of hemorrhage in a given individual assuming that, for that individual, the risk of hemorrhage is constant over time. According to their calculations, the lifetime risk of hemorrhage can be estimated using the following formula:

$$1 - (\text{risk of no hemorrhage})^{\text{expected years of remaining life}}$$

This formula would assume, for example, that for a patient with a life expectancy of 60 years and a yearly risk of hemorrhage of 4%, the lifetime risk of AVM bleed would be the following:

$$1 - (0.96)^{60} \approx 91\%$$

A simpler model assuming a constant 3% yearly risk of hemorrhage can also be used and still maintains a similar sensitivity:

$$\text{Lifetime risk of hemorrhage} = 105 - \text{patient age in years}$$

For example, a 15-year-old boy with an AVM would have a lifetime risk of hemorrhage of

$$105 - 15 = 90\%$$

Although most studies report clinically relevant AVM ruptures, subclinical episodes of hemorrhage seem to occur more frequently than previously thought.[19] Magnetic resonance imaging (MRI) frequently shows signs of hemosiderin deposits on T1- and T2-weighted sequences, a finding suggesting prior episodes of microbleeding.

### Rehemorrhage rate
Although AVMs are classically reported to carry a lower risk of hyperacute rebleeding compared with intracranial aneurysms,[10,20–22] the risk of recurrent hemorrhage seems to increase temporarily after the initial episode and then subsequently renormalize.[15,23–26] In a retrospective series of 191 patients harboring AVMs whereby 102 patients presented with hemorrhage and were followed for up to 37 years, Graf and colleagues[15] found that the risk of rehemorrhage increased to 6% during the first year and then renormalized to 2% per year for up to 20 years. Forster and colleagues,[24] in their retrospective series of 150 patients with AVMs, identified 106 patients who presented with acute rupture and followed them for an average of 15 years. After a single episode of bleeding, the risk of rehemorrhage increased to 25% in the 4 years following the episode. That same risk quadrupled after an additional hemorrhage to reach 25% per year. In their retrospective analysis of 43 patients with AVM who survived their first hemorrhage, Fults and Kelly[23] found that 67.4% suffered from an additional bleed. The risk of rehemorrhage was evaluated at 17.9% during the first year following the hemorrhage and declined to 3% per year after 5 years and 2% per year after 10 years. Mast and colleagues[25] provided even higher risks of hemorrhage in their prospective cohort. They followed a series of 281 consecutive patients with AVM whereby 142 presented with hemorrhage for a mean duration of 8.5 months (0.1–96.4). The average annual risk of hemorrhage was determined to be 17.8%, with a 32.9% risk of rerupture during the first year that declined to 11.3% in subsequent years. In comparison, patients who did not present with acute hemorrhage had a 0% risk of bleeding 1 year after presentation and a 2.9% risk for subsequent years. It should be noted, though, that only 20 untreated patients were still being followed 1 year after their hemorrhage. This finding should be contrasted with Ondra and colleagues'[27] retrospectively analyzed series of 114 untreated patients with AVM that were followed over a duration of

approximately 23.7 years. The rate of major re-bleed was estimated at 4% per year, which surprisingly showed little difference compared with the 2% to 3% per year classically reported rate.

## Risk factors for AVM hemorrhage

Evidence describing predictors of AVM hemorrhage is largely derived from anecdotal case series or nonrandomized cohort studies using historical controls (levels of evidence V and IV).[12] Most studies only retrospectively examine features related to hemorrhage and many convey conflicting results. Radiological parameters predicting hemorrhage can be categorized into (1) morphological, (2) arterial, and (3) venous factors.

AVM nidal size or volume has been inconsistently reported as a risk factor for hemorrhage.[15,28–32] Although smaller AVMs may tend to have higher pressure in their feeding arteries and, thus, a higher propensity to bleed, it has been suggested that although large and giant AVMs most frequently present with steal or seizures because of their size, smaller AVMs were more likely to be detected in the context of hemorrhage, with size actually being a confounding factor. A prospective analysis of 73 consecutive patients with Spetzler-Martin grade (SMG) IV and V AVMs estimated a 1.5% annual bleeding risk, a number lower than those classically reported for grades I through III.[33] On the other hand, a prospective study of 390 patients by Stefani and colleagues[34] found that large AVMs tended to bleed more frequently than smaller lesions (odds ratio: 2.5, 1.41–4.35, $P<.0001$). Similarly, Jayaraman and colleagues[35] suggested, after the retrospective examination of the medical records of 61 patients with SMG IV and V lesions, that the annual hemorrhage risk for these lesions could be as high as 10.4%, a number substantially higher than that reported for all other AVMs.[16] Diffuse AVM morphology has also been suggested as a possible factor for rupture.[36] Intraventricular, periventricular, basal ganglia, and deep brain AVM locations have also been suggested[12,13,32,37] as predisposing factors for hemorrhage.

Second, on the arterial side, increased feeding artery pressure, the presence of intranidal aneurysms, and a perforator origin for arterial supply have all been postulated as potential risks factors for AVM rupture.[12,24,36,38,39]

Finally, venous predictors of hemorrhage include the presence of deep venous drainage, a single draining vein, draining vein stenosis, or other causes of impaired venous drainage.[36,40,41] A deep venous component has also been linked to subsequent episodes of hemorrhage.[14]

Suggested clinical predictors of AVM hemorrhage include patient presentation with seizures[15,42]; male sex; increasing age, especially the fourth, fifth, and sixth decades[15]; and, most importantly, a history of prior hemorrhage.[13,14,43] Increasing age has also been linked to the risk of rehemorrhage.[15]

Although individual risk factors for AVM hemorrhage have been suggested, it seems that organizing findings into a personalized risk profile may provide an optimized model for predicting the risk of rupture and rerupture. Olivecrona and colleagues[44] used the history of prior hemorrhage, angiographic findings of a single draining vein, and the presence of diffuse AVM morphology to define a high-risk patient population. They found that these patients had an 8.9% yearly risk of rupture compared with 1% in triple-negative controls.[12] Similarly, in a prospectively collected cohort of 622 consecutive patients with AVM, Stapf and colleagues[13] identified initial hemorrhagic AVM presentation, deep brain location, and exclusive deep venous drainage as individual risk factors for subsequent AVM bleed, with respective hazard ratios of 5.38, 3.25, and 3.25. When these 3 factors were found in combination, the annual risk of hemorrhage increased dramatically to 34.4% compared with 0.9% in individuals who had none of these 3 factors.

## Natural History of AVM Hemorrhage

Although considerable information related to cerebral AVM pathophysiology and management is available, surprisingly scarce publications address the issue of morbidity and mortality from repeat bleeds. Most available studies have produced level V data and provide assumptions from the analysis of small anecdotal case series or retrospective chart reviews of patients with AVM.[14,26,45]

Mortality from a first hemorrhage is thought to range from 10% to 30%,[12,14,26,46] although lower rates have been reported.[14] Overall morbidity is generally estimated at around 50%,[26] with a long-term permanent disability rate of 10% to 20%.[12] Fults and Kelly,[23] in a retrospective analysis of 131 patients with AVM, discovered a tendency of increasing mortality with subsequent episodes of hemorrhage from 13.6% to 20.7% to 25.0%, after the first, second, and third episodes respectively, although statistical significance was not reached. Svien and McRae[47] also found that the mortality rate from AVM rupture doubled from 3% to 6% after subsequent hemorrhages.[48] This trend was not found in the analysis by Hartmann and colleagues[14,49] of 115 prospectively enrolled patients with AVM who presented with hemorrhage as part of the Columbia-Presbyterian Medical

Center AVM Study Project. In that study, 84% of the patients did not suffer from any neurological deficit or were independent in their daily activities (modified Rankin score of 1) after a single episode of hemorrhage, with only 16% severely disabled (modified Rankin score ≥4). Of the 27 patients who had recurrent hemorrhages, 74% were neurologically intact or independent in their daily activities, with only 4% severely disabled. These findings seem to go against the hypothesis of a cumulative impact of recurrent hemorrhage on prognosis. Interestingly, no fatalities were recorded after either episode. Although this data may seem reassuring, it does go against observations from many other studies and anecdotal observations.[12,14,26,45] The lower morbidity of AVM rupture compared with intracranial hemorrhage attributed to other causes, such as hypertensive or aneurysmal bleeds, may be attributed to several factors.[49] Although small AVMs with high intranidal pressure may lead to extensive bleedings, larger lesions with low-resistance arteriovenous shunts and low feeding artery pressure would tend to cause less damage. AVMs also rarely tend to cause vasospasm after they rupture. Rupture of deep draining veins often results in purely intraventricular hemorrhage.[15] Additionally, bleeding limited to the nidus tends to spare normal brain parenchyma and minimally disrupt functional neuronal tissue. On the other hand, parenchymal AVM hemorrhages have been shown to have the highest rate of associated focal deficits (51.9%), followed by exclusively subarachnoid (41.2%) or purely intraventricular (27.8%) locations. Finally, patients with AVM tend to be younger,[27] a fact that may contribute positively to recovery.[50,51]

## Medical Management of Acute AVM Hemorrhage

Recommendations for secondary intracranial hemorrhage management have been detailed in the American Heart Association–American Stroke Association guidelines.[52] Although a thorough discussion of these recommendations is beyond the scope of this article, the authors briefly present available evidence.

All patients should be admitted in an intensive care unit where they can be monitored for erratic variations in intracerebral and systemic pressures and where ventilator support is available (class I, level of evidence B). Antiepileptic treatment should be administered promptly at the first sign of clinical seizures (class I, level of evidence B) and may be continued for a brief period after the onset of intracerebral hemorrhage because it may reduce the risk of subsequent epileptic episodes, especially in cases of lobar hemorrhage (class IIb, level of evidence C). Fever and hyperthermia of any cause should be appropriately treated, and antipyretics should be administered to prevent additional brain injury because elevated cerebral temperature has been shown to increase ischemic brain damage (class I, level of evidence C). Persisting early hyperglycemia is associated with poor outcome and should be managed with insulin administration if levels go more than 185 mg/dL (class IIa, level of evidence C). Incomplete evidence is available on blood pressure management in the setting of intracranial hemorrhage, but intravenous drug administration to reduce extremely high variations and maintain cerebral perfusion pressure more than 60 to 80 mm Hg is recommended (class IIB, level of evidence C). Medical treatment of elevated intracranial pressure should start with simple measures, such as elevating the patient's head and appropriate analgesia, but may include sedation, osmotic diuretics, hyperventilation, and cerebrospinal fluid drainage (class IIa, level of evidence B). Early mobilization of clinically stable patients is recommended to prevent deep vein thrombosis and pulmonary embolism (class I, level of evidence C), and hemiparetic/hemiplegic individuals should have intermittent pneumatic compression of their lower limbs (class I, level of evidence B). Subcutaneous heparin should only be administered after cessation of bleeding has been documented (class IIB, level of evidence B).

## Acute Surgical Management After AVM Rupture

### Early versus delayed surgical removal

Although most intracranial aneurysms are operated on acutely because of the high risk and morbid consequences of early rerupture, surgeons have been classically reluctant to operate acutely on patients with AVM presenting with hemorrhage unless the hemorrhage is aneurismal in origin or the hematoma is life threatening.[8] Reports in the literature suggest that acute surgical removal of ruptured AVMs may be hazardous and lead to persistent and possibly preventable neurological deficits.[8] AVMs are reported to have a lower risk and morbidity from acute rerupture compared with intracranial aneurysms,[8,10,20] a fact that lead to recommendations to defer surgery weeks or even months after the initial bleed to allow brain swelling to subside and patients to recover.[20] Ruptured AVMs often result in intraparenchymal clots and brain edema that is most severe during the first days after the hemorrhage, a fact that may require retraction and manipulation of noncompliant brain tissue to improve visualization.[21]

Compression of the AVM by the hematoma may also partially mask parts of the lesion that may not be evident using digital subtraction angiography[53] because contrast may not completely fill the nidus causing incongruence between the radiological image and operative surgical anatomy. Waiting 3 to 6 weeks for the hematoma to resolve or liquefy may improve visualization of the AVM, with the resulting hematoma cavity usually creating a well-defined dissection plane between the lesion and normal brain parenchyma.[10,20] An exception to this principle may be extremely superficial and small AVMs whereby the anatomy necessary for lesion access and removal is straightforward.[10,11]

Early surgery for intraparenchymal brain hemorrhage can quickly reduce mass effect and potentially spare healthy neuronal tissue from a prolonged exposure to toxic blood degradation products.[54] Kuhmonen and colleagues[8] reported a large series of 45 patients with AVM presenting acutely with hemorrhage who were treated with surgery within 4 days. Although two-thirds of the patients were admitted with a Hunt-Hess score of 4 to 5, 55% had good functional outcome 2 to 3 months after surgery. It was the investigator's conclusion that aggressive and early surgical management of the lesions with evacuation of the hematoma can lead to favorable outcomes and accelerated rehabilitation compared with the natural history of the disease or delayed surgical management. One should consider, though, that 60% of the AVMs that were treated were classified as SMG I and II. Pavesis and colleagues[21] retrospectively reviewed 27 SMG I and II AVMs that presented acutely with hemorrhage and were surgically treated within 6 days and came to the same conclusions: early surgery with hematoma evacuation provided complete lesion excision, immediate decompression, bleeding control, shorter hospital stay, and favorable functional outcome. Acute surgery for lesions with SMG greater than or equal to III may require further study before any conclusions are reached because the risk of direct surgery increases in that population and because careful planning of multimodal therapy is more likely needed.

All this being said, it should be noted that instances of ultra-early rebleeding have been reported.[55] In cases whereby the origin of bleeding can be determined with certainty (eg, obvious intranidal or prenidal ruptured aneurysms), early embolization can provide security against rehemorrhage. Microsurgical or endovascular repair of a proximal saccular aneurysm should also be considered early when indicated.

## Perioperative anesthetic considerations

Although AVM surgery is usually not emergent and allows for the optimization of patient parameters and careful operative planning, acute resection often requires strict blood pressure control, placing patients in a barbiturate-induced coma with vasopressor administration in cases of myocardial depression as well as invasive monitoring of systemic and intracranial pressures.[20] Increases in intracranial pressure have been associated with higher morbidity and mortality in patients with intracranial hemorrhage. Close monitoring and control of intracranial pressure with hyperventilation, hyperosmotic treatment, and barbiturate administration is, therefore, essential to ensure good postoperative functional outcome. Intracranial pressure monitoring is also essential during a barbiturate coma because an increase in intracranial pressure may be the only sign of a postoperative hematoma and impending herniation. In their series of 10 patients who underwent emergency AVM surgery in the context of hemorrhage, Jafar and colleagues concluded that the 2 conditions necessary to ensure good surgical results were prompt decompression with hematoma evacuation and aggressive perioperative management of intracranial pressure.[20]

## Predictors of outcome after acute surgery

Although some risk factors for elective AVM surgery have been identified,[56] such as increasing patient age, lesion size, and eloquent location, little data are available on predictors of good functional outcome in the acute surgical setting. In their 3-month follow-up of 49 patients with ruptured AVMs that were operated within 4 days of hemorrhage, Kuhmonen and colleagues[8] identified the severity of the hemorrhage at presentation reflected by the Hunt-Hess score ($P = .001$), as well as increasing patient age ($P = .006$), as clear predictors of worse postoperative outcome. The concomitant presence of intraventricular hemorrhage also seemed to correlate with increasing morbidity and mortality ($P = .049$).

## Clinical Case Presentations

### Clinical case I

A 50-year-old man presented to the authors' emergency department complaining of headaches. Clinical examination was normal, but computed tomography revealed signs of subarachnoid hemorrhage (**Fig. 1**). An angiogram showed a left inferior/posterior frontal lobe and left basal ganglia AVM, measuring 4.5 × 3.0-cm with superficial venous drainage (**Fig. 2**). Five intracranial aneurysms were also detected, including an 8 × 5-mm flow-related aneurysm (**Fig. 3**A) that was

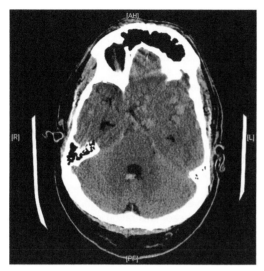

**Fig. 1.** Computed tomography scan revealing intraventricular hemorrhage.

discovered at the posterior communicating (PCOM)-P1 segment of the posterior cerebral artery junction and was determined to be the cause of the bleeding. The patient underwent immediate coiling of his PCOM aneurysm (see **Fig. 3**B) and was discharged home in normal neurological condition. Four months later, the patient was readmitted and underwent surgical clipping of his 4 remaining aneurysms (a 2-mm aneurysm of the anterior communicating artery, a 3-mm aneurysm adjacent to an enlarged left choroidal artery infundibulum, a 4-mm wide-necked aneurysm on the M1 segment of the left middle cerebral artery, and a 3-mm left medial paraclinoid aneurysm). Subsequently, the patient elected to undergo staged embolization sessions followed by staged radiosurgery over 2 sessions. Thirty months later, he was neurologically intact, and his AVM was completely obliterated on digital subtraction angiography (see **Fig. 3**C).

*Clinical case II*
A 30-year-old woman was brought unresponsive to our emergency department. She had complained of headaches before losing consciousness. Her computed tomography scan showed a 3-cm intraparenchymal cerebellar and vermian hemorrhage, with blood in the fourth ventricle (**Fig. 4**). She was taken to the operating room for an immediate posterior fossa craniectomy and underwent partial hematoma evacuation. An external ventricular drain was placed initially and opened once the posterior fossa dura was exposed. An AVM was noted but not removed because of significant brain swelling. Postoperatively, a vermian AVM was determined to be the

source of the bleeding (**Fig. 5**). She was discharged home complaining only of mild gait incoordination and left-hand apraxia, with plans to be later readmitted for AVM resection. Three months later, the AVM was uneventfully resected microsurgically and she made a full recovery.

*Clinical case III*
A 51-year-old woman was transferred to the authors' institution from a peripheral hospital unresponsive, with intracranial bleeding and acute hydrocephalus, which was treated with external ventricular drain placement. Her computed tomography scan revealed a large vermian and cerebellar hematoma with mass effect (**Fig. 6**). A vertebral angiogram revealed a small (<1 cm) AVM in the midportion of the vermis with a single cortical draining vein (**Fig. 7**). Her posterior fossa was decompressed with a craniectomy and partial hematoma evacuation (**Fig. 8**). Two months later, the AVM was resected uneventfully and she made an excellent recovery.

*Clinical case IV*
A 32-year-old woman was diagnosed with a right frontoparietal parasagittal 4-cm AVM (**Fig. 9**) when she was 13 years old.[57] The AVM was managed conservatively. She was left with spastic hyperreflexic paresis on her left side after her lesion ruptured. Ultimately, she was referred for evaluation of her AVM and possible treatment. After careful counseling, the patient and family elected to have the AVM managed with staged embolization followed by microsurgical resection. The initial angiogram and embolization were uneventful, and multiple small intranidal aneurysms were noted (**Fig. 10**). The second embolization took place 2 weeks later without any notable clinical changes. The following day, however, she quickly became unresponsive and her computed tomography scan revealed a diffuse intraventricular hemorrhage with fourth ventricle dilation (**Fig. 11**). An external ventricular derivation drain was placed, and she underwent embolization to secure the intranidal aneurysm that was deemed responsible of her hemorrhage (**Fig. 12**). Recombinant tissue plasminogen activator was then administered through her ventricular drain for a total of 9 injections and gradually started to improve her coma with the resolution of her hemorrhage (**Fig. 13**). She was discharged 20 days after her hemorrhage and was clinically at her preadmission baseline.

*Key Messages*

- A key principle in the surgical management of patients with AVM presenting with

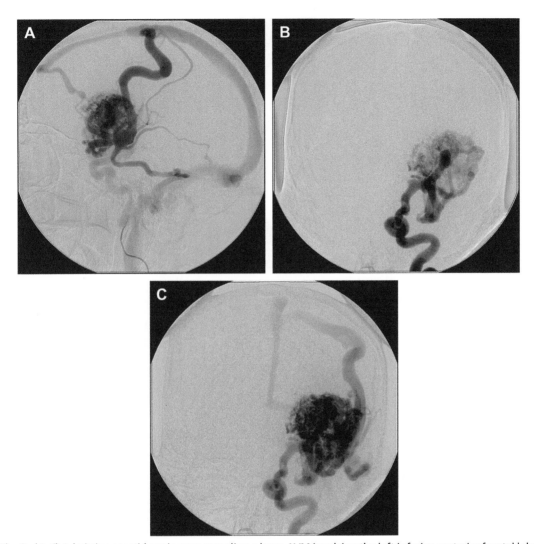

**Fig. 2.** (*A–C*) Admission carotid angiogram revealing a large AVM involving the left inferior-posterior frontal lobe and the anterior basal ganglia.

hemorrhage that require surgical decompression is to evacuate hematoma and defer AVM treatment by several weeks to months.

- If the source of hemorrhage can be clearly attributed to an accessible intranidal aneurysm, endovascular embolization of the rupture site may be indicated. Ruptured prenidal aneurysms should be treated microsurgically or endovascularly if they are determined to be the cause of the hemorrhage and if access can be achieved safely.
- Approximately 50% of AVMs present with hemorrhage, with an estimated mortality that can be as high as 30%.
- The risk of AVM rehemorrhage can increase by a factor of 3 for a duration of up to 1 year after the initial hemorrhage.

- Increasing age (especially the fourth, fifth, and sixth decades of life) has been linked to a higher risk of rehemorrhage and worse postoperative outcomes.

## DURAL ARTERIOVENOUS FISTULAS

Dural arteriovenous fistulas (DAVFs), also known as dural arteriovenous malformations or dural arteriovenous fistulous malformations,[26,58] are uncommon lesions of the central nervous system that compose approximately 10% to 15% of all intracranial AVMs.[29] They are described as isolated or a multitude of dural-based arteriovenous fistulas, often without the presence of a well-defined nidus.[26,58] Postulations about their origin vary from congenital to acquired after traumatic injury or venous sinus thrombosis.[31,55,59–61] These

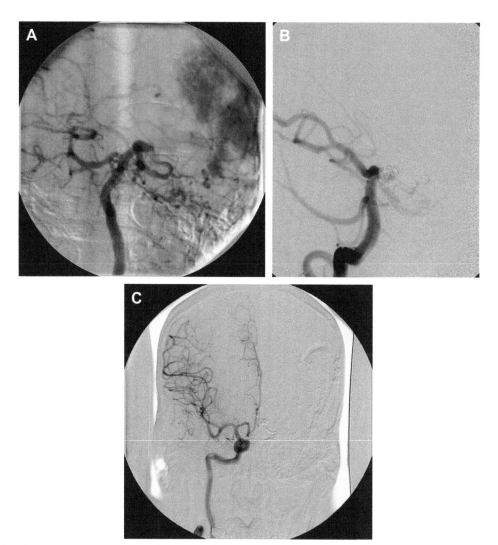

**Fig. 3.** (*A*) An 8 × 5-mm aneurysm of the posterior communicating-P1 segment of the posterior cerebral artery junction that was the likely cause of hemorrhage, before (*A*) and after (*B*) coiling. Follow-up carotid angiogram (*C*) showed complete angiographic occlusion of the AVM.

complex lesions can either remain asymptomatic for an extended period of time, lead to minor discomfort and be managed conservatively, or cause debilitating intracranial hemorrhage,[26,60–63] with a reported estimated mortality rate as high as 19% per year.[60,64]

Although several studies address the risk of initial hemorrhage from DAVFs and the radiological risk factors for hemorrhage, literature describing rebleeding rates is exceedingly sparse.[26,65] Available natural history data on morbidity rates and predictors of outcome after hemorrhage are also lacking, likely because of the rarity of these lesions because most reports only reach class V level of evidence.

## Epidemiology of DAVF Hemorrhage

Although the incidence of DAVFs may be lower than that of other central nervous system lesions, such as AVMs or aneurysms, they, nevertheless, significantly contribute to the incidence of secondary intracerebral hemorrhage and especially to the resulting mortality. In a prospective analysis of 141 adults presenting with intracranial hemorrhage caused by an underlying intracranial vascular malformation, Cordonnier and colleagues[66] found DAVFs to be responsible for the bleed in 6.4% of cases. Mortality rates after an initial episode of hemorrhage have been reported to be as high as 20% to 30%.[26,60,64,67] As with

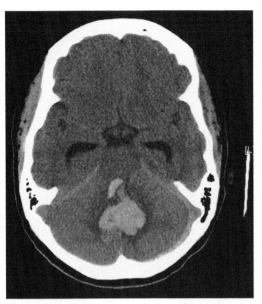

**Fig. 4.** Computed tomography scan showing a 3.5-cm hemorrhage in the cerebellar vermis.

AVMs, thorough knowledge of the classification, behavior, natural history, and treatment complication rates of these often complex lesions is essential to a neurosurgeon's ability to correctly advise his or her patients and provide them with viable therapeutic options.

### Initial and recurrent hemorrhage

The hemorrhage rate of DAVFs has been extensively studied by many investigators,[26,39,67–73] with an overall estimated yearly rate of around 1.8%.[26,67] Considerably higher risk is associated with specific anatomical and radiological features,

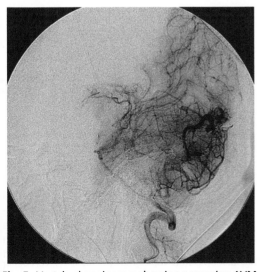

**Fig. 5.** Vertebral angiogram showing a vermian AVM.

particularly cortical venous drainage, a fact that lead to the creation of multiple DAVFs classification systems in an attempt to predict clinical lesion behavior.[58,61,72] The Borden[58] and Cognard[72] systems are currently most widely used to determine a lesion's natural history and grossly group DAVFS into benign versus aggressive lesions. Aggressive lesions all have retrograde cortical reflux filling in common, with a reported overall hemorrhage rate ranging between 20%[26] and 66%[62] and an annual bleeding rate between 8.1%[60] and 19.2%.[60] Even benign DAVFs have a 2% risk of developing cortical venous reflux and consequently pose a risk for brain hemorrhage.[73] The location of hemorrhage secondary to DAVF, as is the case with AVMs, is most frequently parenchymal, accounting for the high mortality rate associated with a hemorrhagic presentation but could also involve the ventricles and the subdural or subarachnoid spaces. The incidence of rehemorrhage has been less extensively studied. Duffau and colleagues[65] reported a series of 20 patients with Cognard type III and type IV DAVF who presented with hemorrhage and did not receive early surgical treatment; 35% of the patients suffered from radiologically proven rebleeding within an interval of 2 weeks after diagnosis. Borden and colleagues[58] found similar results in their series of 14 patients, with 20% to 35% of radiologically proven recurrent hemorrhages within 2 weeks. Davies and colleagues[60] also saw the risk of hemorrhage increase to 19.2% per lesion year in patients who refused treatment. Furthermore, the second hemorrhage had a heavier clinical toll on these patients compared with their initial bleed. In light of these findings, many investigators advocate early and definitive treatment of lesions with cortical venous drainage presenting with hemorrhage.

### Risk factors for DAVF hemorrhage

The presence of retrograde cortical venous drainage seems to be the main predictor of malignant DAVF behavior reported in the literature. It is also at the foundation of the Borden[58] and Cognard[72] classification scales, which are frequently used to predict lesional natural history and either encourage or defer surgical management. Additional risk factors have been identified and are often related to cortical drainage. These factors include variceal or aneurysmal venous dilations, galenic vein drainage, and stenosis or occlusion of associated venous sinuses.[63,74–76] Awad and colleagues,[63] in a comparison of 100 aggressive with 227 benign DAVFs, concluded that although aggressive lesions could occur at any intracranial location, the floor of the anterior

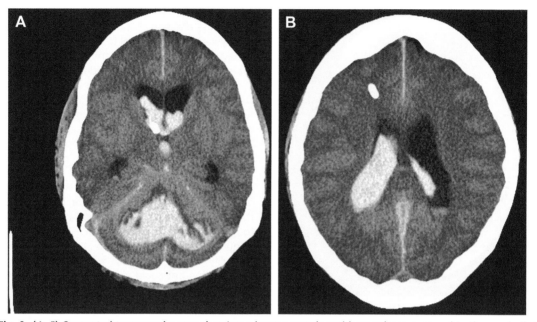

**Fig. 6.** (*A, B*) Computed tomography scan showing a large parenchymal hemorrhage centered in the cerebellar vermis with ventricular extension (*A*). Significant ventricular hemorrhage with moderate ventricular enlargement can also be seen (*B*).

cranial fossa, the tentorial incisura, and associations with the transverse-sigmoid sinuses and the cavernous sinus were more likely to behave malignantly. This finding can be partially explained by the fact that DAVFs of the floor of the anterior fossa and of the tentorial incisura are often drained by cortical vein and, therefore, are constitutionally more prone to bleed.

*Natural history of DAVF hemorrhage*

As is the case with AVMs, scarce data are found in the literature on mortality rates after intracerebral hemorrhage secondary to DAVFs and even less on the associated morbidity. Mortality rates after an initial hemorrhagic episode range between 10.0% and 19.3% per year, depending on the

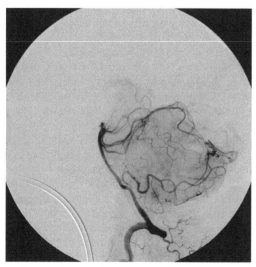

**Fig. 7.** Vertebral angiogram showing a small AVM of the vermis.

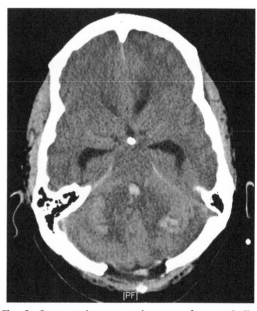

**Fig. 8.** Computed tomography scan after cerebellar hematoma evacuation.

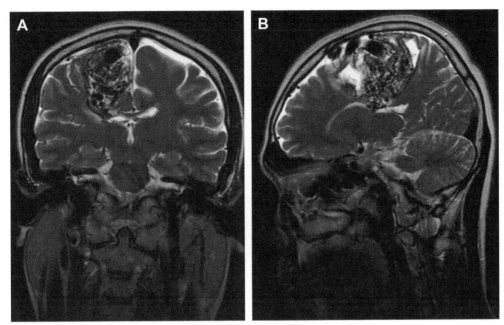

**Fig. 9.** (A, B) MRI of the brain revealing a large right frontal parasagittal AVM.

persistence of cortical drainage and on lesion grade.[60,62,64] The overall estimated mortality rate reported by some series can be as high as 45%.[64] Clinical course is reported to be even more morbid in the setting of early rebleeding.[65]

## Medical Management of Acute DAVF Hemorrhage

As is the case with AVMs, the recommendations for the management of DAVF bleeds follow the American Heart Association–American Stroke Association guidelines[52] that were reported in the previous section.

## Microsurgical and Endovascular Management of DAVF

As discussed earlier in this article, malignant DAVFs are characterized by an abnormal retrograde filling of leptomeningeal veins with fragilization, increased tortuosity, and possible variceal dilation of cortical draining veins and have a high propensity of causing cerebral bleeding and nonhemorrhagic

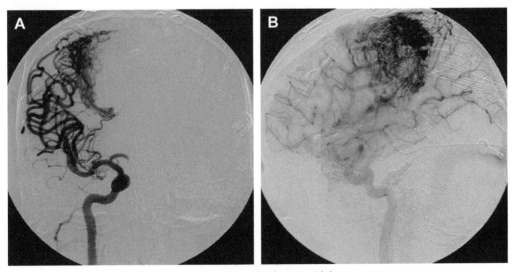

**Fig. 10.** (A, B) Preembolization angiogram showing multiple intranidal aneurysms.

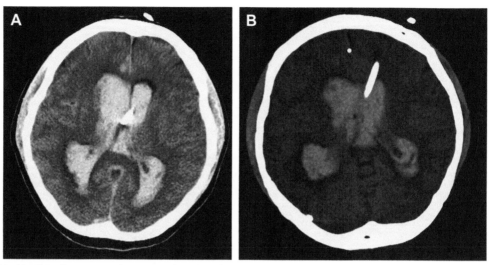

**Fig. 11.** (*A, B*) Brain computed tomography scan after hemorrhage.

neurological deterioration. Cortical drainage in malignant DAVFs is further classified as direct (non–sinus-type) or indirect (sinus-type), depending on the involvement of venous sinuses in retrograde venous drainage. Although there is currently no consensus about preferred absolute treatment modality, with open surgical, endovascular, and hybrid approaches described in the literature, experts unanimously agree that these high-risk lesions need to be treated because of their inherent morbidity and mortality. In the following sections, the authors provide a general overview of available surgical and endovascular treatment options, discussing the technical advantages, success rate, and morbidity/mortality of each technique, as well as specific recommendations depending on the location of the DAVF, based on available evidence. Stereotactic radiosurgery and gamma knife are not discussed because these options are not usually appropriate in an emergent setting because of the significant 1- to 3-year lag[64] between the initiation of treatment and the observation of a clinically and radiologically significant response.

### Microsurgical treatment
**General considerations** Surgical management with or without prior embolization has evolved considerably since its description by Sundt and

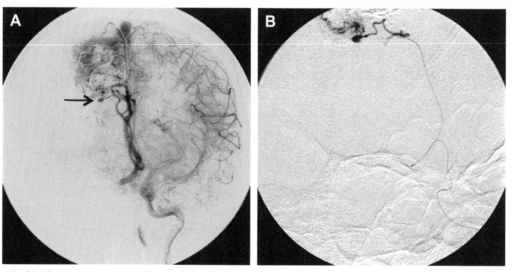

**Fig. 12.** (*A, B*) Anteroposterior left carotid angiogram showing the aneurysm (*black arrow*) (*A*). Microselective catheter angiography (*B*).

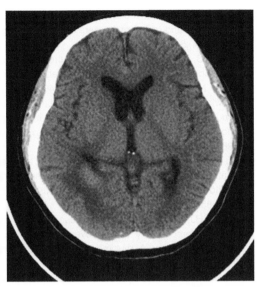

**Fig. 13.** Brain computed tomography after 5 days of tissue plasminogen activator administration.

Piepgras in 1983[77] and is considered to be both a versatile and effective therapeutic option.[26] It is particularly useful in cases of acute hemorrhage whereby parenchymal hematomas cannot be managed medically or expectantly. Early surgical reports advocated ligating the feeding arteries, but cure rates were very low (0%–8%) with frequent recurrence because of new feeder recruitment and exposed the patient to perilesional hemodynamic disturbances with the potential for an increased risk of rupture.[26,62,78] Although definitive cure historically required complete surgical excision, extensive blood loss with reported rates as high as 300 mL/min[77] lead to the innovation of new but effective surgical concepts. Currently adopted techniques differ for sinus-type fistulas and fistulas with direct cortical drainage (non–sinus-type)[79] but can provide highly satisfactory and definitive results.

*DAVFs with sinus involvement (sinus-type)* Excision of the diseased sinus segment can be effective and provide definitive cure, but care should be taken not to remove patent sinuses or sinuses without prominent collateral venous drainage to avoid the morbid consequences of edema and venous infarction.[26,62] In surgically accessible sinuses, direct access and incision with packing using oxidized cellulose, or catheterization followed by coiling, can efficiently stop DAVF arterial blood flow. Reported occlusion rates with this technique approach 100%, with acceptable morbidity and mortality.[54,79,80] Alternatively, Van Djik and colleagues[38] advocated disconnecting the sinus cortical reflux while preserving the integrity of the

arterialized sinus, thus, converting aggressive DAVFs into more benign lesions with a lower risk of hemorrhage.

*DAVFs with direct cortical drainage (non–sinus-type)* In non–sinus-type DAVFs, the discontinuation of the cortical draining vein at its entry point at the dura without interfering with the nidus, arterialized dura, or feeding arteries seems to be a safe and highly effective method.[60,79] Normal hemodynamic flow resumes in the cortical vessels, and the draining vein spontaneously thromboses. Reported success rates for this procedure can be as high as 97.6%, with minimal morbidity and mortality.

### Endovascular embolization

**General considerations** New endovascular techniques and embolic materials and increasing operator expertise have transformed the endovascular approach from a palliative means of treating surgically inaccessible DAVFs to an effective therapeutic option. Transvenous embolization with coils of the nidus or the arterialized sinus was classically the preferred approach and provided the best chance of complete cure, although success rates were significantly lower than those reported today. Stenting of a stenosed sinus to reduce venous congestion and obliterate the DAVF by engaging its pathophysiological mechanism has also been reported in a few case illustrations, but long-term patency and efficacy has not been adequately presented. The transarterial route was classically avoided because older generation embolic materials, such as silk sutures, coils, collagen, and particles, failed to completely obliterate the lesion, and were often dislodged over time with consequential recanalization of the fistula.[81] These materials also tended to block the feeding arteries, preventing further access to the lesion.[17] New-generation embolic materials, such as Onyx (Microtherapeutics, Inc, Irvine, California) and N-butyl-cyanoacrylate (NBCA, Codman Neurovascular, Inc, Irvine, California), have radically changed these outdated concepts. The rapid precipitation of NBCA makes it highly effective in obliterating high-flow lesions, whereas the distal penetration and diffusion of Onyx is ideal for transarterial embolization of the nidus and the draining veins. These advances have made the endovascular approach as effective as surgery, with occlusion rates as high as 100%[79] and many investigators advocating it as a first-line treatment.

*DAVFs with sinus involvement (sinus-type)* Retrograde transvenous sinus embolization can be as effective as surgical packing, with low mortality and reported obliteration rates of 81.0% to 87.5%. Transarterial administration of Onyx has also been advocated, with occlusion as high as 78%.[79,82,83] Positioning of the microcatheter in a dural feeder close to the nidus is the most important factor that determines the likelihood of lesion obliteration.

***DAVFs with direct cortical drainage (non–sinus-type)*** As the authors previously mentioned, new-generation embolic materials, such as NBCA and Onyx, have revolutionized the treatment of fistulas with leptomeningeal drainage. Retrograde venous access in non–sinus-type DAVF is usually avoided because of the fragility and tortuosity of cortical veins, but transarterial embolization using Onyx has been reported to be effective in a high percentage of cases (68.4%–100%).[79,84–87] It should be noted that complication rates ranging from 9% to 21%, and cases of morbidity have been reported in recent series,[49,82,88–90] making microsurgical interruption of the draining vein the procedure of choice of some investigators for this type of lesion.[79]

## Key Messages

- The risk of hemorrhage from DAVFs is approximately 1.8% per year but can increase significantly from patient to patient based on specific anatomical features.
- Cortical venous lesion drainage is correlated with an increased risk for brain hemorrhage.
- Cortical venous drainage is the single most important factor affecting the natural history of DAVFs.
- For high-grade dural fistulas that present with hemorrhage, rehemorrhage rates are high within the first 2 weeks, hence, justifying aggressive early intervention.
- Transarterial embolization has become more effective at lesion obliteration since the introduction of Onyx.
- Microsurgical disconnection of the arterialized draining vein may be all that is needed to eliminate the dural fistula or at least its high-risk feature.
- The choice between an endovascular and a microsurgical approach in DAVF management depends in great part on the anatomical features of the lesion.
- Disconnection of the arterialized veins may be addressed at the time of hematoma evacuation if an adequate understanding of the anatomy was achieved preoperatively.

## REFERENCES

1. Lobato RD, Perez C, Rivas JJ, et al. Clinical, radiological, and pathological spectrum of angiographically occult intracranial vascular malformations. Analysis of 21 cases and review of the literature. J Neurosurg 1988;68(4):518–31.
2. Hsieh PC, Awad IA, Getch CC, et al. Current updates in perioperative management of intracerebral hemorrhage. Neurosurg Clin N Am 2008;19(3):401–14, v.
3. Crawford PM, West CR, Chadwick DW, et al. Arteriovenous malformations of the brain: natural history in unoperated patients. J Neurol Neurosurg Psychiatry 1986;49(1):1–10.
4. Cunha e Sa MJ, Stein BM, Solomon RA, et al. The treatment of associated intracranial aneurysms and arteriovenous malformations. J Neurosurg 1992;77(6):853–9.
5. Steiger HJ, Schmid-Elsaesser R, Muacevic A, et al, editors. Neurosurgery of arteriovenous malformations and fistulas. A multimodal approach. Wien (NY): Springer; 2002.
6. Perret G, Nishioka H. Report on the cooperative study of intracranial aneurysms and subarachnoid hemorrhage. Section VI. Arteriovenous malformations. An analysis of 545 cases of cranio-cerebral arteriovenous malformations and fistulae reported to the cooperative study. J Neurosurg 1966;25(4):467–90.
7. Drake CG. Cerebral arteriovenous malformations: considerations for and experience with surgical treatment in 166 cases. Clin Neurosurg 1979;26:145–208.
8. Kuhmonen J, Piippo A, Vaart K, et al. Early surgery for ruptured cerebral arteriovenous malformations. Acta Neurochir Suppl 2005;94:111–4.
9. Gonzalez-Duarte A, Cantu C, Ruiz-Sandoval JL, et al. Recurrent primary cerebral hemorrhage: frequency, mechanisms, and prognosis. Stroke 1998;29(9):1802–5.
10. Ashley WW Jr, Charbel FT, Amin-Hanjani S. Surgical management of acute intracranial hemorrhage, surgical aneurysmal and arteriovenous malformation ablation, and other surgical principles. Neurol Clin 2008;26(4):987–1005, ix.
11. Starke RM, Komotar RJ, Hwang BY, et al. Treatment guidelines for cerebral arteriovenous malformation microsurgery. Br J Neurosurg 2009;23(4):376–86.
12. Ogilvy CS, Stieg PE, Awad I, et al. Recommendations for the management of intracranial arteriovenous malformations: a statement for healthcare professionals from a special writing group of the Stroke Council, American Stroke Association. Circulation 2001;103(21):2644–57.
13. Stapf C, Mast H, Sciacca RR, et al. Predictors of hemorrhage in patients with untreated brain arteriovenous malformation. Neurology 2006;66(9):1350–5.
14. Hartmann A, Mast H, Mohr JP, et al. Morbidity of intracranial hemorrhage in patients with cerebral arteriovenous malformation. Stroke 1998;29(5):931–4.
15. Graf CJ, Perret GE, Torner JC. Bleeding from cerebral arteriovenous malformations as part of their natural history. J Neurosurg 1983;58(3):331–7.

16. Nakagawa H, Kubo S, Nakajima Y, et al. Shifting of dural arteriovenous malformation from the cavernous sinus to the sigmoid sinus to the transverse sinus after transvenous embolization. A case of left spontaneous carotid-cavernous sinus fistula. Surg Neurol 1992;37(1):30–8.

17. Stapf C, Mast H, Sciacca RR, et al. The New York Islands AVM Study: design, study progress, and initial results. Stroke 2003;34(5):e29–33.

18. Kondziolka D, McLaughlin MR, Kestle JR. Simple risk predictions for arteriovenous malformation hemorrhage. Neurosurgery 1995;37(5):851–5.

19. Kucharczyk W, Lemme-Pleghos L, Uske A, et al. Intracranial vascular malformations: MR and CT imaging. Radiology 1985;156(2):383–9.

20. Jafar JJ, Rezai AR. Acute surgical management of intracranial arteriovenous malformations. Neurosurgery 1994;34(1):8–12.

21. Nowak K, Luniak N, Witt C, et al. Peroxisomal localization of sulfite oxidase separates it from chloroplast-based sulfur assimilation. Plant Cell Physiol 2004;45(12):1889–94.

22. Choi JH, Mast H, Sciacca RR, et al. Clinical outcome after first and recurrent hemorrhage in patients with untreated brain arteriovenous malformation. Stroke 2006;37(5):1243–7.

23. Fults D, Kelly DL Jr. Natural history of arteriovenous malformations of the brain: a clinical study. Neurosurgery 1984;15(5):658–62.

24. Forster DM, Steiner L, Hakanson S. Arteriovenous malformations of the brain. A long-term clinical study. J Neurosurg 1972;37(5):562–70.

25. Mast H, Young WL, Koennecke HC, et al. Risk of spontaneous haemorrhage after diagnosis of cerebral arteriovenous malformation. Lancet 1997; 350(9084):1065–8.

26. Schmid-Elsaesser R, Steiger HJ, Yousry T, et al. Radical resection of meningiomas and arteriovenous fistulas involving critical dural sinus segments: experience with intraoperative sinus pressure monitoring and elective sinus reconstruction in 10 patients. Neurosurgery 1997;41(5):1005–16 [discussion: 1016–8].

27. Ondra SL, Troupp H, George ED, et al. The natural history of symptomatic arteriovenous malformations of the brain: a 24-year follow-up assessment. J Neurosurg 1990;73(3):387–91.

28. Duong DH, Young WL, Vang MC, et al. Feeding artery pressure and venous drainage pattern are primary determinants of hemorrhage from cerebral arteriovenous malformations. Stroke 1998;29(6): 1167–76.

29. Arnautovic KI, Al-Mefty O, Angtuaco E, et al. Dural arteriovenous malformations of the transverse/sigmoid sinus acquired from dominant sinus occlusion by a tumor: report of two cases. Neurosurgery 1998;42(2):383–8.

30. Hoops JP, Rudolph G, Schriever S, et al. Dural carotid-cavernous sinus fistulas: clinical aspects, diagnosis and therapeutic intervention. Klin Monbl Augenheilkd 1997;210(6):392–7 [in German].

31. Davies MA, Saleh J, Ter Brugge K, et al. The natural history and management of intracranial dural arteriovenous fistulae. Part 1: benign lesions. Interv Neuroradiol 1997;3(4):295–302.

32. Kim MS, Han DH, Kwon OK, et al. Clinical characteristics of dural arteriovenous fistula. J Clin Neurosci 2002;9(2):147–55.

33. Vinuela F, Fox AJ, Pelz DM, et al. Unusual clinical manifestations of dural arteriovenous malformations. J Neurosurg 1986;64(4):554–8.

34. Stefani MA, Porter PJ, terBrugge KG, et al. Large and deep brain arteriovenous malformations are associated with risk of future hemorrhage. Stroke May 2002;33(5):1220–4.

35. Jayaraman MV, Marcellus ML, Do HM, et al. Hemorrhage rate in patients with Spetzler-Martin grades IV and V arteriovenous malformations: is treatment justified? Stroke 2007;38(2):325–9.

36. Larsson EM, Desai P, Hardin CW, et al. Venous infarction of the spinal cord resulting from dural arteriovenous fistula: MR imaging findings. AJNR Am J Neuroradiol 1991;12(4):739–43.

37. Debrun GM, Vinuela F, Fox AJ, et al. Indications for treatment and classification of 132 carotid-cavernous fistulas. Neurosurgery 1988; 22(2):285–9.

38. van Dijk JM, TerBrugge KG, Willinsky RA, et al. Selective disconnection of cortical venous reflux as treatment for cranial dural arteriovenous fistulas. J Neurosurg 2004;101(1):31–5.

39. Orabi AA, Ramsden R. Spontaneous resolution, after superselective angiography, of pulsatile tinnitus resulting from dural arteriovenous fistula. Int Tinnitus J 2004;10(1):51–3.

40. Waragai M, Takeuchi H, Fukushima T, et al. MRI and SPECT studies of dural arteriovenous fistulas presenting as pure progressive dementia with leukoencephalopathy: a cause of treatable dementia. Eur J Neurol 2006;13(7):754–9.

41. Halbach VV, Higashida RT, Hieshima GB, et al. Treatment of dural arteriovenous malformations involving the superior sagittal sinus. AJNR Am J Neuroradiol 1988;9(2):337–43.

42. Cuvinciuc V, Viguier A, Calviere L, et al. Isolated acute nontraumatic cortical subarachnoid hemorrhage. AJNR Am J Neuroradiol 2010;31(8): 1355–62.

43. Arnaout OM, Gross BA, Eddleman CS, et al. Posterior fossa arteriovenous malformations. Neurosurg Focus 2009;26(5):E12.

44. Olivecrona H, Riives J. Arteriovenous aneurysms of the brain: their diagnosis and treatment. Arch Neurol Psychiatry 1948;59:567–603.

45. Mahmood A, Malik GM. Dural arteriovenous malformations of the skull base. Neurol Res 2003;25(8): 860–4.

46. Lawton MT, Kim H, McCulloch CE, et al. A supplementary grading scale for selecting patients with brain arteriovenous malformations for surgery. Neurosurgery 2010;66(4):702–13 [discussion: 713].

47. Svien HJ, McRae JA. Arteriovenous anomalies of the brain. Fate of patients not having definitive surgery. J Neurosurg 1965;23:23–8.

48. Lawton MT, Arnold CM, Kim YJ, et al. Radiation arteriopathy in the transgenic arteriovenous fistula model. Neurosurgery 2008;62(5):1129–38 [discussion: 1138–9].

49. Tomak PR, Cloft HJ, Kaga A, et al. Evolution of the management of tentorial dural arteriovenous malformations. Neurosurgery 2003;52(4):750–60 [discussion: 760–2].

50. Saran R, Elder SJ, Goodkin DA, et al. Enhanced training in vascular access creation predicts arteriovenous fistula placement and patency in hemodialysis patients: results from the Dialysis Outcomes and Practice Patterns Study. Ann Surg 2008; 247(5):885–91.

51. Tamhankar MA, Liu GT, Young TL, et al. Acquired, isolated third nerve palsies in infants with cerebrovascular malformations. Am J Ophthalmol 2004; 138(3):484–6.

52. Broderick J, Connolly S, Feldmann E, et al. Guidelines for the management of spontaneous intracerebral hemorrhage in adults: 2007 update: a guideline from the American Heart Association/American Stroke Association Stroke Council, High Blood Pressure Research Council, and the Quality of Care and Outcomes in Research Interdisciplinary Working Group. Circulation 2007;116(16):e391–413.

53. Naito I, Iwai T, Shimaguchi H, et al. Percutaneous transvenous embolisation through the occluded sinus for transverse-sigmoid dural arteriovenous fistulas with sinus occlusion. Neuroradiology 2001;43(8):672–6.

54. Endo S, Kuwayama N, Takaku A, et al. Direct packing of the isolated sinus in patients with dural arteriovenous fistulas of the transverse-sigmoid sinus. J Neurosurg 1998;88(3):449–56.

55. Brown RD Jr, Flemming KD, Meyer FB, et al. Natural history, evaluation, and management of intracranial vascular malformations. Mayo Clin Proc 2005; 80(2):269–81.

56. Luo CB, Chang FC, Wu HM, et al. Transcranial embolization of a transverse-sigmoid sinus dural arteriovenous fistula carried out through a decompressive craniectomy. Acta Neurochir (Wien) 2007; 149(2):197–200 [discussion: 200].

57. Pollock GA, Shaibani A, Awad I, et al. Intraventricular hemorrhage secondary to intranidal aneurysm rupture-successful management by arteriovenous malformation embolization followed by intraventricular

58. Borden JA, Wu JK, Shucart WA. A proposed classification for spinal and cranial dural arteriovenous fistulous malformations and implications for treatment. J Neurosurg 1995;82(2):166–79.

59. Costakos DM, Bennett JL. Dural fistulas. Curr Treat Options Neurol 2001;3(4):377–82.

60. Davies MA, Ter Brugge K, Willinsky R, et al. The natural history and management of intracranial dural arteriovenous fistulae. Part 2: aggressive lesions. Interv Neuroradiol 1997;3(4):303–11.

61. Barrow DL, Spector RH, Braun IF, et al. Classification and treatment of spontaneous carotid-cavernous sinus fistulas. J Neurosurg 1985;62(2):248–56.

62. Steiger HJ, Hanggi D, Schmid-Elsaesser R. Cranial and spinal dural arteriovenous malformations and fistulas: an update. Acta Neurochir Suppl 2005;94: 115–22.

63. Awad IA, Little JR, Akarawi WP, et al. Intracranial dural arteriovenous malformations: factors predisposing to an aggressive neurological course. J Neurosurg 1990;72(6):839–50.

64. van Dijk JM, terBrugge KG, Willinsky RA, et al. Clinical course of cranial dural arteriovenous fistulas with long-term persistent cortical venous reflux. Stroke 2002;33(5):1233–6.

65. Duffau H, Lopes M, Janosevic V, et al. Early rebleeding from intracranial dural arteriovenous fistulas: report of 20 cases and review of the literature. J Neurosurg 1999;90(1):78–84.

66. Cordonnier C, Al-Shahi Salman R, Bhattacharya JJ, et al. Differences between intracranial vascular malformation types in the characteristics of their presenting haemorrhages: prospective, population-based study. J Neurol Neurosurg Psychiatry 2008;79(1):47–51.

67. Brown RD Jr, Wiebers DO, Nichols DA. Intracranial dural arteriovenous fistulae: angiographic predictors of intracranial hemorrhage and clinical outcome in nonsurgical patients. J Neurosurg 1994;81(4): 531–8.

68. Enker SH. Progression of a dural arteriovenous malformation resulting in an intracerebral hematoma. A case report. Angiology 1979;30(3):198–204.

69. Fardoun R, Adam Y, Mercier P, et al. Tentorial arteriovenous malformation presenting as an intracerebral hematoma. Case report. J Neurosurg 1981;55(6):976–8.

70. Halbach VV, Higashida RT, Hieshima GB, et al. Transvenous embolization of dural fistulas involving the transverse and sigmoid sinuses. AJNR Am J Neuroradiol 1989;10(2):385–92.

71. Harding AE, Kendall B, Leonard TJ, et al. Intracerebral haemorrhage complicating dural arteriovenous fistula: a report of two cases. J Neurol Neurosurg Psychiatry 1984;47(9):905–11.

72. Cognard C, Gobin YP, Pierot L, et al. Cerebral dural arteriovenous fistulas: clinical and angiographic

tissue plasminogen activator: case report. Neurosurgery 2011;68(2):E581–6 [discussion: E586].

correlation with a revised classification of venous drainage. Radiology 1995;194(3):671–80.

73. Satomi J, van Dijk JM, Terbrugge KG, et al. Benign cranial dural arteriovenous fistulas: outcome of conservative management based on the natural history of the lesion. J Neurosurg 2002;97(4):767–70.

74. Houser OW, Campbell JK, Campbell RJ, et al. Arteriovenous malformation affecting the transverse dural venous sinus–an acquired lesion. Mayo Clin Proc 1979;54(10):651–61.

75. Lasjaunias P, Chiu M, ter Brugge K, et al. Neurological manifestations of intracranial dural arteriovenous malformations. J Neurosurg 1986;64(5):724–30.

76. Malik GM, Pearce JE, Ausman JI, et al. Dural arteriovenous malformations and intracranial hemorrhage. Neurosurgery 1984;15(3):332–9.

77. Sundt TM Jr, Piepgras DG. The surgical approach to arteriovenous malformations of the lateral and sigmoid dural sinuses. J Neurosurg 1983;59(1):32–9.

78. Harrigan MR, Deveikis JP. Handbook of cerebrovascular disease and neurointerventional technique. Handbook of cerebrovascular disease and neurointerventional technique. New York (NY): Humana Press; 2009.

79. Wachter D, Hans F, Psychogios MN, et al. Microsurgery can cure most intracranial dural arteriovenous fistulae of the sinus and non-sinus type. Neurosurg Rev 2011;34(3):337–45 [discussion: 345].

80. Houdart E, Saint-Maurice JP, Chapot R, et al. Transcranial approach for venous embolization of dural arteriovenous fistulas. J Neurosurg 2002;97(2):280–6.

81. Narayanan S. Endovascular management of intracranial dural arteriovenous fistulas. Neurol Clin 2010;28(4):899–911.

82. Kirsch M, Liebig T, Kuhne D, et al. Endovascular management of dural arteriovenous fistulas of the transverse and sigmoid sinus in 150 patients. Neuroradiology 2009;51(7):477–83.

83. Roy D, Raymond J. The role of transvenous embolization in the treatment of intracranial dural arteriovenous fistulas. Neurosurgery 1997;40(6):1133–41 [discussion: 1141–4].

84. Carlson AP, Taylor CL, Yonas H. Treatment of dural arteriovenous fistula using ethylene vinyl alcohol (onyx) arterial embolization as the primary modality: short-term results. J Neurosurg 2007;107(6):1120–5.

85. Nogueira RG, Dabus G, Rabinov JD, et al. Preliminary experience with onyx embolization for the treatment of intracranial dural arteriovenous fistulas. AJNR Am J Neuroradiol 2008;29(1):91–7.

86. Rossitti S. Transarterial embolization of intracranial dural arteriovenous fistulas with direct cortical venous drainage using ethylene vinyl alcohol copolymer (Onyx). Klin Neuroradiol 2009;19(2):122–8.

87. Wachter D, Psychogios M, Knauth M, et al. IvACT after aneurysm clipping as an alternative to digital subtraction angiography–first experiences. Cen Eur Neurosurg 2010;71(3):121–5.

88. van Lindert E, Hassler W, Kuhne D, et al. Combined endovascular-microsurgical treatment of tentorial-incisural dural arteriovenous malformations. Report of five cases. Minim Invasive Neurosurg 2000;43(3):138–43.

89. van Rooij WJ, Sluzewski M, Beute GN. Dural arteriovenous fistulas with cortical venous drainage: incidence, clinical presentation, and treatment. AJNR Am J Neuroradiol 2007;28(4):651–5.

90. Jiang C, Lv X, Li Y, et al. Endovascular treatment of high-risk tentorial dural arteriovenous fistulas: clinical outcomes. Neuroradiology 2009;51(2):103–11.

# Surgical Treatment of Cranial Arteriovenous Malformations and Dural Arteriovenous Fistulas

Gustavo Pradilla, MD, Alexander L. Coon, MD, Judy Huang, MD, Rafael J. Tamargo, MD*

**KEYWORDS**

- Arteriovenous malformations • Dural arteriovenous fistulas
- Microsurgical resection • Surgical outcomes

Microsurgical resection remains the treatment of choice for more than half of all patients with arteriovenous malformations (AVMs). It compresses the treatment window into a span of a few weeks and is curative. Careful patient selection, meticulous surgical planning, and painstaking technical execution of the surgery are typically rewarded with excellent outcomes. The techniques for AVM resection have improved steadily over the past 80 years since the first report of the complete resection of an AVM. Five milestones in this surgical field have been: (1) the introduction of cerebral angiography in 1927 by Antonio Caetano de Abreu Freire Egas Moniz from Portugal,[1] (2) the first reported complete resection of a posterior fossa AVM in 1932 by Herbert Olivecrona from Sweden,[2] (3) the first reported embolization of an intracranial AVM in 1960 by Luessenhop and Spence,[3] (4) the introduction of the operating microscope in neurosurgery in the mid-1960s,[4] and (5) the first large microsurgical series of AVM resections reported in 1988 by M. Gazi Yasargil (414 patients).[5] In the case of dural arteriovenous fistulas (DAVFs), microsurgical obliteration is often reserved for cases in which endovascular therapy either cannot be pursued or fails. When performed, however, microsurgical obliteration of DAVFs is associated with excellent outcomes as well. This article reviews the current state of microsurgical treatment of AVMs and DAVFs.

## ARTERIOVENOUS MALFORMATIONS
### Case Selection

In general terms, the angioarchitecture of the AVM as well as the patient's age and medical/neurologic condition are the major determinants of whether a patient is a candidate for surgery. Age is the major determinant of the patient's risk of hemorrhage and also of how well he or she can tolerate surgery. To calculate the actuarial lifetime risk of hemorrhage for a specific patient, one of two methods can be used. The simple method is to subtract the patient's age from 105.[6] This method assumes a 3% annual risk of hemorrhage. The more accurate, but also more complex method, is to use the formula for the multiplicative law of probability ($1 - [1 -$ annual risk of hemorrhage$]^{\text{expected years remaining of life}}$), which assumes a constant annual risk of hemorrhage and independent event behavior each year.[7] Older patients and those with debilitating medical conditions are obviously poor surgical candidates.

Division of Cerebrovascular Neurosurgery, Department of Neurosurgery, The Johns Hopkins University School of Medicine, Johns Hopkins Hospital, Meyer Building, Suite 8-181, 600 North Wolfe Street, Baltimore, MD 21287, USA
* Corresponding author.
E-mail address: rtamarg@jhmi.edu

Neurosurg Clin N Am 23 (2012) 105–122
doi:10.1016/j.nec.2011.10.002
1042-3680/12/$ – see front matter © 2012 Elsevier Inc. All rights reserved.

Determining whether a particular AVM is suitable for surgery, on the other hand, is a more complex issue, given the numerous anatomic variations associated with these lesions. This analysis, however, was simplified by the introduction in 1986 of the Spetzler-Martin scale[8] and by its modification in 2003 by Lawton.[9] The Spetzler-Martin scale reduces the analysis of an AVM to its size (S), pattern of venous drainage (V), and eloquence of adjacent brain (E), and has proved to be predictive of surgical outcomes. In the large Finnish series of 623 AVM cases accrued over 55 years (1951–2005), 13% were Grade I, 29% were Grade II, 32% were Grade III, 19% were Grade IV, and 4% were Grade V.[10] Grade I and II AVMs, which comprise about 42% of all AVMs, are generally considered favorable for surgery. In their original series of 100 cases, Spetzler and Martin[8] reported no morbidity in 23 Grade I AVMs and a 5% morbidity in 21 Grade II AVMs. By contrast, they reported 27% and 31% morbidity in Grade IV and Grade V AVMs, respectively. Therefore, Grade I and II AVMs are favorable for surgery, but Grade IV and V AVMs are not. Han and colleagues[11] as well as Heros[12] have gone on to recommend no treatment for most Grade IV and V AVMs.

Grade III AVMs are a varied group at the boundary between favorable and unfavorable surgical outcomes, and also happen to be the most common type of AVM. In the original Spetzler-Martin series, all Grade III AVMs were associated with 16% morbidity. Lawton studied in detail 76 Grade III AVMs (out of 174 total AVMs) and proposed a modification of the Spetzler-Martin system that has proved valuable in terms of surgical selection.[9] Of the 76 Grade III AVMs, 46.1% were small (S1V1E1), 18.4% were medium/deep (S2V1E0), and 35.5% were medium/eloquent (S2V0E1). (Lawton did not encounter any S3V0E0 AVMs.) In this series of Grade III AVMs, the combined surgical morbidity/mortality was 2.9% for small AVMs, 7.1% for medium/deep AVMs, and 14.8% for medium/eloquent AVMs. Therefore, whereas a small Grade III AVM (<3 cm) with deep drainage and in an eloquent location is still a favorable surgical lesion, a medium Grade III AVM (3–6 cm) in an eloquent location is not. Deep venous drainage alone does not seem to be associated with poor surgical outcomes.

It follows that because Grade I and II AVMs make up about 42% of all AVMs, and Grade III AVMs make up about 32% of all AVMs,[10] and because S1V1E1 and S1V1E0 lesions combined make up about 64% of all Grade III AVMs,[9] the total proportion of AVMs that are favorable for surgery is about 62% (42% + [32% × 64%]).

Although these two scales provide helpful guidelines for surgical selection, many other factors will affect this decision. Lawton and colleagues[13] have proposed a further refinement of their selection criteria by considering older age, hemorrhagic presentation, nidal diffuseness, and a deep perforating arterial supply as negative predictive features. Patients with Grade I and II AVMs but with serious medical conditions, such as severe coronary disease, are best treated radiosurgically. By contrast, a patient with a Grade IV AVM previously treated with serial embolizations and several rounds of radiosurgery, who presents with recurrent hemorrhages, then becomes a reasonable surgical candidate. Incidentally, the authors continue to favor the original formulation of the Spetzler-Martin scale over its recent 3-tier modification.[14]

## Preoperative Imaging

Conceptually, AVMs are best approached as both vascular lesions and mass lesions. As such, they should be imaged with computed tomography (CT) and magnetic resonance imaging (MRI) scans, as well as full catheter angiography, which should include external carotid artery circulation injections. The CT scan is best for identifying acute and resolving hemorrhages, calcifications, and the location of embolic material. The MRI, particularly the T2 sequence, provides an excellent correlation of the AVM components with the surrounding parenchyma. The angiogram obviously provides detailed imaging of the arterial feeders and the draining veins. One should recognize that the angiogram typically shows only the major arterial feeders and anticipate that more will be encountered during surgery as the dissection proceeds, especially in the deepest portions of the AVM. The venous phase of the angiogram is particularly important because once the surface of the brain is exposed at the time of surgery, one will use the surface veins to become oriented to the location of the nidus. The benefits of functional MRI in the planning of AVM resection remain to be established.[15,16]

## Preoperative Embolization

Preoperative embolization of an AVM should be considered strategically, keeping in mind that each embolization carries approximately 3% morbidity and 1% mortality.[17] AVM embolization has dramatically changed the surgery of complex AVMs. Deep arterial feeders likely to be encountered late in the dissection are excellent candidates for embolization. Embolization can also be used to demarcate an arterial boundary of an AVM in eloquent cortex, or to reduce flow through a hyperdynamic AVM. From the perspective of surgical manipulation, both n-butyl-2-cyanoacrylate (NBCA; Cordis Microvascular Inc, New Brunswick, NJ) and ethylene vinyl alcohol copolymer (Onyx; ev3 Inc, Irvine, CA) are easy to displace and cut. In general, the authors prefer to dissociate the risks of embolization from those of surgery by allowing 7 to 10 days between the two interventions.

## Associated Aneurysms

Approximately 7% to 8% of AVM patients have at least one intracranial aneurysm.[18,19] Nidal aneurysms are an integral part of the AVM and do not require separate surgical consideration. Prenidal aneurysms, by contrast, are potentially treacherous and should be treated at the time of AVM resection, preferably before occlusion of the main arterial feeders (**Fig. 1**) or before surgery if they are distant from the surgical field. The concern is that serial occlusion of the AVM arterial feeders can result in an increase in pressure and rupture of a prenidal aneurysm.

## Intraoperative Adjuvants

Electrophysiologic monitoring, in the form of electroencephalography, somatosensory evoked potentials and, in the case of posterior fossa AVMs, brainstem auditory evoked responses, is essential during AVM surgery.[20] Although motor evoked potentials (MEPs) have been advocated by some groups,[21] the muscular contractions during MEP runs are inconvenient during

microsurgical dissection. MRI-guided or CT-guided intraoperative navigation can be helpful in centering the craniotomy over small or medium convexity AVMs. For very small convexity AVMs, the authors use intraoperative angiography for localization.[22] Intraoperative angiography is essential to confirm complete resection of the nidus and detect inadvertent compromise of a normal vessel. A recent review of 14 series (330 patients) of intraoperative angiography in AVM surgery showed that in 15% of cases management was changed by the angiogram results.[23] The benefits of microscope-integrated indocyanine green angiography during intracranial AVM surgery remain to be established, although its usefulness in DAVFs is becoming apparent.[24]

## Staged AVM Surgery

Up until the early 1990s, the authors treated 3 large AVMs in two scheduled surgical sessions. During that time they were still operating on many Grade IV and a few Grade V AVMs while assessing the efficacy of combined treatment with serial embolizations followed by radiosurgery. At present the authors rarely use this option, but staged surgeries should be kept in mind in the case of a large and complex AVM that may require more than 12 hours of surgery or one that has arterial feeders that cannot be reached through a single exposure. In the Andrews and Wilson[25] series of 319 AVMs, 9 (3%) were treated in two staged surgeries without apparent adverse effects from the staging itself. In the authors' 3 cases the first surgery was limited to

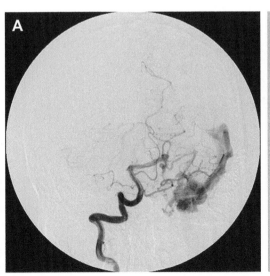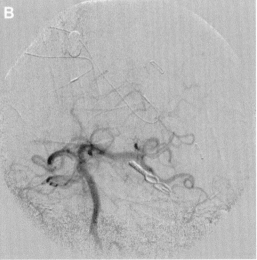

**Fig. 1.** Left temporal lobe AVM associated with a left posterior cerebral artery (PCA) aneurysm. Both were treated at the same time during surgery. (*A*) Preoperative image; (*B*) intraoperative image after AVM resection and aneurysm clipping.

occlusion of the major feeders and taking even minor draining veins was avoided. At the conclusion of the first surgery, the dissection plane was marked with oxidized regenerated cellulose sheets (Surgicel; Ethicon SARL, Neuchatel, Switzerland). The patients were extubated and kept sedated in the intensive care unit. Their mean arterial pressure (MAP) was kept below 100. The two surgeries were separated by 1 to 3 days. The day before the second surgery, a catheter angiogram was obtained to update the anatomy of the AVM. No adverse sequelae from the staging itself were found.

### Surgical Approach

From an angioarchitectonic perspective, AVMs are highly variable and each lesion requires an individualized surgical strategy that builds on the 4 basic steps described below. Surgically AVMs can be divided into cortical (surface) lesions, which are visible on the surface, or subcortical (deep) lesions. Cortical AVMs can be limited to the cortex, or can traverse the cortex and white matter, and breach the subependymal layer into the ventricle (**Fig. 2**). Subcortical AVMs can be found within the deep white matter with or without extension

into the ventricular surface, within the deep gray matter structures, or, in rare instances, exclusively within the ventricle (choroidal AVMs).[26]

In almost all cases, the basic strategy for microsurgical AVM resection consists of: (1) creating a wide craniotomy centered over the nidus and comfortably encompassing the arterial feeders and all the draining veins, (2) gradually devascularizing the AVM by occluding the arterial feeders, (3) circumferentially separating the AVM from the adjacent parenchyma, and (4) finally dividing the draining veins (**Fig. 3**). Early compromise of a major draining vein should be avoided at all costs. When properly executed, an AVM resection is one of the most elegant and satisfying procedures in neurosurgery. With the exception of life-threatening hematomas, AVM surgery should be scheduled electively.

### Positioning

The authors use either the supine or the lateral decubitus ("park bench") position for AVM surgery. The head should always be above the level of the heart. Whenever possible it is ideal to keep the head straight (in relation to the chest) and

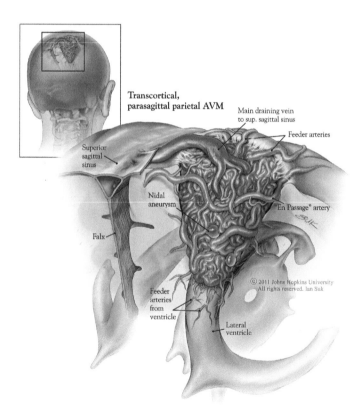

Transcortical, parasagittal parietal AVM

Main draining vein to sup. sagittal sinus

Feeder arteries

Superior sagittal sinus

Nidal aneurysm

"En Passage" artery

Falx

© 2011 Johns Hopkins University All rights reserved. Ian Suk

Feeder arteries from ventricle

Lateral ventricle

**Fig. 2.** Typical angioarchitecture of a transcortical parasagittal parietal AVM. The major arterial feeders, en passage artery, nidal aneurysms, deep ventricular arterial feeders, and major draining vein are highlighted. (*Courtesy of* Ian Suk, Johns Hopkins University; with permission.)

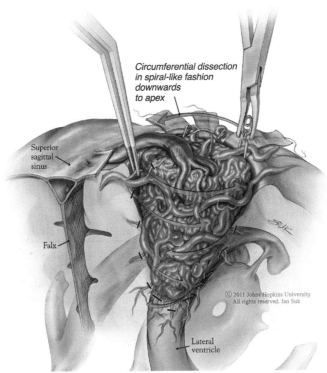

Circumferential dissection
in spiral-like fashion
downwards
to apex

Superior
sagittal
sinus

Falx

© 2011 Johns Hopkins University
All rights reserved. Ian Suk

Lateral
ventricle

**Fig. 3.** The basic steps in the resection of an AVM include temporary clipping and division of the major arterial feeders, circumferential dissection and isolation of the nidus, placement of cottonoids on the parenchymal wall for gravity retraction and protection of the brain, dissection of en passage arteries and division of their feeder arterioles, division of deep ependymal feeders, and finally division of the major draining veins. (*Courtesy of Ian Suk, Johns Hopkins University; with permission.*)

slightly extended to maximize venous return in the neck (the "sniffing position"). The authors avoid extreme head rotation in the supine position, which can compromise contralateral venous drainage, and prefer the lateral decubitus position in such cases. The authors rarely use the prone or Concorde position because it compromises venous return in both chest cavities, requires marked flexion of the neck, and often causes brain swelling and increased venous pressure intracranially. Chi and Lawton[27] have discussed the advantages of the lateral versus prone positions in 46 patients (23 lateral and 23 prone) who underwent the posterior interhemispheric approach for vascular lesions. The authors have found that interhemispheric and posterior midline AVMs can be reached comfortably with the patient in the lateral decubitus position. Whether the patient is placed in the right lateral or left lateral position depends on how far off the midline the lesion lies (keeping in mind the advantages of the contralateral interhemispheric transcallosal or transcingulate approach[28]), and on maximizing gravity retraction on the dependent lobe or hemisphere. An additional advantage of the lateral position for interhemispheric lesions is that the surgeon can work with his hands side by side as opposed to one on top of the other, as required in interhemispheric cases positioned either supine or prone.

The authors use lumbar drains intraoperatively for AVM locations in which large cisterns will not be accessible in the early stages of the surgery, such as interhemispheric (parafalcine, callosal, cingulate) or occipital AVMs. In such cases, lumbar cerebrospinal fluid (CSF) drainage can be used for relaxation early on in the case until a large cistern or the ventricle is reached for removal of larger quantities of CSF. The authors no longer use the sitting position because of the risks of hypotension and venous air embolism.

### Craniotomy and Dural Opening

The craniotomy should be wide enough to comfortably expose the normal brain surrounding the AVM. The entire superficial draining venous system should be exposed, including the superior sagittal sinus in the case of parafalcine, callosal, cingulate, or convexity AVMs, or the transverse sinus in the case of posterior temporal, inferior parietal, or occipital AVMs. If external carotid circulation feeders are present, they should be incorporated into the flap to occlude them early in the approach. When making and connecting the burr holes, one should be mindful of the course of the major draining veins to avoid inadvertent injury or compression of bulging veins. In general, more burr holes and short passes between burr holes are preferable (**Figs. 4–7**).

The dural opening should be similarly wide. The dural opening should be started away from the draining veins and nidus. The dura overlying the draining veins should be opened carefully, keeping in mind potential adhesions of these to the underside of the dura, which are particularly common after embolization or hemorrhage. In case of injury of a major draining vein, pressure should be applied with cotton and/or oxidized regenerated cellulose (Surgicel) and moderated to allow ongoing drainage until bleeding subsides; occluding a draining vein at this early stage could be disastrous. At times the dura may be densely adherent to a draining vein or the nidus itself, and it is preferable to simply cut this portion of dura and leave it attached to the AVM.

### Initial Exposure and Inspection of the AVM

The superficial draining veins are often the key to orientation regarding the exact location of the nidus. On exposing the AVM, one should take a couple of minutes to correlate the surgical anatomy with that on the angiogram. Feeding arteries, although prominent in the angiogram, are often not visible on the surface. Opening all accessible sulci and fissures allows for better understanding of the surface components of the AVM, relaxes the brain, and often dissociates the surface draining veins from the bulk of the AVM, so that manipulation of the nidus does not torque the draining veins. Obviously, any adjacent arachnoid cisterns should be similarly opened and drained.

Subcortical AVMs may have a single arterialized vein apparent on the surface. In these cases the draining vein can be followed retrogradely as it dives into the brain to reach the nidus. Ultrasonography may also be helpful in finding the nidus in these cases.

### Initial Dissection: Division of Arterial Feeders

Ideally the approach should be planned to allow access to the major feeding arteries early on and to minimize manipulation of the draining veins during the early dissection. Often, however, a compromise has to be reached. The initial dissection should be immediately directed toward the major arterial feeders for early reduction in the flow of the AVM. As these are identified, it is best to temporarily clip them and observe the AVM for a few minutes. Electrophysiologic data are also helpful during this period of temporary occlusion. Alternatively, smaller arteries can be gently pinched with the bipolar forceps and observed. It often can be difficult to distinguish between an arterial feeder and an arterialized draining vein. Arterial feeders should be divided as close to the

**A**                                                                 **B**

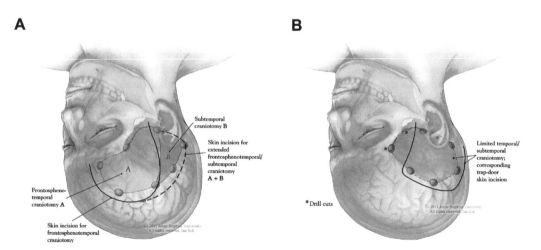

**Fig. 4.** (A) Frontosphenotemporal (pterional) craniotomy and combined pterional/subtemporal craniotomy. In general, for AVM surgery more burr holes and short passes between burr holes are preferable to avoid inadvertent injury of superficial draining veins. (B) Temporal/subtemporal craniotomy for AVMs restricted to the temporal lobe. (*Courtesy of* Ian Suk, Johns Hopkins University; with permission.)

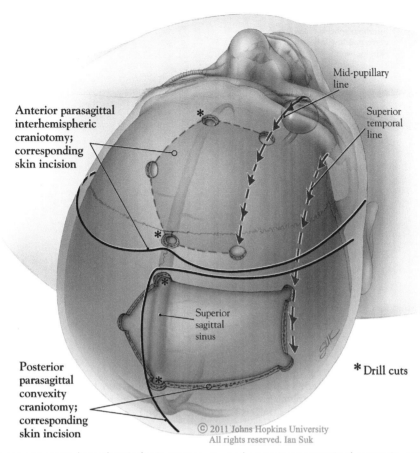

**Fig. 5.** Anterior parasagittal interhemispheric craniotomy and posterior parasagittal convexity craniotomy. The midline burr holes over the superior sagittal sinus are made with the high-speed drill and not the perforator. The parasagittal interhemispheric craniotomy can be shifted depending on the location of the AVM. Similarly, the parasagittal convexity craniotomy can be shifted depending on the location of the AVM. (*Courtesy of* Ian Suk, Johns Hopkins University; with permission.)

nidus as possible. Correct identification and occlusion of a major arterial feeder is often rewarded with an immediate change in color of the blood in the draining veins, which turns darker, as well as decreased pulsation and turgidity of the nidus. By contrast, erroneous temporary occlusion of an arterialized vein often results in increased pulsation, turgidity, and even hemorrhage. Small to medium arterial feeders can simply be coagulated and cut. For permanent occlusion of large arterial feeders, the authors prefer to use hemostatic clips instead of aneurysm clips; as aneurysm clips accumulate in the field, their hubs and bulk interfere with visualization of the deeper planes and with manipulation of the AVM.

"En passage" vessels are arteries that supply the brain surrounding the AVM but give rise to small feeding arterioles to the AVM. Painstaking dissection of these arteries is necessary to understand their anatomy and divide the feeding arterioles without compromising the en passage parent artery.

## Circumferential Dissection

The next stage consists of a spiral dissection around the nidus down to its apex, which in many cases reaches the ventricular surface. In general, large AVMs start wide on the cortical surface and become narrower as they reach the ventricular surface (see **Fig. 2**). These AVMs have the generalized shape of an inverted conical frustum (a geometric figure shaped like a cone but with its tip cut off). Keeping this in mind, one should tighten the radius of the spiral dissection as one proceeds toward the ventricular surface. The objective is to penetrate the parenchyma evenly around the nidus, level by level, and avoid a lopsided dissection in terms of depth. The technique of simultaneous bipolaring and suction is used to separate

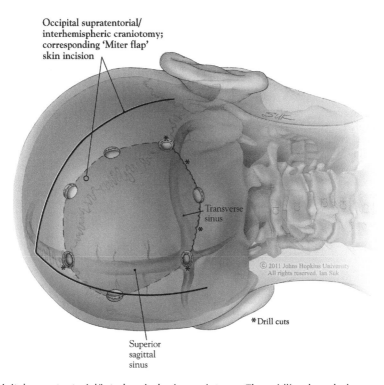

Occipital supratentorial/
interhemispheric craniotomy;
corresponding 'Miter flap'
skin incision

Transverse
sinus

© 2011 Johns Hopkins University
All rights reserved. Ian Suk

*Drill cuts

Superior
sagittal
sinus

**Fig. 6.** Occipital supratentorial/interhemispheric craniotomy. The midline burr holes over the superior sagittal sinus and the lateral burr hole over the transverse sinus are made with the high-speed drill and not the perforator. (*Courtesy of* Ian Suk, Johns Hopkins University; with permission.)

the nidus from the parenchyma. This boundary is often gliotic and feels slightly firmer than normal white matter. It also can have a darker, yellowish color in comparison with normal white matter. In cases of a prior hemorrhage, this boundary can be clear-cut with a porencephalic plane between the nidus and the brain. When working in a noneloquent boundary, one may intentionally drift away from the AVM slightly and avoid the small venous or arteriovenous loops (Hashimoto's U-shaped channels[29]) that protrude from the nidus. Although injury of any single venous or arteriovenous loop does not much change the hemodynamics of the AVM, the cumulative effect of occlusion of many of these loops can be equivalent to taking a major draining vein, and could result in increased nidal turgidity and hemorrhage. By contrast, when working in an eloquent boundary one should stay close to the AVM, which often results in more entries into the nidus as the dissection proceeds. In general, the spiral dissection weaves in and out of the AVM plane; bleeding indicates that one should correct the trajectory and dissect further out into the white matter, but complete absence of bleeding suggests that one has strayed away from the nidus and should dissect back into the direction of the nidus.

Progress in the spiral dissection around the nidus should be marked by placing cottonoids (Premium Americot strips; American Surgical Sponges, Lynn, MA) on the brain side at the newly defined nidus-parenchyma interface. These cottonoids will mark this region of the dissection as "completed," will retract the brain tissue away from the nidus cavity, and will eventually create a cottonoid surface around the dissection cavity that protects the brain from injury and desiccation under the hot microscope light. Gravity retraction with cottonoids often obviates use of a brain retractor.

AVMs with subependymal and ventricular extension present a special problem during the final stages of the dissection. These AVMs have periventricular arterial feeders that are extremely friable. A lower bipolar setting, broader bipolar tips, coating of the tips with wax, repeated irrigation, and rapid entry into the ventricle to eliminate the small ventricular feeders are all techniques that can help during this often frustrating portion of the surgery. It is important to avoid the tendency to tamponade these small feeders because this can result in an intraparenchymal or intraventricular hematoma.

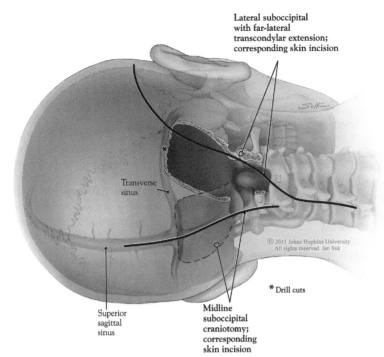

Lateral suboccipital
with far-lateral
transcondylar extension;
corresponding skin incision

Transverse
sinus

© 2011 Johns Hopkins University
All rights reserved. Ian Suk

\* Drill cuts

Superior
sagittal
sinus

Midline
suboccipital
craniotomy;
corresponding
skin incision

**Fig. 7.** The posterior fossa craniotomies: midline suboccipital and lateral suboccipital with far-lateral transcondylar extension. (*Courtesy of* Ian Suk, Johns Hopkins University; with permission.)

### Final Dissection: Division of the Draining Veins

As the circumferential dissection comes to a close, the tips of the cottonoids that have been placed along the wall of the cavity will meet at the apex of the cavity, thus confirming that the AVM is completely separated from the brain and that all feeders have been divided. At this point the AVM should be soft, have only venous flow, and be attached by only one or two major draining veins. If the AVM remains arterialized, one should suspect an arterial feeder hiding immediately below a draining vein. Although it is best to preserve all draining veins until the end of the dissection, smaller veins may obstruct the early dissection and may have to be divided before this final stage, as long as their temporary occlusion does not result in increased nidal turgidity, pulsation, and/or hemorrhage. Major draining veins, however, should not be divided until all arterial feeders have been eliminated. Draining veins should be divided as close as possible to a normal vein or sinus to avoid leaving a blind venous sac in which a thrombus can form and then propagate into the normal venous system, eventually resulting in occlusive hyperemia. Once the AVM is removed, the resection cavity is inspected for any bleeding, which can indicate that there is an AVM remnant. The authors

typically test the resection cavity with two Valsalva maneuvers to peak pressures of 30 to 40 mm Hg and with a 5-minute period of sustained systolic blood pressure to 140 mm Hg. An intraoperative angiogram is always obtained to confirm a complete resection. At times the angiogram may show residual dysplastic vessels that resemble a residual portion of the AVM, but are not associated with an early draining vein. If no shunting into the venous system is noted, no further resection is necessary, as these dysplastic vessels will involute over the next few days or weeks.[30]

In patients with epilepsy and temporal lobe AVMs, strong consideration should be given to removing the amygdala and hippocampus after resection of the AVM, to improve seizure control. This approach has been validated in both AVMs and cavernous malformations.[31,32]

### Routine Postoperative Management

Postoperatively the authors maintain the patient's MAP in the range of 80 to 100 mm Hg, allowing for slightly higher values in hypertensive patients. Patients are kept in a monitored setting for at least 48 hours even if they are doing well, and anticonvulsants are discontinued prior to discharge if the patient does not have a history of seizures and does not have a seizure postoperatively.

The authors are currently routinely loading AVM patients intraoperatively with both fosphenytoin, 15 mg/kg and levetiracetam, 30 mg/kg.

## Complications

The two major idiosyncratic postoperative complications peculiar to AVM resection are hemorrhage and edema of unclear etiology. Such complications are more common after resection of large AVMs, but can occur also after extensive AVM embolization and even after resection of small AVMs. An unrecognized AVM remnant as the source of a postoperative hemorrhage has been practically eliminated by the use of intraoperative angiography. Two mechanisms have been postulated to explain idiopathic hemorrhages and/or edema after AVM resection. The first is occlusive hyperemia, a concept introduced in 1993 by al-Rodhan and colleagues[33] from the Mayo Clinic. These investigators reported that of 295 patients, 13 (4%) developed hemorrhages and edema and 6 (2%) developed edema alone despite confirmation of complete AVM resection. The investigators proposed that these complications were the result of either obstruction of the venous outflow adjacent to the AVM with hyperemia and engorgement, or stagnant arterial flow in former AVM feeders with worsening of hypoperfusion, ischemia, and hemorrhage or edema in these areas. The second mechanism is normal perfusion pressure breakthrough, a concept introduced in 1978 by Spetzler and colleagues.[34] These investigators postulated that the arterial system surrounding an AVM is chronically dysautoregulated to allow for maximal vasodilatation, and that after resection of the AVM these arteries cannot vasoconstrict, leading to hyperemia, edema, and hemorrhage. It is likely that components of both are present in any given case. The authors currently manage this complication with the administration of hypertonic (3% or 2%) sodium chloride/acetate solutions with serum sodium goals as high as 165 mEq/L titrated to minimizing neurologic deficits or improving the level of consciousness, and wait for the dysautoregulation to subside.[35] This therapy reduces edema while maintaining adequate perfusion in the region at risk.

Other complications include neurologic deficits, seizures, infection, and hydrocephalus. Acute postoperative hydrocephalus can be avoided by placing an intraventricular catheter after resection of ventricular AVMs associated with extensive bleeding.

## Surgical Outcomes

Since 1986, when the Spetzler-Martin system was introduced,[8] surgical outcomes have been reported and compared using this scale. Earlier series reported outcomes in different forms, which have made comparisons difficult. For instance, in the Yasargil series of 414 AVMs operated on between 1967 and 1985 and published in 1988,[5] surgical outcomes were broken down by AVM locations. Since 1986, 8 series have been reported with outcomes broken down by Spetzler-Martin grades.[8,13,36–41] Of these 8 series, 2 are updates of earlier series.[37,40] The cumulative outcomes of 7 of these series have been reviewed by Spetzler and Ponce.[14] (The eighth series consists of an update of Heros' 578 cases in a recent article.[40]) The following 5 series, published between 1994 and 2011, all reported similar results. In 1994, Spetzler and Martin[8] updated their earlier series and reported the following surgical morbidity rates at 1 year in 120 patients: Grade I, 6%; Grade II, 17%; Grade III, 11%; Grade IV, 34%; and Grade V, 42%.[37] In 1998, Schaller and colleagues[41] reported the following rates of late "permanent neurologic major and minor deficit" in 150 patients: Grade I, 3%; Grade II, 0; Grade III, 23%; Grade IV, 38%; and Grade V, 50%. In 2000, Hartmann and colleagues[38] reported the following rates of "any deficit/disabling deficit" morbidity in 124 patients: Grade I, 8%/8%; Grade II, 36%/6%; Grade III, 32%/4%; Grade IV, 65%/4%; and Grade V, 33%/33%. In 2010, Lawton and colleagues[13] reported the following rates of "worse, dead" outcomes in 300 patients treated between 2000 and 2007: Grade I, 9%; Grade II, 24%; Grade III, 30%; Grade IV, 31%; and Grade V, 100%. In 2011, Heros and colleagues[39] updated their earlier series and reported the following rates of "fair, poor, or dead" outcomes in 578 patients treated between 1981 and 2008: Grade I, 3%; Grade II, 7%; Grade III, 22%; Grade IV, 29%; and Grade V, 67%.[40] There was no mortality associated with AVM resection in most of these series.

Therefore, after microsurgical resection favorable outcomes can be expected in most Grade I and II AVMs (91%–97% and 76%–100%, respectively), in many Grade III AVMs (70%–89%), but only a reduced proportion of Grade IV and particularly Grade V AVMs (62%–71% and 0%–58%, respectively).[13,37,40,41] Death as a consequence of AVM surgery, however, is exceedingly rare.

## Overview of AVMs by Location

This section provides a tabular summary of the different types of AVMs by anatomic location (Table 1). Given that AVMs can be found anywhere in the brain parenchyma, ependymal surfaces, or choroid plexus, listing AVMs by anatomic location is no less complex a task than describing the entire anatomy of the brain itself. Nevertheless, an overview of common locations is helpful. Although a comprehensive discussion of each type of AVM is beyond the scope of this article, **Table 1** summarizes the typical anatomic features of each type of AVM as well as its preferred surgical approach. The fact that surgical approaches for lesions such as thalamic/capsular/basal ganglia or brainstem AVMs have been listed does not mean that the authors necessarily favor surgery for most of these lesions, for which radiosurgery is currently the treatment of choice. Anatomically, AVMs can be classified as either supratentorial or infratentorial lesions. Supratentorial and infratentorial lesions in turn can each be subdivided into peripheral or central types, depending on whether they are associated with superficial or deep brain structures, respectively. The subtypes of each of these 4 groups (supratentorial peripheral, supratentorial central, infratentorial peripheral, and infratentorial central) are listed in **Table 1**. Please note that this anatomic classification serves a different purpose to that of the surgical classification described earlier (cortical or surface lesions versus subcortical or deep lesions). The authors' anatomic classification follows closely that proposed by Yasargil and colleagues,[5,26] but modifications by other investigators have also been adopted.[42]

## DURAL ARTERIOVENOUS FISTULAS

DAVFs are anatomically different from AVMs. Whereas AVMs are found at the level of or below the pial layer, DAVFs are "epipial" and are associated with the dura or in the subarachnoid space. In the vast majority of cases, AVMs have a nidus but AVFs do not. Most DAVFs are currently treated endovascularly. On rare occasions, however, surgical treatment of an aggressive DAVF may be indicated. Circumstances that lead to surgical consideration include DAVFs with numerous and/or tortuous arterial feeders not appropriate for embolization, an arterial feeder with prominent branches into normal structures near or at the fistulous connection, a long and tortuous feeder that is difficult to navigate, or a persistent fistula after endovascular or radiosurgical therapy. DAVFs considered for surgery are typically high-grade lesions with retrograde cortical drainage, as determined by either the Merland-Cognard[43] or Borden[44] classification systems. High-grade DAVFs have a higher rate of hemorrhage, approximately 20%.[45] The cumulative experience of surgical treatment of DAVFs is not as extensive as that of AVMs by an order of magnitude; DAVF surgical series typically consist

of 30 to 50 cases, as opposed to hundreds of cases in AVM series.[46–48]

For surgical purposes, one must differentiate between direct or indirect DAVFs. Direct DAVFs (nonsinus type) typically are simple lesions that have a well-defined arterial-feeder-to-draining-vein connection. Indirect DAVFs (sinus type), on the other hand, are more complex lesions that typically have numerous, small arterial feeders that drain into a venous sinus. These arterial feeders travel through the dura. The special case of carotid cavernous fistulas is not considered here and is discussed in detail by Miller elsewhere in this issue.

### Surgical Approaches

With 2 major exceptions, most of the principles described for AVM surgery apply to surgery of DAVFs. The first exception is that whereas with AVMs the nidus has to be removed, with DAVFs there is no nidus and thus simple interruption of the arteriovenous shunt is sufficient to treat the DAVF.[48–50] The second is that whereas in AVM surgery the draining vein is initially avoided and is taken only after the arterial supply is eliminated, in the case of direct DAVFs simple occlusion of the draining vein is often sufficient to treat the lesion.

The authors have used two surgical strategies for DAVFs. In the case of a direct (nonsinus type) DAVF, the draining vein is exposed at the point where it exits or enters the dura and is coagulated, clipped, and divided. If the arterial feeders are readily accessible and are not supplying any important structures, the authors may coagulate and cut them as well. An intraoperative angiogram typically confirms obliteration of the fistula.

In the case of indirect (sinus type) DAVFs, the authors prefer the technique of sinus isolation or skeletonization, as originally described in 1974 by Hugosson and Bergstrom[51] from Sweden and later advocated by Kuhner and colleagues[52] and Lucas and colleagues.[53] For this purpose, the authors expose the entire length of the involved sinus and skeletonize it by cutting the dura along both sides of the sinus, to interrupt the drainage of the feeding arteries into it; they then bipolar both edges of the dura on both sides of the sinus, and place hemostatic clips along them to prevent recanalization. This action preserves patency of the sinus. An intraoperative angiogram is then performed. In the case of indirect DAVFs, the authors have found often that new segments of the DAVF become apparent and thus the skeletonization of the sinus has to be extended. Several repeat angiograms during these cases are not

**Table 1**
AVM classification by anatomic location

| AVM Location | Structures Involved | Arterial Supply | Venous Drainage | Position, Surgical Approach |
|---|---|---|---|---|
| **SUPRATENTORIAL** | | | | |
| **Supratentorial Peripheral** | | | | |
| **Lobar** | | | | |
| *Frontal* | | | | |
| Paramedian | Superior and medial frontal gyri | ACA, secondarily MCA | Superior sagittal sinus | Supine, interhemispheric |
| Dorsolateral | Middle and inferior frontal gyri | MCA, secondarily ACA | Middle cerebral vein, sphenoparietal sinus | Supine, pterional |
| Frontobasal | Orbital gyrus, gyrus rectus | A1 and A2 segments, M1 perforators, ethmoidal arteries | Superior sagittal sinus, sphenoparietal sinus | Supine, pterional |
| Frontopolar | Frontal pole | A1 and A2 segments, M1 perforators, ethmoidal arteries | Superior sagittal sinus, sphenoparietal sinus | Supine, pterional |
| *Temporal* | | | | |
| Temporopolar | Superior and middle temporal gyri | MCA | Sphenoparietal sinus | Supine, pterional |
| Dorsal | Superior temporal gyrus | MCA | Sphenoparietal sinus, vein of Labbe | Supine, pterional |
| Laterobasal anterior | Middle and inferior temporal gyri | MCA and secondarily PCA | Vein of Labbe, Sphenoparietal sinus | Supine, pterional |
| Laterobasal posterior | Middle and inferior temporal gyri | MCA and PCA | Vein of Labbe | Lateral decubitus, temporal/subtemporal |
| *Parietal* | | | | |
| Paramedian | Postcentral gyrus, precuneal region | ACA and MCA | Superior sagittal sinus | Supine, interhemispheric |
| Dorsolateral anterior | Postcentral gyrus | ACA and MCA | Sylvian veins, vein of Labbe | Lateral decubitus, parietal |
| Dorsolateral posterior | Superior and inferior parietal lobules | ACA, MCA, and PCA | Sylvian veins, vein of Labbe | Lateral decubitus, parietal |
| *Occipital* | | | | |
| Paramedian | Cuneus, lingual gyrus | PCA, secondarily ACA | Superior sagittal sinus, tentorial vein | Lateral decubitus, interhemispheric |

| | | | | |
|---|---|---|---|---|
| Dorsolateral | Lateral occipital gyri | MCA and PCA | Tentorial veins, transverse sinus | Lateral decubitus, occipital |
| Inferolateral | Lateral occipital gyri | MCA and PCA | Tentorial veins, transverse sinus | Lateral decubitus, occipital |
| Mediobasal | Occipitotemporal gyrus | MCA and PCA | Tentorial veins, transverse sinus | Lateral decubitus, occipital |
| Occipitopolar | Lateral occipital gyri | PCA | Tentorial veins, transverse sinus | Lateral decubitus, occipital |
| **Sylvian** | | | | |
| Opercular | Frontal, temporal, and parietal opercula | MCA | Vein of Labbe | Supine, pterional |
| Insular | Insula, opercula, basal ganglia | MCA | Vein of Labbe | Supine, pterional |
| **Supratentorial Central** | | | | |
| **Callosal/Cingulate** | | | | |
| Anterior corpus callosum and anterior cingulate gyrus | Rostrum and genu, cingulate gyrus | ACA, thalamoperforators | Internal cerebral vein, inferior or superior sagittal sinuses | Supine, interhemispheric |
| Middle corpus callosum and middle cingulate gyrus | Body of corpus callosum, cingulate gyrus | ACA | Internal cerebral vein, inferior or superior sagittal sinuses | Supine, interhemispheric |
| Posterior corpus callosum and posterior cingulate gyrus | Splenium, cingulate gyrus | ACA, PCA | Medial atrial vein, basilar veins, inferior or superior sagittal sinuses | Lateral decubitus, interhemispheric |
| **Ventricular** | | | | |
| Frontal horn/body of lateral ventricle | Caudate, fornix, choroid plexus, corpus callosum | ACA, lenticulostriates | Internal cerebral vein | Supine, interhemispheric |
| Trigone/occipital horn | Fornix, basal ganglia, corpus callosum | Lateral posterior choroidal artery, thalamoperforators, anterior choroidal artery | Internal cerebral vein | Supine, interhemispheric or lateral decubitus, parietal |
| Temporal horn | Stria terminalis, tail of caudate, fimbria | Anterior choroidal artery, thalamoperforators of posterior communicating artery | Basal vein of Rosenthal | Supine, pterional |

(continued on next page)

**Table 1**
*(continued)*

| AVM Location | Structures Involved | Arterial Supply | Venous Drainage | Position, Surgical Approach |
|---|---|---|---|---|
| Third ventricle | Fornix, thalamus, hypothalamus | Posterior choroidal arteries, thalamoperforators, thalamogeniculates | Internal cerebral veins | Supine, interhemispheric |
| **Mesial Temporal (Amygdalohippocampal)** | | | | |
| Anterior | Amygdala/uncus | Anterior choroidal artery, PCA | Amygdalar vein, inferior ventricular vein, longitudinal hippocampal vein, basal vein of Rosenthal | Supine, pterional |
| Posterior | Hippocampus | Anterior choroidal artery, PCA | Amygdalar vein, inferior ventricular vein, longitudinal hippocampal vein, basal vein of Rosenthal | Lateral decubitus, temporal |
| **Thalamic–capsular–basal ganglia** | | | | |
| | Thalamus, internal capsule, caudate, putamen/globus pallidus, hypothalamus | ACA and MCA, lenticulostriates, thalamoperforators | Anterior thalamic vein, septal vein, basilar vein, sphenoparietal sinus | (Preferred treatment is radiosurgery) Supine, interhemispheric or supine, pterional |
| **INFRATENTORIAL** | | | | |
| **Infratentorial Peripheral** | | | | |
| **Cerebellar** | | | | |
| **Hemisphere** | | | | |
| Superior | Cerebellum superior to great horizontal fissure | SCA, secondarily AICA, PICA | Superior cerebellar, precentral cerebellar, superior vermian, lateral mesencephalic veins, or single paramedian vein, straight sinus | Lateral decubitus, lateral suboccipital |

| | | | | |
|---|---|---|---|---|
| Inferior | Cerebellum inferior to great horizontal fissure | PICA, secondarily AICA | Median cerebellar, vermian veins | Lateral decubitus, lateral suboccipital |
| **Vermis** | | | | |
| Superior | Superior vermis, fourth ventricle | SCA | Superior vermian vein | Lateral decubitus, midline suboccipital |
| Inferior | Inferior vermis, fourth ventricle | PICA, secondarily AICA | Inferior vermian vein | Lateral decubitus, midline suboccipital |
| Tonsillar | Cerebellar tonsil | PICA | Inferior vermian vein | Lateral decubitus, midline suboccipital and C1 laminectomy |
| **Cerebellopontine Angle** | | | | |
| Extrinsic | Epipial, choroid plexus of Luschka (?) | PICA, AICA, SCA | Vein of the lateral recess, lateral pontine vein, petrosal vein | Lateral decubitus, lateral suboccipital |
| Intrinsic | Ventral cerebellum | AICA | Vein of the lateral recess, lateral pontine vein, petrosal vein | Lateral decubitus, lateral suboccipital |
| **Infratentorial Central** | | | | |
| **Brainstem** | | | | |
| Mesencephalon | Collicular plate, dorsolateral midbrain | Vertebrobasilar perforators, SCA, AICA | Dorsal mesencephalic vein | (Preferred treatment is radiosurgery) Lateral decubitus, lateral suboccipital |
| Pons | Pons | Vertebrobasilar perforators, AICA, PICA | Basal vein of Rosenthal, petrosal sinus | (Preferred treatment is radiosurgery) Lateral decubitus, lateral suboccipital |
| Fourth ventricle | Fourth ventricular floor | AICA, PICA | Intraventricular ependymal veins | Lateral decubitus, midline suboccipital |

Surgical approaches are listed even for lesions for which radiosurgery is the treatment of choice, such as thalamic/capsular/basal ganglia or brainstem AVMs. The purpose of the summary is to record the surgical approaches that would be used if surgery were to be pursued in these lesions. This anatomic classification follows closely that proposed by Yasargil, but the authors have adopted modifications by other investigators as well.

*Abbreviations:* ACA, anterior cerebral artery; AICA, anterior inferior cerebellar artery; MCA, middle cerebral artery; PCA, posterior cerebral artery; PICA, posterior inferior cerebellar artery; SCA, superior cerebellar artery.

*Data from* Refs.[5,26,42]

unusual. The drawbacks of sinus skeletonization, however, have been discussed by D'Aliberti and colleagues.[54]

## Surgical Outcomes

Surgical treatment of DAVFs is generally associated with favorable outcomes. It must be recognized that surgical DAVF series include highly selected patients, and that their results may be difficult to generalize and compare. Wachter and colleagues[48] reported a series of 42 patients with a transient surgical morbidity of 11.9% and permanent surgical morbidity of 7.1%. Kakarla and colleagues[47] reported a series of 54 patients in which 92% had good or excellent outcomes and 6% died. Five patients had a residual fistula. Collice and colleagues[46] reported a series of 34 patients with no lasting morbidity, no mortality, and complete radiographic obliteration in all cases.

## SUMMARY

Careful patient selection, meticulous surgical planning, and painstaking technical execution of AVM and DAVF surgery are typically rewarded with excellent outcomes. Surgery remains the treatment of choice for about 60% of all AVMs. By contrast, DAVFs are generally treated endovascularly, but a few require surgery. With the exception of life-threatening hematomas, AVM and DAVF surgery should be scheduled electively. When properly executed, an AVM resection is one of the most elegant and satisfying procedures in neurosurgery. Surgery for AVMs and DAVFs has evolved considerably over the past 80 years, since the first report in 1932 of the complete resection of an intracranial AVM. Improved imaging of these lesions with angiography, MRI, and CT has clarified their angioarchitecture and relationships to other brain structures. The Spetzler-Martin/Lawton scales for AVMs and Merland-Cognard/Borden scales for DAVFs have simplified the selection of favorable surgical candidates. Increasingly sophisticated endovascular embolization techniques have reduced the surgical risks of complex lesions. The combination of embolization and radiosurgery has provided an alternative treatment for AVMs and DAVFs, which were previously associated with poor surgical outcomes, and has removed them from surgical consideration. Most importantly, the introduction of the microscope, increasingly sophisticated microsurgical techniques, and improved understanding of the microsurgical anatomy of AVMs and DAVFs have resulted in extremely low mortality and morbidity rates in carefully selected patients.

## REFERENCES

1. Egas Moniz AC. L'encephalographie artérielle: Sor importance dans la localisation des tumeurs céré brales. Rev Neurol (Paris) 1927;2:72–90 [in French]
2. Olivecrona H, Riives J. Arteriovenous aneurysms o the brain, their diagnosis and treatment. Arch Neuro Psychiatry 1948;59:567–602.
3. Luessenhop AJ, Spence WT. Artificial embolizatior of cerebral arteries. Report of use in a case of arteriovenous malformation. J Am Med Assoc 1960;172 1153–5.
4. Pool JL, Colton RP. The dissecting microscope fo intracranial vascular surgery. J Neurosurg 1966;25 315–8.
5. Yasargil MG, Curcic M, Kis M, et al. AVM of the brain, clinical considerations, general and specia operative techniques, surgical results, nonoperatec cases, cavernous and venous angiomas, neuroanesthesia (IIIB). Stuttgart (Germany), New York Georg Thieme Verlag/Thieme medical Publishers Inc; 1988.
6. Brown RD Jr. Simple risk predictions for arteriovenous malformation hemorrhage. Neurosurgery 2000;46:1024.
7. Kondziolka D, McLaughlin MR, Kestle JR. Simple risk predictions for arteriovenous malformatior hemorrhage. Neurosurgery 1995;37:851–5.
8. Spetzler RF, Martin NA. A proposed grading system for arteriovenous malformations. J Neurosurg 1986; 65:476–83.
9. Lawton MT. Spetzler-Martin Grade III arteriovenous malformations: surgical results and a modification of the grading scale. Neurosurgery 2003;52:740–8 [discussion: 748–9].
10. Laakso A, Dashti R, Seppanen J, et al. Long-term excess mortality in 623 patients with brain arteriovenous malformations. Neurosurgery 2008;63:244–53 [discussion: 253–5].
11. Han PP, Ponce FA, Spetzler RF. Intention-to-treat analysis of Spetzler-Martin grades IV and V arteriovenous malformations: natural history and treatment paradigm. J Neurosurg 2003;98:3–7.
12. Heros RC. Spetzler-Martin grades IV and V arteriovenous malformations. J Neurosurg 2003;98:1–2 [discussion: 2].
13. Lawton MT, Kim H, McCulloch CE, et al. A supplementary grading scale for selecting patients with brain arteriovenous malformations for surgery. Neurosurgery 2010;66:702–13 [discussion: 713].
14. Spetzler RF, Ponce FA. A 3-tier classification of cerebral arteriovenous malformations. Clinical article. J Neurosurg 2011;114:842–9.
15. Latchaw RE, Hu X, Ugurbil K, et al. Functional magnetic resonance imaging as a management tool for cerebral arteriovenous malformations. Neurosurgery 1995;37:619–25 [discussion: 625–6].

16. Maldjian J, Atlas SW, Howard RS 2nd, et al. Functional magnetic resonance imaging of regional brain activity in patients with intracerebral arteriovenous malformations before surgical or endovascular therapy. J Neurosurg 1996;84:477–83.

17. Ledezma CJ, Hoh BL, Carter BS, et al. Complications of cerebral arteriovenous malformation embolization: multivariate analysis of predictive factors. Neurosurgery 2006;58:602–11 [discussion: 602–11].

18. Deruty R, Mottolese C, Soustiel JF, et al. Association of cerebral arteriovenous malformation and cerebral aneurysm. Diagnosis and management. Acta Neurochir (Wien) 1990;107:133–9.

19. Thompson RC, Steinberg GK, Levy RP, et al. The management of patients with arteriovenous malformations and associated intracranial aneurysms. Neurosurgery 1998;43:202–11 [discussion: 211–2].

20. Chang SD, Lopez JR, Steinberg GK. The usefulness of electrophysiological monitoring during resection of central nervous system vascular malformations. J Stroke Cerebrovasc Dis 1999;8:412–22.

21. Ichikawa T, Suzuki K, Sasaki T, et al. Utility and the limit of motor evoked potential monitoring for preventing complications in surgery for cerebral arteriovenous malformation. Neurosurgery 2010;67: ons222–8 [discussion: ons228].

22. Germanwala AV, Thai QA, Pradilla G, et al. Simple technique for intraoperative angiographic localization of small vascular lesions. Neurosurgery 2010; 67:818–22 [discussion: 822–3].

23. Lefkowitz MA, Vinuela F, Martin N. Intraoperative and postoperative angiography. In: Stieg PE, Batjer HH, Samson D, editors. Intracranial arteriovenous malformations. New York: Informa Healthcare; 2007.

24. Killory BD, Nakaji P, Gonzales LF, et al. Prospective evaluation of surgical microscope-integrated intraoperative near-infrared indocyanine green angiography during cerebral arteriovenous malformation surgery. Neurosurgery 2009;65:456–62 [discussion: 462].

25. Andrews BT, Wilson CB. Staged treatment of arteriovenous malformations of the brain. Neurosurgery 1987;21:314–23.

26. Yasargil MG, Teddy PJ, Valvanis A, et al. AVM of the brain, history, embryology, pathological considerations, hemodynamics, diagnostic studies, microsurgical anatomy (IIIA). Stuttgart (Germany), New York: Georg Thieme Verlag/Thieme Medical Publishers, Inc; 1987.

27. Chi JH, Lawton MT. Posterior interhemispheric approach: surgical technique, application to vascular lesions, and benefits of gravity retraction. Neurosurgery 2006;59:ONS41–9 [discussion: ONS41–9].

28. Lawton MT, Golfinos JG, Spetzler RF. The contralateral transcallosal approach: experience with 32 patients. Neurosurgery 1996;39:729–34 [discussion: 734–5].

29. Hashimoto N, Nozaki K, Takagi Y, et al. Surgery of cerebral arteriovenous malformations. Neurosurgery 2007;61:375–87 [discussion: 387–9].

30. Solomon RA, Connolly ES Jr, Prestigiacomo CJ, et al. Management of residual dysplastic vessels after cerebral arteriovenous malformation resection: implications for postoperative angiography. Neurosurgery 2000;46:1052–60 [discussion: 1060–2].

31. Upchurch K, Stern JM, Salamon N, et al. Epileptogenic temporal cavernous malformations: operative strategies and postoperative seizure outcomes. Seizure 2010;19:120–8.

32. Yeh HS, Kashiwagi S, Tew JM Jr, et al. Surgical management of epilepsy associated with cerebral arteriovenous malformations. J Neurosurg 1990;72: 216–23.

33. al-Rodhan NR, Sundt TM Jr, Piepgras DG, et al. Occlusive hyperemia: a theory for the hemodynamic complications following resection of intracerebral arteriovenous malformations. J Neurosurg 1993;78: 167–75.

34. Spetzler RF, Wilson CB, Weinstein P, et al. Normal perfusion pressure breakthrough theory. Clin Neurosurg 1978;25:651–72.

35. Suarez JI, Qureshi AI, Parekh PD, et al. Administration of hypertonic (3%) sodium chloride/acetate in hyponatremic patients with symptomatic vasospasm following subarachnoid hemorrhage. J Neurosurg Anesthesiol 1999;11:178–84.

36. Davidson AS, Morgan MK. How safe is arteriovenous malformation surgery? A prospective, observational study of surgery as first-line treatment for brain arteriovenous malformations. Neurosurgery 2010; 66:498–504 [discussion: 504–5].

37. Hamilton MG, Spetzler RF. The prospective application of a grading system for arteriovenous malformations. Neurosurgery 1994;34:2–6 [discussion: 6–7].

38. Hartmann A, Stapf C, Hofmeister C, et al. Determinants of neurological outcome after surgery for brain arteriovenous malformation. Stroke 2000;31: 2361–4.

39. Heros RC, Korosue K, Diebold PM. Surgical excision of cerebral arteriovenous malformations: late results. Neurosurgery 1990;26:570–7 [discussion: 577–8].

40. Kretschmer T, Heros RC. Microsurgical management of arteriovenous malformations. In: Winn H, editor. Youman's neurological surgery. Philadelphia: Elsevier; 2011. p. 4072–87.

41. Schaller C, Schramm J, Haun D. Significance of factors contributing to surgical complications and to late outcome after elective surgery of cerebral arteriovenous malformations. J Neurol Neurosurg Psychiatry 1998;65:547–54.

42. Stieg PE, Batjer HH, Samson D. Intracranial arteriovenous malformations. New York: Informa Healthcare; 2007.

43. Cognard C, Gobin YP, Pierot L, et al. Cerebral dural arteriovenous fistulas: clinical and angiographic correlation with a revised classification of venous drainage. Radiology 1995;194:671–80.

44. Borden JA, Wu JK, Shucart WA. A proposed classification for spinal and cranial dural arteriovenous fistulous malformations and implications for treatment. J Neurosurg 1995;82:166–79.

45. Steiger HJ, Hanggi D, Schmid-Elsaesser R. Cranial and spinal dural arteriovenous malformations and fistulas: an update. Acta Neurochir Suppl 2005;94: 115–22.

46. Collice M, D'Aliberti G, Arena O, et al. Surgical treatment of intracranial dural arteriovenous fistulae: role of venous drainage. Neurosurgery 2000;47:56–66 [discussion: 66–7].

47. Kakarla UK, Deshmukh VR, Zabramski JM, et al. Surgical treatment of high-risk intracranial dural arteriovenous fistulae: clinical outcomes and avoidance of complications. Neurosurgery 2007;61:447–57 [discussion: 457–9].

48. Wachter D, Hans F, Psychogios MN, et al. Microsurgery can cure most intracranial dural arteriovenous fistulae of the sinus and non-sinus type. Neurosurg Rev 2011;34:337–45 [discussion: 345].

49. Davies MA, Ter Brugge K, Willinsky R, et al. The natural history and management of intracranial dura arteriovenous fistulae. Part 2: aggressive lesions. Interv Neuroradiol 1997;3:303–11.

50. van Dijk JM, TerBrugge KG, Willinsky RA, et al. Selective disconnection of cortical venous reflux as treatment for cranial dural arteriovenous fistulas. J Neurosurg 2004;101:31–5.

51. Hugosson R, Bergstrom K. Surgical treatment of dural arteriovenous malformation in the region of the sigmoid sinus. J Neurol Neurosurg Psychiatry 1974;37:97–101.

52. Kuhner A, Krastel A, Stoll W. Arteriovenous malformations of the transverse dural sinus. J Neurosurg 1976;45:12–9.

53. Lucas CP, De Oliveira E, Tedeschi H, et al. Sinus skeletonization: a treatment for dural arteriovenous malformations of the tentorial apex. Report of two cases. J Neurosurg 1996;84:514–7.

54. D'Aliberti G, Talamonti G, Collice M. Sinus skeletonization. J Neurosurg 1996;85:738–40.

# Endovascular Treatment of Cranial Arteriovenous Malformations and Dural Arteriovenous Fistulas

Martin G. Radvany, MD*, Lydia Gregg, MA, CMI

## KEYWORDS

- Endovascular treatment
- Cranial arteriovenous malformation
- Dural arteriovenous fistulas

Pial arteriovenous malformations (AVMs) and dural arteriovenous fistulas (DAVFs) are high-flow vascular lesions with abnormal communications between the arterial and venous system. AVMs are congenital lesions, whereas DAVFs are considered acquired lesions. Both can cause significant morbidity and mortality if they rupture and result in intracranial hemorrhage. The primary goal of treatment is to eliminate the risk of bleeding or at least decrease it. Because the epidemiology, clinical presentation, and classification of AVMs and DAVFs have been covered in previous articles in this issue, the authors only briefly touch on these subjects as they relate to endovascular treatment.

## ENDOVASCULAR THERAPY FOR AVMS

When considering the treatment of an AVM, it is useful to distinguish between those that have hemorrhaged from those that have not. The annual risk of AVM rupture ranges between 2% and 4%[1–6]; however, the risk of repeat hemorrhage increases to between 7% and 17%[5,7] during the first year following the initial event. It is because of this increased risk that prompt treatment of ruptured AVMs is recommended.

The main determinant for the role of endovascular therapy is the location of the AVM with regard to tissue eloquence. If a lesion is within eloquent tissue, the role of endovascular therapy may be limited because the risk of stroke may be unacceptable. For superficial lesions near the motor cortex or deep lesions near the corona radiata or the internal capsule, the intraoperative monitoring of somatosensory-evoked potentials and muscle motor–evoked potentials in combination with pharmacologic provocative testing with amobarbital (Amytal) and lidocaine[8,9] can increase the safety of such procedures.

For unruptured AVMs, it is important to properly select patients in whom therapy is indicated. Initial evaluation of patients with an unruptured AVM should attempt to determine if the patients' clinical symptoms are related to the AVM. AVMs with high-flow shunts may present in childhood with signs of cardiac insufficiency[10] or developmental delay.[11] Venous congestion may also be present secondary to stenosis of the outflow vein or increased vascular resistance secondary to a long draining vein and may result in dementia.[12] Venous varices have been associated with seizures.[13] The supplying arteries and draining veins of an AVM

The authors have nothing to disclose.
Division of Interventional Neuroradiology, The Johns Hopkins University School of Medicine, 600 North Wolfe Street, Radiology B-100, Baltimore, MD 21287, USA
* Corresponding author.
E-mail address: mradvan2@jhmi.edu

Neurosurg Clin N Am 23 (2012) 123–131
doi:10.1016/j.nec.2011.09.009
1042-3680/12/$ – see front matter © 2012 Published by Elsevier Inc.

should be further evaluated for anatomic features that may predispose patients to intracranial hemorrhage (**Fig. 1**) (ie, intranidal aneurysms, venous ectasias, venous stenosis, and exclusive deep venous drainage).[14,15]

The angioarchitecture of the AVM must also be evaluated to determine whether endovascular therapy is technically feasible. On the arterial side, the number and size of the feeding vessels will determine the feasibility of endovascular treatment. Catheterization of a large number of small, minimally dilated feeding vessels is more technically demanding than the treatment of a single, large feeding artery. Feeding arteries may be further categorized as direct arterial feeders that end in the AVM and indirect feeders that supply the normal cortex with small branches to the AVM, so-called en passant vessels. The treatment of direct feeding vessels is relatively safe because the injection of liquid embolic agents with the catheter tip distal to the arterial branches supplying

normal brain tissue can usually be achieved. there is reflux of the embolic material around the catheter tip, it is usually inconsequential. If there is not sufficient purchase of the catheter tip into an indirect feeding vessel, reflux of embolic material into the parent vessel may occur with distal embolization into normal brain tissue with catastrophic consequences, (ie, stroke).

The connection between the feeding arteries and the draining veins should be evaluated to determine the nature of the connection, nidal or fistulous, and the number of compartments in the AVM.[16] This evalutaion may be difficult if the AVM is large and there is rapid shunting. The venous outflow should be scrutinized for features that increase the risk of endovascular therapy Multiple draining veins have a decreased risk as compared with a single vein with a stenosis Embolization of the outflow vein without treatment of the feeding arteries may lead to a sudden increase in pressure within the AVM with

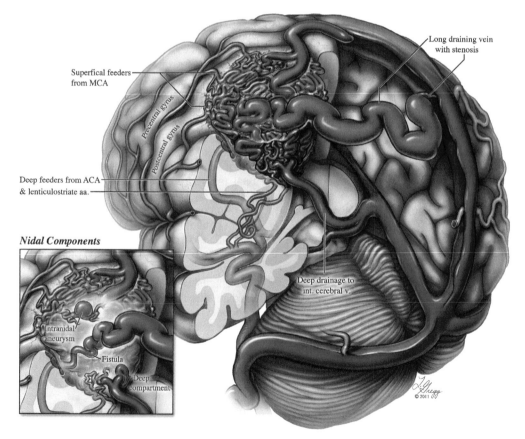

**Fig. 1.** Various features of AVMs are associated with clinical presentations, including hemorrhage, seizures, and dementia. Venous congestion in an AVM may be caused by stenosis of an outflow vein or increased vascular resistance secondary to a long draining vein with patients presenting with dementia. Venous ectasia has been associated with seizures and hemorrhage. Other features that predispose AVMs to hemorrhage include deep venous drainage and intranidal aneurysms. ACA, anterior cerebral artery; MCA, middle cerebral artery. (Copyright © 2011, Lydia Gregg.)

subsequent rupture and catastrophic results.[17] By studying the angioarchitectue on the AVM, one can begin to understand the underlying pathophysiology and appropriately select patients for treatment.

Complete cure of an AVM by endovascular means is only possible in approximately 20% of cases.[18,19] Those AVMs that exhibit an angioarchitecture favorable for complete cure are those that are small and have a single feeding artery and a single compartment. As the size of the AVM nidus increases, the success of embolization as a single mode of treatment decreases and the risk of complication increases. In these cases, partial targeted embolization[17,20] becomes a much more reasonable option. Partial targeted embolization may be used alone or in conjunction with surgery or radiosurgery (**Fig. 2**). In the case of radiosurgery, the periphery of the AVM may be the target of embolization with the goal of reducing the size of the AVM to limit the area and, thus, the radiation dose required to treat the residual AVM and to secure focal weak areas within the AVM while the AVM undergoes complete occlusion. When combined with microsurgery, the goal is to secure those regions that will be more difficult for surgical access, which are the deep feeding vessels that are more difficult for the surgeon to directly visualize and control. Because no two AVMs are the same, every patient requires a tailored, team approach that takes into account the specifics of each case.

## Endovascular Therapy for DAVFs

As with AVMs, the location, drainage pattern, and symptoms attributable to a DAVF dictate treatment strategies. The risk of hemorrhagic complications from a DAVF is related to its drainage pattern. This relationship between drainage pattern and risk of hemorrhage has been studied,[21,22] and it is thought that as the grade increases the risk of intracranial hemorrhage increases. DAVFs with cortical venous reflux have a reported morbidity and mortality rate of 20%[23] and a repeat hemorrhage rate of 35%.[24] As opposed to AVMs in which there is more debate as to the need for treatment, treatment of ruptured and high-grade DAVFs is generally agreed on.

DAVFs of the transverse sinus are the most common type of fistula and have many different approaches to treatment, as such, the authors focus on this specific DAVF for the discussion of endovascular treatment techniques. Within the wall of the transverse sinus there are fistulous connections[25] or pouches, and it is the obliteration of these pathologic connections that must be achieved to treat the DAVF. The treatment of an AVMs is almost exclusively via a transarterial approach, whereas the treatment of DAVFs from a transvenous approach is feasible in a large percentage of cases and is dictated by the arterial supply as well as the venous drainage of the fistula. When treating a fistula of the transverse sinus, it is the direction of flow in the vein of Labbé that that dictates possible treatment strategies. If

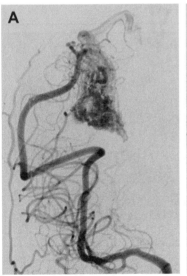
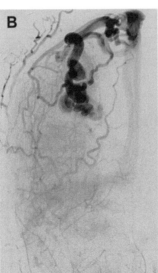
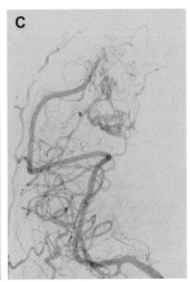

**Fig. 2.** A 32-year-old woman with a right parietal arteriovenous malformation (Spetzler Martin grade III AVM) presented with left-sided seizures. (*A*) The AVM measures approximately 3 cm and is fed primarily by middle cerebral artery branches with (*B*) superficial venous drainage with venous varices. It is located in the primary sensory cortex. (*C*) NBCA embolization with provocative testing was performed in preparation for radiosurgery.

there is antegrade flow in the vein of Labbé, the transverse sinus cannot be sacrificed because there is a risk of venous infarction and transarterial embolization is mandated (**Fig. 3**A). If there is clearly retrograde flow in the vein of Labbé, the transverse sinus is not functioning normally and can be sacrificed without the fear of venous infarction. One can consider sacrificing the transverse sinus from a venous approach provided that the contralateral transverse sinus is widely patent. If the transverse sinus distal to the fistula is patent, the microcatheter used for coil placement can be advanced in a retrograde manner (see **Fig. 3**B). If the sinus is occluded, the microcather used for coiling may be advanced through the contralateral transverse sinus (see **Fig. 3**C). In either case, a microcatheter is advanced into the sinus and a balloon catheter inflated to provide support so that a dense coil pack can be created to compress and occlude the pouches in the wall of the transverse sinus. If the antegrade and retrograde transvenous approaches are not feasible because of vessel occlusion, there is still the possibility of a transarterial approach into the transverse sinus with coil embolization to obliterate the remaining portion or the transverse sinus (see **Fig. 3**D). Endovascular occlusion of the sinus is often successful in curing these lesions.[26,27]

## Embolic Agents

Successful transarterial treatment of AVMs and DAVFs entails the deposition of an embolic agent in the nidus/venous pouches of the respective lesions. If this cannot be achieved, there will be recanalization or recruitment of alternate arteries that will often be more difficult to engage and navigate with a catheter than the initially treated vessels. Although many agents, including calibrated particles,[28] silk,[29] and absolute alcohol

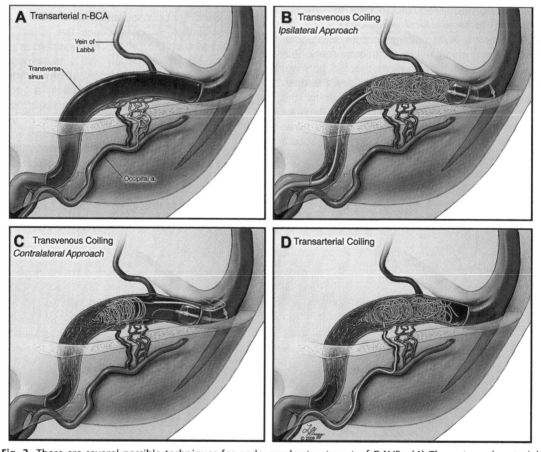

**Fig. 3.** There are several possible techniques for endovascular treatment of DAVFs. (*A*) The antegrade arterial approach may be required when the cortical veins have a normal drainage pattern and cannot be sacrificed. If the transverse sinus is no longer functioning properly and there is cortical venous reflux, a (*B*) retrograde approach through a stenotic sinus may be performed. If the sinus is occluded, a (*C*) contralateral approach across the torcular may be advantageous. If the sinus is isolated, it may be possible to occlude the sinus via a (*D*) transarterial approach. (Copyright © 2009 Lydia Gregg.)

ETOH),[30] have been used in the treatment of cerebral AVMs and DAVFs, it is the liquid embolic agents n-butyl-2-cyanoacrylate (NBCA) and ethylene vinyl alcohol copolymer (EVOH) that are the most successful at achieving this goal. Both agents are approved for the preoperative embolization of AVMs and other uses are considered off label, although they are standard of practice. Detachable coils are sometimes used in conjunction with liquid embolics in the treatment of high-flow AMVs or as a single agent in the treatment of DAVFs.

## NBCA

Cyanoacrylates have a long track record for the treatment of cerebral AVMs and DAVFs. NBCA (Trufil, Codman) is a liquid adhesive monomer that polymerizes on contact with hydroxyl ions in blood. It induces a chronic inflammatory response in the embolized vessel,[31,32] which is thought to play an important role in the durability of vessel occlusion obtained with NBCA. It is the penetration of the nidus and not just the feeding vessels that is required,[33] and recanalization can occur when the nidus is not filled.[34] However, when nidal penetration is achieved, the durability of embolization with NBCA has been demonstrated at a mean follow-up of 5 years (Fig. 4).[35]

NBCA may be mixed with lipiodol in varying concentrations (1:1–1:3) to vary the rate at which it polymerizes. Tanatalum power can be added to it to improve opacification; however, this is typically not required unless the concentration of NBCA to lipiodol is less than 1:1. Tantalum can cause clumping, which makes it difficult to use. The addition of glacial acetic acid has also been described as a means to delay the polymerization of NBCA.[36]

Because NBCA polymerizes when in contact with an ionic solution, operators must take extreme care to keep the equipment free of blood and other ionic solutions. The glue is typically prepared on a separate sterile table after changing gloves. The catheter is then prepared by flushing with a 5% dextrose solution before the injection of the NBCA.

The key is to have the catheter as distal and close to the nidus as possible. Once injection of NBCA begins, it should no be stopped before the NBCA reaches the nidus or the NBCA may polymerize and occlude the artery proximally, without penetrating the nidus. If the catheter cannot be advanced distally in a small vessel but it can be wedged proximally so that no blood can flow around it, the dextrose solution will replace the blood distal to the catheter, which will effectively promote deposition of the NBCA into the nidus.[37] Another technique that can be used to improve penetration of NBCA when the catheter cannot be wedged is the D5 push technique in which 5% dextrose in injected with a large syringe through the guiding catheter, helping to promote the penetration of the nidus.[38]

## EVOH

EVOH is a new liquid embolic agent. As opposed to NBCA, it solidifies by precipitation and not polymerization when it is exposed to an aqueous solution. It has a much longer working time than NBCA and, as such, can be injected over a longer period of time. Because of its longer working time and lack of adherence to devices, it is easier for less-experienced operators to work with. However, higher morbidity rates have been reported with the use of EVOH because of embolization-induced hemorrhages and arterial ischemic complications.[39]

EVOH is dissolved in dimethyl-sulfoxide (DMSO) and mixed with tantalum powder to make it radiopaque. It is approved by the Food and Drug Administration for the preoperative embolization of cerebral AVMs and is available in 2 predetermined viscosities (Onyx, EV3): Onyx 18 (6% EVOH) and Onyx 34 (8% EVOH). EVOH forms a cast of the vessel as it is injected. It must be injected slowly, using a DMSO-compatible microcatheter. Injection of DMSO can cause angionecrosis when performed too quickly.[40] After slowly flushing the catheter with DMSO, the operator injects the EVOH to form a plug at the catheter tip. Some operators will begin with Onyx 34 to create a plug and then switch to Onyx 18 to promote penetration into the AVM nidus.[41] EVOH can be injected over a prolonged period of minutes to hours.[42] Experience with EVOH is growing; however, there is evidence that recanalization can occur with EVOH.[43]

## EQUIPMENT

There are many combinations of catheters and guidewires that can be used for endovascular treatment of DAVFs and AVMs, and every operator should have a set of tools that they are familiar with. The basic starting point for an endovascular procedure is a stable platform. This platform consists of advancing a guiding catheter or a long sheath into a more proximal vessel in the cervical region. If the path to the lesion is exceedingly tortuous, it may be difficult to advance the microcatheter because it may displace the platform or prolapse into a proximal branch vessel. Recently a series

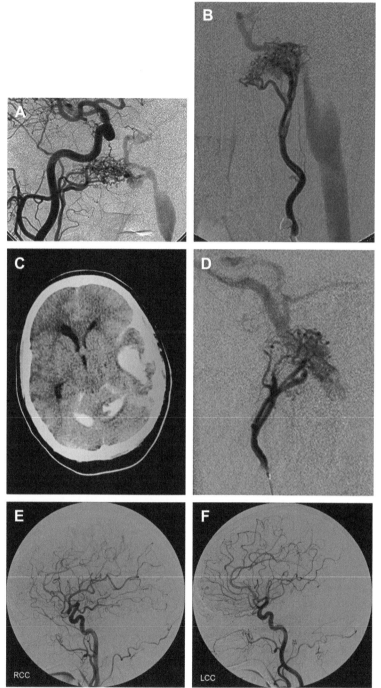

**Fig. 4.** A 60-year-old woman with left-sided tinnitus and a condylar canal vascular anomaly by magnetic reso-nance (MR) imaging and MR angiography. Diagnostic angiography demonstrated a Cognard type IIB DAVF of the condyal canal confluence supplied primarily by branches of the right ascending pharyngeal artery (APA). (*A*) Anteroposterior view and (*B*) lateral projection from selective right APA angiogram. The patient was sched-uled to return for treatment; however, she had a sudden onset of headache. (*C*) CT demonstrated hemorrhage in the left temporal lobe. (*D*) Selective angiography of the right APA, lateral projection, demonstrates spontaneous occlusion of the condylar venous outflow. The fistula was treated with NBCA embolization of the fistula. Follow-up angiography at 5 years demonstrates persistent occlusion of the fistula. (*E*) Right common carotid (RCC) and (*F*) left common carotid (LCC) artery angiograms. (*Courtesy of* Philippe Gailloud, MD.)

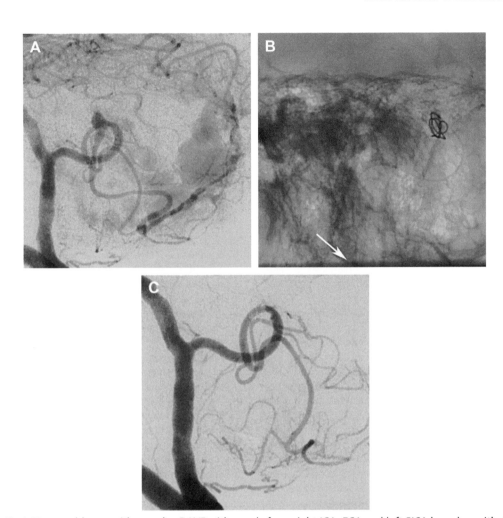

**Fig. 5.** A 68-year-old man with complex DAVF with supply from right ICA, ECA and left PICA branches with deep venous drainage. (*A*) There is a feeding artery aneurysm on the left PICA. During treatment the guiding catheter was displaced from the vertebral artery despite advancing the guiding catheter into the left vertebral artery. (*B*) A distal access catheter (*white arrow*) was advanced to the V3 segment of the vertebral artery providing support for coiling of the aneurysm and gluing of the artery feeding the DAVF. (*C*) Control angiogram demonstrating no flow in the aneurysm or residual supply to DAVF. ECA, external carotid artery; ICA, internal carotid artery; PICA, posterior inferior cerebellar artery.

of catheters have been developed, distal access catheters (Concentric Medical, Mountain View, CA, USA), that can be used in conjunction with traditional microcatheters and guiding catheters to provide additional support[44] for complex cases. Although this coaxial approach increases the complexity of the procedure, the additional support provided by these catheters may be essential to the success of an individual case (**Fig. 5**).

## SUMMARY

Endovascular treatment of AVMs and DAVFs is technically challenging and requires experience with a variety of endovascular techniques as well as a thorough understanding of the unique vascular anatomy associated with each lesion. Continuing development of techniques and equipment is increasing the number of patients who can be successfully treated. Each patient is different and a team approach is necessary to treat these complex lesions, with some cases requiring multimodality treatment or possibly no treatment at all.

## REFERENCES

1. Brown RD Jr, Wiebers DO, Forbes G, et al. The natural history of unruptured intracranial arteriovenous malformations. J Neurosurg 1988;68:352.
2. Crawford PM, West CR, Chadwick DW, et al. Arteriovenous malformations of the brain: natural history in

unoperated patients. J Neurol Neurosurg Psychiatr 1986;49:1.

3. Forster DM, Steiner L, Håkanson S. Arteriovenous malformations of the brain. A long-term clinical study. J Neurosurg 1972;37:562.

4. Graf CJ, Perret GE, Torner JC. Bleeding from cerebral arteriovenous malformations as part of their natural history. J Neurosurg 1983;58:331.

5. Itoyama Y, Uemura S, Ushio Y, et al. Natural course of unoperated intracranial arteriovenous malformations: study of 50 cases. J Neurosurg 1989;71:805.

6. Ondra SL, Troupp H, George ED, et al. The natural history of symptomatic arteriovenous malformations of the brain: a 24-year follow-up assessment. J Neurosurg 1990;73:387.

7. Mast H, Young WL, Koennecke HC, et al. Risk of spontaneous haemorrhage after diagnosis of cerebral arteriovenous malformation. Lancet 1997;350:1065.

8. Niimi Y, Sala F, Deletis V, et al. Neurophysiologic monitoring and pharmacologic provocative testing for embolization of spinal cord arteriovenous malformations. AJNR Am J Neuroradiol 2004;25:1131.

9. Sala F, Beltramello A, Gerosa M. Neuroprotective role of neurophysiological monitoring during endovascular procedures in the brain and spinal cord. Neurophysiol Clin 2007;37:415.

10. Hara H, Burrows PE, Flodmark O, et al. Neonatal superficial cerebral arteriovenous malformations. Pediatr Neurosurg 1994;20:126.

11. Lazar RM, Connaire K, Marshall RS, et al. Developmental deficits in adult patients with arteriovenous malformations. Arch Neurol 1999;56:103.

12. Geibprasert S, Pongpech S, Jiarakongmun P, et al. Radiologic assessment of brain arteriovenous malformations: what clinicians need to know. Radiographics 2010;30:483.

13. Turjman F, Massoud TF, Sayre JW, et al. Epilepsy associated with cerebral arteriovenous malformations: a multivariate analysis of angioarchitectural characteristics. AJNR Am J Neuroradiol 1995;16:345.

14. Hernesniemi JA, Dashti R, Juvela S, et al. Natural history of brain arteriovenous malformations: a long-term follow-up study of risk of hemorrhage in 238 patients. Neurosurgery 2008;63:823.

15. Stapf C, Mast H, Sciacca RR, et al. Predictors of hemorrhage in patients with untreated brain arteriovenous malformation. Neurology 2006;66:1350.

16. Yamada S, Brauer FS, Colohan AR, et al. Concept of arteriovenous malformation compartments and surgical management. Neurol Res 2004;26:288.

17. Krings T, Hans FJ, Geibprasert S, et al. Partial "targeted" embolisation of brain arteriovenous malformations. Eur Radiol 2010;20:2723.

18. Abud DG, Riva R, Nakiri GS, et al. Treatment of brain arteriovenous malformations by double arterial catheterization with simultaneous injection of Onyx: retrospective series of 17 patients. AJNR Am J Neuroradiol 2011;32:152.

19. Yu SC, Chan MS, Lam JM, et al. Complete obliteration of intracranial arteriovenous malformation with endovascular cyanoacrylate embolization: initial success and rate of permanent cure. AJNR Am J Neuroradiol 2004;25:1139.

20. Le Feuvre D, Taylor A. Target embolization of avms: identification of sites and results of treatment. Interv Neuroradiol 2007;13:389.

21. Borden JA, Wu JK, Shucart WA. A proposed classification for spinal and cranial dural arteriovenous fistulous malformations and implications for treatment. J Neurosurg 1995;82:166.

22. Cognard C, Gobin YP, Pierot L, et al. Cerebral dural arteriovenous fistulas: clinical and angiographic correlation with a revised classification of venous drainage. Radiology 1995;194:671.

23. Davies MA, TerBrugge K, Willinsky R, et al. The validity of classification for the clinical presentation of intracranial dural arteriovenous fistulas. J Neurosurg 1996;85:830.

24. Duffau H, Lopes M, Janosevic V, et al. Early rebleeding from intracranial dural arteriovenous fistulas: report of 20 cases and review of the literature. J Neurosurg 1999;90:78.

25. Hamada Y, Goto K, Inoue T, et al. Histopathological aspects of dural arteriovenous fistulas in the transverse-sigmoid sinus region in nine patients. Neurosurgery 1997;40:452.

26. Endo S, Kuwayama N, Takaku A, et al. Direct packing of the isolated sinus in patients with dural arteriovenous fistulas of the transverse-sigmoid sinus. J Neurosurg 1998;88:449.

27. Roy D, Raymond J. The role of transvenous embolization in the treatment of intracranial dural arteriovenous fistulas. Neurosurgery 1997;40:1133.

28. Sorimachi T, Koike T, Takeuchi S, et al. Embolization of cerebral arteriovenous malformations achieved with polyvinyl alcohol particles: angiographic reappearance and complications. AJNR Am J Neuroradiol 1999;20:1323.

29. Schmutz F, McAuliffe W, Anderson DM, et al. Embolization of cerebral arteriovenous malformations with silk: histopathologic changes and hemorrhagic complications. AJNR Am J Neuroradiol 1997;18:1233.

30. Yakes WF, Krauth L, Ecklund J, et al. Ethanol endovascular management of brain arteriovenous malformations: initial results. Neurosurgery 1997;40:1145.

31. Kish KK, Rapp SM, Wilner HI, et al. Histopathologic effects of transarterial bucrylate occlusion of intracerebral arteries in mongrel dogs. AJNR Am J Neuroradiol 1983;4:385.

32. Klara PM, George ED, McDonnell DE, et al. Morphological studies of human arteriovenous malformations. Effects of isobutyl 2-cyanoacrylate embolization. J Neurosurg 1985;63:421.

33. Vinuela F, Fox AJ, Pelz D, et al. Angiographic follow-up of large cerebral AVMs incompletely embolized with isobutyl-2-cyanoacrylate. AJNR Am J Neuroradiol 1986;7:919.

34. Gruber A, Mazal PR, Bavinzski G, et al. Repermeation of partially embolized cerebral arteriovenous malformations: a clinical, radiologic, and histologic study. AJNR Am J Neuroradiol 1996;17:1323.

35. Wikholm G. Occlusion of cerebral arteriovenous malformations with N-butyl cyano-acrylate is permanent. AJNR Am J Neuroradiol 1995;16:479.

36. Gounis MJ, Lieber BB, Wakhloo AK, et al. Effect of glacial acetic acid and ethiodized oil concentration on embolization with N-butyl 2-cyanoacrylate: an in vivo investigation. AJNR Am J Neuroradiol 2002; 23:938.

37. Nelson PK, Russell SM, Woo HH, et al. Use of a wedged microcatheter for curative transarterial embolization of complex intracranial dural arteriovenous fistulas: indications, endovascular technique, and outcome in 21 patients. J Neurosurg 2003;98:498.

38. Moore C, Murphy K, Gailloud P. Improved distal distribution of n-butyl cyanoacrylate glue by simultaneous injection of dextrose 5% through the guiding catheter: technical note. Neuroradiology 2006;48:327.

39. Valavanis A, Pangalu A, Tanaka M. Endovascular treatment of cerebral arteriovenous malformations with emphasis on the curative role of embolisation. Interv Neuroradiol 2005;11:37.

40. Murayama Y, Vinuela F, Ulhoa A, et al. Nonadhesive liquid embolic agent for cerebral arteriovenous malformations: preliminary histopathological studies in swine rete mirabile. Neurosurgery 1998;43:1164.

41. De Keukeleire K, Vanlangenhove P, Kalala Okito JP, et al. Transarterial embolization with ONYX for treatment of intracranial non-cavernous dural arteriovenous fistula with or without cortical venous reflux. J Neuro Intervent Surg 2011;3:224–8.

42. Gemmete JJ, Ansari SA, Gandhi D. Endovascular treatment of carotid cavernous fistulas. Neuroimaging Clin N Am 2009;19:241.

43. Natarajan SK, Ghodke B, Britz GW, et al. Multimodality treatment of brain arteriovenous malformations with microsurgery after embolization with onyx: single-center experience and technical nuances. Neurosurgery 2008;62:1213.

44. Spiotta AM, Hussain MS, Sivapatham T, et al. The versatile distal access catheter: the Cleveland Clinic experience. Neurosurgery 2011;68(6):1677–86.

# Stereotactic Radiosurgery of Cranial Arteriovenous Malformations and Dural Arteriovenous Fistulas

Alfred P. See, BS, Shaan Raza, MD, Rafael J. Tamargo, MD, Michael Lim, MD*

## KEYWORDS

- Arteriovenous malformations • Arteriovenous fistulas
- Stereotactic radiosurgery

Cranial arteriovenous malformations (AVM) are collections and anastomoses of arterial and venous vasculature.[1] These are nonneoplastic and are distinguished from hemangiomas, which have increased endothelial cell turnover. In some cases, they may demonstrate slow growth, but this is caused by hypertrophy and not increased cell cycle.[2] Left untreated, 3% to 5% of AVMs bleed each year, with higher rates of bleeding in AVMs that have previously ruptured or contain intranidal aneurysms.[3–5] High flow rate and venous outflow stenosis have also been proposed to increase the risk of hemorrhage, but these variables have not been reported because they are difficult to measure. In AVMs with no history of bleeding, the annual risk is slightly lower at 2%, but after the first bleed, the annual risk of bleed is nearly 18%.[1,6] A total of 1% to 1.5% of AVM patients die each year, most commonly because of hemorrhage.[1,7,8] Although hemorrhage contributes to significant morbidity and mortality in AVM patients, about 1% also develop new seizures each year.[1] Management of AVMs is a delicate balance of the morbidity and mortality of treatment versus the symptoms of the patient, risk of recurrent hemorrhages, seizure risk, and quality of life.

Dural arteriovenous fistulas (AVFs) are abnormal connections between meningeal arteries and a dural venous sinus, or subarachnoid veins. AVFs have a variable natural history, and not all cases may require intervention. The natural history of AVFs is predicted by the Borden classification scale, which describes AVFs based primarily on the draining veins and the direction of flow (**Table 1**). Risks for hemorrhage can vary from 2% (Borden Grade I) to 19.2% (Borden Grade II or III).[9,10] Furthermore, higher-grade AVFs have increased morbidity and mortality. For example, Borden Grade II and III AVFs have a 10.9% annual neurologic deficit incidence, and a 19.3% annual mortality rate.[10] In addition, AVFs that present with cortical venous drainage are thought to have an increased chance of hemorrhage, and are typically treated regardless of clinical presentation, but this opinion continues to evolve.[11,12] In a similar manner to AVMs, the risks of treatment and the natural history of AVFs must be considered in developing a treatment plan.[13–17]

## STEREOTACTIC RADIOSURGERY

Stereotactic radiosurgery (SRS) is a technique in radiosurgery that delivers a conformal dose of

Department of Neurosurgery, The Johns Hopkins University, 600 North Wolfe Street, Neurosurgery Phipps 123, Baltimore, MD 21287, USA
* Corresponding author.
E-mail address: mlim3@jhmi.edu

Neurosurg Clin N Am 23 (2012) 133–146
doi:10.1016/j.nec.2011.09.011
1042-3680/12/$ – see front matter © 2012 Elsevier Inc. All rights reserved.

**Table 1**
**Borden AVF classification**

| Type | Arterial Supply | Venous Drainage | Direction of Flow |
|------|-----------------|-----------------|-------------------|
| Type I | Meningeal artery | Dural venous sinus or meningeal vein | Anterograde |
| Type II | Meningeal artery | Venous sinus | Retrograde flow into subarachnoid veins |
| Type III | Meningeal artery | Subarachnoid veins or isolated segment of dural venous sinus draining into subarachnoid veins | Retrograde flow into subarachnoid veins |

intense radiation on a target, such as an AVM. A number of different technologies have been developed to achieve this result: Gamma Knife; linear accelerators (LINACs; e.g., CyberKnife, Synergy S, and Trilogy); and proton-beam. Gamma Knife uses a radioactive source (cobalt) and aims radiation through a circular array of ports to focus the beams at a single point. LINACs, which are made by a number of different companies with different designs and implementations, do not have a radioactive source but rather accelerate electrons, which either directly interact with the target tissue or produce an X-ray beam directed at the tissue. Proton-beam therapy uses a synchrotron to accelerate protons to interact with the target tissue. Proton-beam therapy is often distinguished from the Gamma Knife and LINAC by the use of protons, which have more mass. As a result, the steep radiation dose fall-off allows for treatment of larger lesions and use of higher doses to minimize damage to neighboring tissue.[18,19]

By definition, in addition to the radiation source, SRS involves a navigation system that allows the radiation to be delivered accurately and precisely. The original solution developed for the Gamma Knife was a stereotactic frame that was fixed to the skull, providing a set of reference coordinate axes. Other SRS systems, such as the CyberKnife, use frameless guidance involving a thermoplastic mask to minimize movement; built-in imaging systems update the position of the patient in real-time to improve the accuracy.

## MECHANISM AND TECHNIQUES OF RADIOSURGERY FOR AVMs AND AVFs

Radiosurgery works to obliterate the AVM through two stages. Initially, radiosurgery damages the endothelial cells.[20] The intimal layer thickens because of smooth muscle proliferation and deposits of hyaline, calcium, and collagen in the extracellular matrix.[20–22] Ultimately, radiosurgery effects thrombosis and necrosis of AVM vessels

resulting in a durable response that lasts at least a decade after radiosurgery.[21,23] It is important to note that this process can take years to work. The exact mechanism of action for obliteration of AVFs is unknown; however, given the observed time course of obliteration, we believe that the mechanism of endothelial cell damage and thrombosis are likely applicable in AVFs.

Radiosurgery requires a median of 20 months to achieve subtotal (>95%) obliteration in AVMs.[3,24] As a result, radiosurgery is not typically used in AVMs that present with hemorrhage.[25] There is a significantly increased incidence of repeat hemorrhage (18% per 12 months) in these patients, so the immediate effect of microsurgery is a significant benefit compared with radiosurgery.

The important technical point for treating AVMs and AVFs is localization. In appropriately selected patients, radiosurgery obliteration depends on accurate targeting of the nidus or the fistula. Although digital subtraction angiography (DSA) serves as the gold standard for detection of AVM and AVF before and after radiosurgery, the two-dimensional study alone cannot be used for treatment planning.[26,27] Therefore, thin-slice magnetic resonance imaging (MRI) and computed tomography (CT) are used to determine nidus geometry and neighboring at-risk structures for generating radiosurgery treatment plans.[28] However, even MRI and CT have an average of 1-mm difference in stereotactic coordinates.[29]

Technologic advancements in MRI and CT may eventually obviate the need for confirmatory DSA, but they are still insufficiently sensitive. As an example, patients can be followed with MRI or CT while an AVM nidus is visible, but a negative MRI or CT is followed by DSA to confirm AVM obliteration.[30–32] Concurrently, advancements in DSA techniques offer the possibility of three-dimensional information needed for radiosurgery at the high resolution and sensitivity of DSA.[33]

In terms of the actual machines, studies have suggested that the various radiosurgical systems are likely to be equivalent. One comparison of LINAC at 16 Gy the 70% isodose line with Gamma Knife at 20 Gy at the 50% isodose line found angiography-confirmed obliteration rates of 60% and 72%, respectively.[34] Toxicity was observed in 8% of patients in both groups.[34] The subsequent studies for the Gamma Knife and LINAC have also suggested no difference in efficacy.[34–36] However, these studies are small and further comparative studies are necessary.

## CHOOSING THE APPROPRIATE AVM AND AVF FOR RADIOSURGERY

In determining the role of SRS for AVM patients, various scales are used to guide treatment. In unhemorrhaged AVMs, case selection can be guided by a number of AVM grading scales, such as the Spetzler-Martin scale (SM), modified Spetzler-Martin scale (mSM), and Pittsburgh radiosurgery-based AVM grading scale (**Table 2**).[37,38] Key components shared by these scales are AVM size and location. Although the SM scale was developed for predicting surgical morbidity and mortality, its role in guiding surgery has led to its use in guiding SRS.[39] General recommendations are microsurgery for mSM Grades I to IIIA, whereas SRS or multimodal therapies are applied

for mSM Grades IIIB to V.[39,40] It is important to note that SM and mSM grading does not reflect the degree of protection from AVM hemorrhage, which is nearly 100%, but is dependent on extent of resection.[41] Microsurgery remains the gold standard for AVM treatment; therefore, typical cases that are considered for SRS are SM Grade III or higher: greater than 3 cm involving eloquent cortex or deep drainage, or greater than 6 cm.[41–43]

In SRS, successful obliteration of the AVM nidus has been found to depend on nidus volume, marginal dose, age, and gender, in addition to the SM grade.[37,43] The Radiosurgery Based AVM Scale (RBAS) captures the effect of nidus volume, age, and location (hemisphere, corpus callosum, and cerebellum vs basal ganglia, thalamus, or brainstem). The location is closely related to the marginal dose, because the location determines the maximum dose deliverable to the nidus without clinically significant damage to neighboring structures.[44] The RBAS score is calculated as follows: (0.1) (volume, mL) + (0.02) (age, yr) + (0.5) (location). Cases scoring less than 1 have 90% chance of AVM obliteration without a new neurologic deficit, whereas cases scoring greater than 2 have greater than 50% chance of such an outcome. For lesions greater than 15 cm$^3$, nearly half have new neurologic deficits or incompletely

## Table 2
## AVM grading scales

**Modified Pittsburgh radiosurgery-based AVM grading scale**

| | Volume | | Age | | | Location |
|---|---|---|---|---|---|---|
| AVM score = | 0.1 x volume (cc) | + | 0.02 x age (years) | + | 0.5 x | 0 (frontal, temporal, parietal, occipital, intraventricular, corpus callosum, cerebellar) 1 (basal ganglia, thalamus, brainstem) |

**Spetzler-Martin grading scale for AVM**

| | Size | | Eloquence of adjacent brain | | Venous drainage |
|---|---|---|---|---|---|
| | 1 (<3cm) | | 0 (noneloquent) | | 0 (superficial only) |
| Score = | 2 (3-6cm) | + | 1 (sensorimotor, language, or visual cortex; hypothalamus or thalamus; internal capsule; brain stem; cerebellar peduncles, or nuclei) | + | 1 (deep) |
| | 3 (>6cm) | | | | |

**Modified Spetzler-Martin AVM grading scale**

| | Size | | Eloquence of adjacent brain | | Venous drainage | Modifier (if Grade 3) |
|---|---|---|---|---|---|---|
| | 1 (<3cm) | | 0 (noneloquent) | | 0 (superficial only) | A (>3cm) |
| Score = | 2 (3-6cm) | + | 1 (sensorimotor, language, or visual cortex; hypothalamus or thalamus; internal capsule; brain stem; cerebellar peduncles, or nuclei) | + | 1 (deep) | B (<3cm) |
| | 3 (>6cm) | | | | | |

obliterated AVMs when treated with SRS. In eloquent locations, such as the basal ganglia, brainstem, and the optic nerve, SRS can be challenging for lesions as small as 10 cm$^3$.[44]

Because the variables that predict radiosurgical success overlap with the criteria used for selecting microsurgery patients, some patients are not suitable candidates for either treatment alone. Giant AVMs (>25 cm$^3$) may require a combination of surgery, embolization, and SRS.[45,46] Moderately sized lesions in challenging locations, such as the brainstem, may also necessitate combination therapy.[47]

AVMs in pediatric patients present a distinct risk–benefit balance. Pediatric patients are exposed to a longer posttreatment at-risk period, increasing the cumulative lifetime risk.[48,49] Therefore, successful obliteration and reduction of hemorrhage risk is very important. Many groups have resorted to a multidisciplinary treatment team delivering combination therapy.[50]

Patients who present with a history of a prior bleed may not be good candidates for SRS. Studies have reported an increase in the relative risk of hemorrhage: the annual incidence of AVM hemorrhage is 2%, but the incidence of recurrent AVM hemorrhage is 18%. This is reflected in a 9.09 (confidence interval [CI], 5.44–15.19; P<.001) relative risk of recurrent hemorrhage.[3,25] However, sometimes SRS can be an appropriate choice in patients who present with a prior hemorrhage if the risks of microsurgery or observation are also high.

In addressing AVFs, some AVFs have been reported to spontaneously resolve, particularly cavernous sinus AVFs.[9,51] Therefore, some AVFs that present incidentally may not require intervention.[51] In addition, up to 81% of patients receiving conservative treatment may have improvement or resolution of their symptoms.[9] However, AVFs presenting with hemorrhage or severe neurologic deficit are likely to require treatment. Embolization or surgery, which both achieve immediate obliteration of the nidus, is the treatment of choice for cases with high risk of bleeding or with severe symptoms.[13,52] Surgery can also be used as an adjunct to embolization for large AVFs that are incompletely obliterated by embolization or that are not amenable to embolization.[13,15,16] Therefore, SRS monotherapy is most often used to treat small AVFs that are difficult to access surgically and present with significant but not severe symptoms.[53] Larger lesions that are not amenable to surgery may also be responsive to combined embolization and SRS.[53] Treatment of AVFs can be complicated by venous sinus thrombosis, which leads to increasing venous hypertension

and edema after occlusive therapies, such as embolization or SRS.[16,54,55] These patients can also be treated with SRS, but may require adjunctive therapies to restore cerebral drainage before SRS.[54]

## FACTORS IMPACTING OUTCOME OF RADIOSURGERY IN AVMs AND AVFs

To determine the factors that affect the outcome of SRS, one must acknowledge that there are varying opinions on the definition of successful treatment of an AVM or AVF. Success of SRS has been defined in terms of hemorrhage prevention and symptom management, or nidus obliteration. Typically, the most severe consequence of AVMs and AVFs is morbidity and mortality from hemorrhage, so seizure control is less well studied. However, only a subset of AVMs and AVFs hemorrhage each year, which limits statistical power. Therefore, many studies also define success as nidus or fistula obliteration. The likelihood of SRS success is associated with the patient's clinical history, characteristics of the AVMs and AVFs, and the SRS technique.

History of embolization decreases the likelihood of SRS-induced AVM obliteration by an estimated 86%.[56,57] This has not been shown to be a result of direct interaction between embolization therapy and SRS.[58] Rather, embolization has an associated failure rate, either from inadequate penetration or from local recanalization; one study found this in 18.2% of embolizations.[59] A nidus may develop where the prior embolization site is thought to be obliterated, and is therefore excluded from the radiation plan. Persistence of this nidus is referred to as an "out-of-field nidus."[57] Embolization may also create multiple segments of AVM, complicating SRS treatment design, but this has not been studied.[58] This may be resolved by including the embolized region in the SRS plan. SRS has been shown to reduce local angiogenesis, which may decrease recanalization.[60] However, this may not be feasible in cases where embolization is used to obliterate nidus that is near radiation-sensitive structures.

Characteristics of the AVM (size, venous drainage, and location) are associated with success of SRS.[56] AVM size is often measured by maximum linear dimension or by nidus volume. A common threshold is maximum linear dimension of 3 and 6 cm, but studies have used numerous different thresholds for their statistical analysis. Increased AVM size is consistently associated with decreased obliteration rates or increased treatment-associated deficits.[36,56,61] For example, AVMs greater than 10 cm$^3$ may have as much as a fivefold increase (7%–35.7%) in posttreatment hemorrhage rate.[62] The number of draining veins and pattern of venous drainage are associated with microsurgical success, but are unclear factors for hemorrhage after SRS.[37] One study observed that a single draining vein increases the relative risk of hemorrhage (relative risk, 1.66; P<.01), but another study found no difference in AVMs: 5 of 66 (7.6%) single draining vein AVMs hemorrhaged, compared with 8 (7%) of 115 in the overall population.[62] Deep venous drainage was associated with double the odds of hemorrhage, but another study suggests that this may be confounded by an association with the location of the AVM.[25,62] Proximity to eloquent structures is associated with decreased obliteration rates, but is not associated with hemorrhage rates.[44,63] Lower nidus density, as defined on CT, is associated with a decreased obliteration rate (odds ratio, 0.246; P = .008),[63] and as defined on MRI, is associated with an increased hemorrhage rate (relative risk, 1.64; P<.01).[25] A history of AVM hemorrhage and prior treatment are not included in the common scoring systems, but are strongly associated with SRS success. RBAS and SM scales classify AVMs by characteristics of the patient and AVM at presentation.

Scales such as the RBAS and mSM may be used to help predict the success for SRS in AVMs because they incorporate the aforementioned clinical characteristics. RBAS and mSM scales are designed for ease of use and incorporate significant, clinically applicable predictive variables. The RBAS score is a simple method of determining the likelihood of obliteration without new neurologic deficits, but only considers the AVM size, patient age, and location.[44] In the RBAS, the likelihood of obliteration without new neurologic deficit is 91.7% for less than 1, 74.1% for 1 to 1.5, 60% for 1.5 to 2, and 33.3% for greater than 2.[64] Although designed for assessing microsurgery success, the mSM scale evaluates based on size (<3, 3–6, and >6 cm); location (eloquent or not); and venous drainage (superficial or deep). It approximately correlates with the RBAS score: 88.9% for Grade 1, 69.6% for Grade 2, 61.5% for Grade IIIB, and 44.8% for Grades IIIA and IV.[64]

Finally, hemorrhage and nidus obliteration are also associated with radiation marginal dose, dose homogeneity, and fraction of nidus treated, but are not associated with the system used to deliver SRS. Increasing marginal dose of radiation correlates with increasing rates of nidus obliteration, as measured on MRI. At a threshold of 15 Gy, the odds ratio of successful obliteration is 3.743.[63] A detailed study of dose-response suggests that this is a logistical function, with the

inflection point near 16 Gy, and the plateau between 18 and 25 Gy, with a maximum obliteration rate of about 88% (**Fig. 1**).[57] However, it is also important to note that increasing dose can also lead to increased complications, such as radiation necrosis, and dose selection should also take into account the various regions of the brain. For example, the dose tolerance of surrounding brain tissue is significantly lower in the area around the thalamus than around the frontal lobe. The homogeneity index is another measure of radiation delivered. It is a ratio of the maximum dose to the prescribed dose. Increased homogeneity index is associated with slower nidus obliteration.[24]

Although the natural history of AVF is unpredictably variable, AVF outcomes in patients receiving treatment are known to depend on the pattern of drainage. The Borden Classification system classifies AVFs into three types (see **Table 1**).[65] It associates lower rehemorrhage rates for drainage into a dural venous sinus or meningeal vein versus a cortical vein, and also with anterograde flow versus retrograde flow. The Cognard system further distinguishes AVFs based on dilation of the draining vein and considers spinal perimedullary veins as a separate type.[66] Because higher-grade lesions more often present with hemorrhage and acute risk of rehemorrhage, they are typically treated with surgical or endovascular techniques, limiting the statistical power of studies that report SRS outcomes to identify differences between grades.[12] Of note, AVFs involving the cavernous sinus are associated with better obliteration

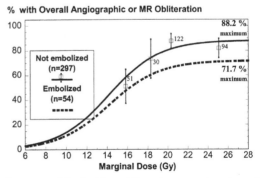

% with Overall Angiographic or MR Obliteration

Fig. 1. Model of nidus obliteration as a function of marginal dose in patients without prior embolization. This illustrates the dramatic increase in obliteration rate observed around 15 GY, and the flattening of the curve around 18 GY, which is the approximate dose typically used in AVM SRS. (*From* Flickinger JC, Kondziolka D, Maitz AH, et al. An analysis of the dose-response for arteriovenous malformation radiosurgery and other factors affecting obliteration. Radiother Oncol 2002; 63(3):347–54; with permission.)

rates.[53] However, this may be confounded by a higher rate of spontaneous resolution in cavernous sinus AVFs.[51]

## RADIOSURGERY OUTCOMES IN TREATMENT OF AVMs AND AVFs

SRS may aim to control AVM symptoms or prevent morbidity and mortality from AVM hemorrhage, but many studies focus on the prevention of hemorrhage. In addition to hemorrhage events, studies also measure AVM nidus or AVF obliteration, which is typically very strongly associated and is thought to be causatively related to hemorrhage.

### Hemorrhage Prevention

Hemorrhage occurs after SRS, particularly during the latent period, before complete obliteration by the initial SRS, repeat SRS, or other definitive treatment (Tables 3 and 4). Although a number of conflicting studies have analyzed the risk of hemorrhage in the latent period, a recently published large retrospective study of 500 patients found that the risk is unchanged or slightly decreased (hazard ratio, 0.26; 95% CI, 0.10–0.68).[67] After SRS but before nidus obliteration, annual hemorrhage rates are estimated at 4.8% to 7.9% per year for the first 2 years, then 2.2% to 5% per year in the third, fourth, and fifth years.[68,69] However, after the nidus is obliterated, the risk of hemorrhage is near zero.[68,69] In one large study where post-obliteration hemorrhage was observed, the risk of hemorrhage is estimated at 0.12 (hazard ratio; CI, 0.1–0.68) of the pretreatment risk.[67]

### AVM Nidus Obliteration

In the ideal AVMs (RBAS <1: small nidus, young patient, and in an uncomplicated location), total nidus obliteration is achieved in 75% of cases (see Tables 3 and 4).[35,57,70] However, this decreases to 33% in AVMs that are larger than 20 $cm^3$ (2.7-cm length cube, or 3.4-cm diameter sphere), or are larger than 10 $cm^3$ in a complex location. The RBAS was developed based on a mix of MRI and angiogram follow-up imaging to assess posttreatment nidus volume.

Comparison of MRI and angiogram for detecting residual AVM nidus has shown that MRI has a negative predictive value of 84% to 91%. For example, in one patient set, MRI detected no nidus in 75 (86%) of 87 cases, whereas angiography detected no nidus in 193 (73%) of 264 cases.[71] Clinical studies continue to report obliteration rates from MRI, angiogram, or a mix. A straightforward correction to compare MRI and angiogram success rates is division by the appropriate ratio.[57] However, this remains challenging as technology evolves.

In non-giant AVMs, the radiation dose is a significant predictor of total obliteration rate.[57] The likelihood of final obliteration ranges from 50% to 88% as a function of dose from 16 to 25 Gy.[35,57,72]

### Pediatric AVMs

Although SRS in pediatric patients has a different long-term impact, pediatric AVM SRS case series

## Table 3
Outcomes of SRS in overall AVM case series

| Median Volume (cm³) | Median Marginal Dose (Gy) | Follow-up (mo) | N | Obliteration (%) | Imaging Modality | Hemorrhage (%) | Death (%) | Source |
|---|---|---|---|---|---|---|---|---|
| 3.3 | 20 | 39 | 293 | 68 | MRI or angiography | 6 | 3 | 38 |
| 3.8 | 20 | 38 | 108 | 71 | angiography | 14 | 2 | 96 |
| 4.48 | — | — | 54 | 76 | CT or MRI or angiography | 13 | — | 97 |
| 6.64 | 16 | 26.8 | 62 | 35 | CT or MRI | 5 | — | 98 |
| 7.3 | 18 | 42 | 127 | 64 | MRI or angiography | — | 1 | 36 |
| 9.9 | 15 | — | 330 | 55 | MRI | 8 | — | 99 |
| 17.7 | 18 | — | 75 | 56 | MRI or angiography | 12 | 6 | 100 |
| 48.8 | 13.9 | 109 | 44 | 34 | MRI or angiography | 7 | — | 46 |

**Table 4**
**Outcomes of SRS in AVM of deep or eloquent brain**

| Grade (Mean RBAS, Median SM) | Median Volume (cm³) | Median Marginal Dose (Gy) | Follow-Up (mo) | N | Obliteration (%) | Imaging Modality | Hemorrhage (%) | Death (%) | Source |
|---|---|---|---|---|---|---|---|---|---|
| 1.69 | 5.2 | 18 | 24 | 65 | 55 | CT or angiography | 9 | — | 101 |
| 1.83 | 3.8 | 18 | 45 | 56 | 43 | MRI or angiography | 13 | 9 | 102 |
| 1.63 | 1.5 | 20 | 72 | 45 | 66 | Angiography | 4 | 0 | 103 |
| — | 1.35 | 18.4 | 52.2 | 29 | 41 | Angiography | 17 | 14 | 104 |
| III | 4.3 | 25 | 28 | 19 | 74 | Angiography | — | — | 105 |
| — | 9.1 | 18.75 | 23 | 15 | 47 | Angiography | — | — | 106 |
| 1.51 | 2.8 | 16.2 | 39 | 42 | 62 | MRI or angiography | 14 | 7 | 107 |

report low RBAS grade lesions. These patients have excellent outcomes: AVM obliteration without new neurologic deficits at 24, 36, and 42 months is seen in approximately 45%, 65%, and 68% of patients, respectively.[73,74] Most studies have found overall obliteration rates between 50% and 70% at latest follow-up (Table 5). In addition, SRS in pediatric patients provides excellent seizure control: one series of 13 patients reported 11 patients to be free of seizures and medications over 47 months of follow-up. The remaining two had improvement of seizure management, but still require medication. However, 2 of 72 patients developed new seizures.[75] SRS in selected pediatric patients offers effective control of the nidus volume and seizures associated with AVM.

## Proton-beam Therapy

Proton-beam has been reported to control seizures related to AVM and reduce the AVM nidus. In a small study of AVMs less than 10 cm$^3$, proton-beam achieved complete obliteration in at least 50% and greater than 98% obliteration in another 20%. However, in this study, no AVMs greater than 25 cm$^3$ were obliterated.[18] Another study found 67% of AVMs less than 14 cm$^3$ were obliterated, whereas 43% of AVMs greater than 14 cm$^3$ were obliterated, but included a hypofractionated proton-beam protocol.[76] Proton-beam has also been reported to control up to 78% of AVM-related seizures.

## AVF Obliteration

Success for AVFs is measured primarily through angiographic occlusion, as a surrogate for hemorrhage prevention. Interpretation of reported AVF series are difficult because most reported AVF series combine patients who received SRS monotherapy with those who received combination therapy. In one series, 30 (55%) of 55 patients had demonstrated angiographic obliteration of the AVF, whereas three patients (5%) had post-treatment hemorrhage.[11] Another series reported 67% obliteration with SRS monotherapy, and 75% obliteration in low-risk AVFs treated by SRS alone, but 83% obliteration when SRS was combined with embolization.[53] This series reported one death caused by hemorrhage (3%) 2 months after SRS. Another series reported SRS outcomes where half of the patients had prior surgery or embolization: 11 (58%) of 19 patients had complete obliteration by MRI or magnetic resonance angiography, and no patients hemorrhaged after treatment.[77] Finally, in a series of mixed SRS and combination SRS–embolization, 11 (64%) of 17 patients with angiographic follow-up had complete obliteration.[78]

It is important to interpret these results with consideration for the limitations of these studies: some AVFs are known to spontaneously resolve, although the rate is unknown in the various grades of AVFs; and angiographic follow-up is resource intensive and typically is achieved in only a portion of the treated patients, making the studies prone to selection bias.[9,51]

## LIMITATIONS AND COMPLICATIONS OF RADIOSURGERY

Although SRS is suitable for treating many AVMs, there are specific challenges that limit its application. In addition to adverse effects and

**Table 5**
**Outcomes of SRS in pediatric AVM**

| Grade (Mean RBAS) | Median Volume (cm$^3$) | Median Marginal Dose (Gy) | Follow-Up (mo) | N | Obliteration (%) | Yearly Hemorrhage Risk (%) | Source |
|---|---|---|---|---|---|---|---|
| 1.07 | 4.2 | 18 | 36 | 22 | 54 | 9 (yr 1), 13.6 (yr 2) | 108 |
| 1.08 | 3.4 | — | 42 | 38 | 68 | — | 73 |
| | 1.5 | 20 | 24 | 34 | 47 | — | 109 |
| | 1.7 | 20 | 36 | 53 | 72 | — | 110 |
| | 2.8 | 23 | 26 | 103 | 70 | — | 111 |
| | 2.9 | 18.8 | 24 | 22 | 68 | — | 74 |
| | 3.2 | 21.9 | — | 186 | 50 | 5.4 (yr 0–2), 0.8 (yr 2–5) | 112 |
| | 5.37 | 18 | 60 | 31 | 35 | 3.2–4.3 | 113 |
| | 6.9 | 18 | 21 | 17 | 53 | 0 | 114 |

complications of SRS, the most distinct limitation is the delayed effect of SRS on nidus obliteration.

The time from SRS treatment to maximum nidus obliteration is typically cited as 24 to 36 months. An exponential decay model estimated an average of 44% decrease in volume annually.[79] The obliteration rate of SRS has been found to depend on the dose homogeneity index, and the volume of nidus irradiated to 22 Gy.[24] These two variables can alter the median time to obliteration from 11.6 to 27.8 months.[24]

Although total obliteration eliminates the risk of hemorrhage,[68] the delayed obliteration after SRS exposes the patient to an extended duration of risk. In addition, it is unclear whether the risk of hemorrhage during the latent period is different than before treatment. Studies have found that during the latent period, there is no difference in the hemorrhage risk,[68,80] an increase in hemorrhage risk,[81–83] and a decrease in hemorrhage risk.[46,67,84,85]

In addition to the risks of an AVM, SRS treatment has its own risks. Radiation damage to neighboring healthy tissues can occur when large volumes are irradiated, in about 2% to 10% of cases.[86–88] Resolution of neurologic deficits caused by this damage is dependent on severity of the symptoms (hazard rate ratio, 2.74; $P<.0001$) and prior hemorrhage (hazard rate ratio, 1.65; $P = .0126$). In addition to neurologic deficits, SRS is known to induce hair loss, particularly in superficial lesions, which occurs approximately 3 weeks after treatment, and typically lasts for about 3 months. Although the mechanism is unclear, there have also been reports of increased seizures in up to 1% of patients after SRS.[88,89] Most severely, fatal complications occur in approximately 0.1% of cases.[88]

Similar to SRS in AVMs, there is a latent period in AVF SRS during which the nidus is not obliterated and the patient remains at risk of hemorrhage.[11] This is one of the reasons for considering embolization or surgery as a first option. Likewise, radiation damage to neighboring tissue is also possible in SRS treatment of AVFs. Radiation-induced change in MRI was observed in 33 (63%) of 52 patients in one series, but this did not associate with radiation dose, and did not have clear clinical implications.[11] The series reported one case of hemiparesis.[11] Although not observed in AVMs, venous hypertension and edema may be associated with AVFs, and may be exacerbated after SRS. In cases with complicated venous drainage, a combination of endovascular angioplasty preceding SRS may restore physiologic cerebral perfusion before the occlusion of the AVF.[54]

## NUANCES AND PEARLS IN TREATING PATIENTS WITH AVMs AND AVFs USING RADIOSURGERY

There are situations where radiosurgery may be useful, but where traditional single-dose radiosurgery does not offer a viable solution, such as geometrically complex AVMs or extremely large AVMs. A number of variations have been explored but are less well studied. Because the radiobiology of radiosurgery is not completely understood, it has been difficult to predict which of these modifications will improve obliteration rate or decrease hemorrhage. In addition, the applicable patient population is insufficient for large studies powered to detect complications or demonstrate that the variations do not achieve improved outcomes.

SRS delivers a large number of radiation beams focused at the target to administer a high dose of radiation delivery to the target, compared with a low dose in the neighboring tissue, in one sitting. Even with the optimum SRS treatment plan, at least 12% of AVMs are not entirely obliterated. Some of these have been retreated with SRS. Repeat SRS can achieve obliteration in 34.1% at a median follow-up of 109.4 months.[46]

Large AVMs may require high doses to neighboring tissue or subtherapeutic doses to the AVM nidus. One proposed solution is volume-staged radiosurgery, where the nidus volume is treated in multiple sessions, allowing lower radiation of normal tissue while maintaining therapeutic radiosurgery in the nidus. This has been applied to AVMs greater than 40 $cm^3$, but in some studies the threshold has been as low as 15 $cm^3$. Most studies report less than 50 patients but have found 28% to 50% with total obliteration and 29% with near-total obliteration.[90,91] Critics of this technique suggest that, based on surgical resection of AVMs previously treated by radiosurgery, the interval between the first and second therapy may expose the patient to a higher risk of hemorrhage in the untreated volume; first because of increased time before treatment, and second because of histologic changes, such as angiogenesis and venous stenosis, which may increase the interval bleed risk.[92] Additional investigations in volume-staged radiosurgery in AVMs need to identify the interval risk of hemorrhage and determine a threshold where this risk is balanced with the benefits of volume-staging.

An alternative to volume fractionation is dose fractionation. This has been implemented as a monotherapy, and in combination with follow-up surgery. Interpretation of these studies is challenging because the patients are a heterogeneous population with history of embolization and prior radiosurgery, and because the sample sizes are very small at less than 30.[79,93,94] Critics have questioned whether the radiobiology of AVMs, essentially normal cells that are disordered at the level of tissue organization, may be distinct from the radiobiology of neoplastic cells, which can be treated with fractionated radiosurgery to accomplish a cumulative therapeutic dose.[95]

## SUMMARY

SRS is a complementary treatment option to microsurgery and embolization for AVMs and AVFs. AVM and AVF patient selection needs to be carefully considered given the immediate benefit and high success rate of microsurgery. Cases that are not amenable to surgery may also be poorly suited for monotherapy SRS and combination therapy should be considered. History of hemorrhage or embolization, size of the AVM or AVF, proximity to radiosensitive structures, and patient age are key factors in identifying patients likely to benefit from SRS. After determining SRS as the appropriate therapy, the most significant factor in successfully obliterating the nidus or fistula and reducing hemorrhage risk is accurate definition of the nidus or fistula for treatment planning. SRS failure is often caused by the AVM nidus or fistula falling outside of the treatment volume; therefore, complete obliteration is hightly dependent on the accuracy of the treatment plan in targeting the entire nidus volume. In addition to the well-known risk of hemorrhage during the latent period, dreaded complications of SRS include radiation damage to neighboring structure and ischemic stroke. However, SRS is a viable treatment option with up to 88% success for patients with difficult-to-resect AVMs that are not in imminent risk of hemorrhage. For AVFs, complications are a result of the venous congestion or direct radiation injury. In addition, the success rate of AVFs seems to be lower than the rate of AVMs but the studies are less clearly defined because they include patients who received multimodal therapy.

## REFERENCES

1. Al-Shahi R, Warlow C. A systematic review of the frequency and prognosis of arteriovenous malformations of the brain in adults. Brain 2001;124:1900–26.
2. Mulliken JB, Glowacki J. Hemangiomas and vascular malformations in infants and children: a classification based on endothelial characteristics. Plast Reconstr Surg 1982;69(3):412–20.
3. Barrow D, Reisner A. Natural history of intracrania aneurysms and vascular malformations. Clin Neurosurg 1993;3–39.
4. Laakso A, Dashti R, Juvela S, et al. Risk of hemorrhage in patients with untreated Spetzler-Martir Grade IV and V arteriovenous malformations a long-term follow-up study in 63 patients. Neurosurgery 2011;68(2):372–7.
5. Hernesniemi JA, Dashti R, Juvela S, et al. Natura history of brain arteriovenous malformations a long-term follow-up study of risk of hemorrhage in 238 patients. Neurosurgery 2008;63(5):823–9.
6. Mast H, Young WL, Koennecke HC, et al. Risk o spontaneous haemorrhage after diagnosis of cerebral arteriovenous malformation. Lancet 1997 350(9084):1065–8.
7. Ondra SL, Troupp H, George ED, et al. The natural history of symptomatic arteriovenous-malformations of the brain: a 24-year follow-up assessment. J Neurosurg 1990;73(3):387–91.
8. Crawford PM, West CR, Chadwick DW, et al. Arteriovenous-malformations of the brain: natural-history in unoperated patients. J Neurol Neurosurg Psychiatr 1986;49(1):1–10.
9. Davies MA, Saleh J, Ter Brugge K, et al. The natura history and management of intracranial dural arteriovenous fistulae. Part 1: benign lesions. Interv Neuroradiol 1997;3(4):295–302.
10. Davies MA, Ter Brugge K, Willinsky R, et al. The natural history and management of intracranial dural arteriovenous fistulae. Part 2: aggressive lesions. Interv Neuroradiol 1997;3(4):303–11.
11. Cifarelli CP, Kaptain G, Yen CP, et al. Gamma Knife radiosurgery for dural arteriovenous fistulas. Neurosurgery 2010;67(5):1230–5.
12. Duffau H, Lopes M, Janosevic V, et al. Early rebleeding from intracranial dural arteriovenous fistulas: report of 20 cases and review of the literature. J Neurosurg 1999;90(1):78–84.
13. Katsaridis V. Treatment of dural arteriovenous fistulas. Curr Treat Options Neurol 2009;11(1):35–40.
14. Koebbe CJ, Singhal D, Sheehan J, et al. Radiosurgery for dural arteriovenous fistulas. Surg Neurol 2005;64(5):392–9.
15. OlteanuNerbe V, Uhl E, Steiger HJ, et al. Dural arteriovenous fistulas including the transverse and sigmoid sinuses: results of treatment in 30 cases. Acta Neurochir (Wien) 1997;139(4):307–18.
16. Agid R, TerBrugge K, Rodesch G, et al. Management strategies for anterior cranial fossa (ethmoidal) dural arteriovenous fistulas with an emphasis on endovascular treatment. J Neurosurg 2009;110(1):79–84.
17. Giller CA, Barnett DW, Thacker IC, et al. Multidisciplinary treatment of a large cerebral dural arteriovenous fistula using embolization, surgery, and

radiosurgery. Proc (Bayl Univ Med Cent) 2008; 21(3):255–7.

18. Silander H, Pellettieri L, Enblad P, et al. Fractionated, stereotactic proton beam treatment of cerebral arteriovenous malformations. Acta Neurol Scand 2004;109(2):85–90.

19. Ogilvy CS. Radiation-therapy for arteriovenous-malformations: a review. Neurosurgery 1990; 26(5):725–35.

20. Schneider BF, Eberhard DA, Steiner LE. Histopathology of arteriovenous malformations after Gamma Knife radiosurgery. J Neurosurg 1997; 87(3):352–7.

21. Chang SD, Shuster DL, Steinberg GK, et al. Stereotactic radiosurgery of arteriovenous malformations: pathologic changes in resected tissue. Clin Neuropathol 1997;16(2):111–6.

22. Szeifert GT, Kemeny AA, Timperley WR, et al. The potential role of myofibroblasts in the obliteration of arteriovenous malformations after radiosurgery. Neurosurgery 1997;40(1):61–5.

23. Steinberg GK, Chang SD, Levy RP, et al. Surgical resection of large incompletely treated intracranial arteriovenous malformations following stereotactic radiosurgery. J Neurosurg 1996;84(6):920–8.

24. Wowra B, Muacevic A, Tonn JC, et al. Obliteration dynamics in cerebral arteriovenous malformations after CyberKnife radiosurgery: quantification with sequential nidus volumetry and 3-tesla 3-dimensional time-of-flight magnetic resonance angiography. Neurosurgery 2009;64(2):A102–9.

25. Pollock BE, Flickinger JC, Lunsford LD, et al. Factors that predict the bleeding risk of cerebral arteriovenous malformations. Stroke 1996;27(1):1–6.

26. Buis DR, Lagerwaard FJ, Barkhof F, et al. Stereotactic radiosurgery for brain AVMs: role of interobserver variation in target definition on digital subtraction angiography. Int J Radiat Oncol Biol Phys 2005;62(1):246–52.

27. Hamm KD, Klisch J, Surber G, et al. Special aspects of diagnostic imaging for radiosurgery of arteriovenous malformations. Neurosurgery 2008; 62(5):A44–52.

28. Buis DR, Lagerwaard FJ, Dirven CM, et al. Delineation of brain AVMs on MR-angiography for the purpose of stereotactic radiosurgery. Int J Radiat Oncol Biol Phys 2007;67(1):308–16.

29. Bednarz G, Downes B, Werner-Wasik M, et al. Combining stereotactic angiography and 3D time-of-flight magnetic resonance angiography in treatment planning for arteriovenous malformation radiosurgery. Int J Radiat Oncol Biol Phys 2000; 46(5):1149–54.

30. Zhang XQ, Shirato H, Aoyama H, et al. Clinical significance of 3D reconstruction of arteriovenous malformation using digital subtraction angiography and its modification with CT information in stereotactic radiosurgery. Int J Radiat Oncol Biol Phys 2003;57(5):1392–9.

31. Stancanello J, Cavedon C, Francescon P, et al. Development and validation of a CT-3D rotational angiography registration method for AVM radiosurgery. Med Phys 2004;31(6):1363–71.

32. Gauvrit JY, Oppenheim C, Nataf F, et al. Three-dimensional dynamic magnetic resonance angiography for the evaluation of radiosurgically treated cerebral arteriovenous malformations. Eur Radiol 2006;16(3):583–91.

33. Colombo F, Cavedon C, Francescon P, et al. Three-dimensional angiography for radiosurgical treatment planning for arteriovenous malformations. J Neurosurg 2003;98(3):536–43.

34. Orio P, Stelzer KJ, Goodkin R, et al. Treatment of arteriovenous malformations with linear accelerator-based radiosurgery compared with Gamma Knife surgery. J Neurosurg 2006;105:58–63.

35. Colombo F, Cavedon C, Casentini L, et al. Early results of CyberKnife radiosurgery for arteriovenous malformations. J Neurosurg 2009;111(4): 807–19.

36. Sun DQ, Carson KA, Raza SM, et al. The radiosurgical treatment of arteriovenous malformations: obliteration, morbidities, and performance status. Int J Radiat Oncol Biol Phys 2011;80(2): 354–61.

37. Spetzler RF, Martin NA. A proposed grading system for arteriovenous-malformations. J Neurosurg 1986; 65(4):476–83.

38. Wegner RE, Oysul K, Pollock BE, et al. A modified radiosurgery-based arteriovenous malformation grading scale and its correlation with outcomes. Int J Radiat Oncol Biol Phys 2011;79(4):1147–50.

39. Ogilvy C, Stieg P, Awad I, et al. AHA Scientific Statement: recommendations for the management of intracranial arteriovenous malformations: a statement for healthcare professionals from a special writing group of the Stroke Council, American Stroke Association. Stroke 2001;32:1458–71.

40. Davidson AS, Morgan MK. How safe is arteriovenous malformation surgery? A prospective, observational study of surgery as first-line treatment for brain arteriovenous malformations. Neurosurgery 2010;66(3):498–504.

41. Pikus HJ, Beach ML, Harbaugh RE. Microsurgical treatment of arteriovenous malformations: analysis and comparison with stereotactic radiosurgery. J Neurosurg 1998;88(4):641–6.

42. Friedman WA, Bova FJ, Bollampally S, et al. Analysis of factors predictive of success or complications in arteriovenous malformation radiosurgery. Neurosurgery 2003;52(2):296–307.

43. Starke RM, Komotar RJ, Hwang BY, et al. A comprehensive review of radiosurgery for cerebral arteriovenous malformations: outcomes,

predictive factors, and grading scales. Stereotact Funct Neurosurg 2008;86(3):191–9.

44. Pollock BE, Flickinger JC, Chang SD, et al. Modification of the radiosurgery-based arteriovenous malformation grading system. Neurosurgery 2008;63(2):239–43.

45. Chang SD, Marcellus ML, Marks MP, et al. Multimodality treatment of giant intracranial arteriovenous malformations. Neurosurgery 2003;53(1):1–11.

46. Kim HY, Chang WS, Kim DJ, et al. Gamma Knife surgery for large cerebral arteriovenous malformations. J Neurosurg 2010;113:2–8.

47. Kelly ME, Guzman R, Sinclair J, et al. Multimodality treatment of posterior fossa arteriovenous malformations. J Neurosurg 2008;108(6):1152–61.

48. Niazi TN, Klimo P, Anderson RCE, et al. Diagnosis and management of arteriovenous malformations in children. Neurosurg Clin N Am 2010;21(3):443–56.

49. Mirza B, Monsted A, Harding J, et al. Stereotactic radiotherapy and radiosurgery in pediatric patients: analysis of indications and outcome. Childs Nerv Syst 2010;26(12):1785–93.

50. Zadeh G, Andrade-Souza YM, Tsao MN, et al. Pediatric arteriovenous malformation: University of Toronto experience using stereotactic radiosurgery. Childs Nerv Syst 2007;23(2):195–9.

51. Kiyosue H, Hori Y, Okahara M, et al. Treatment of intracranial dural arteriovenous fistulas: current strategies based on location and hemodynamics, and alternative techniques of transcatheter embolization. Radiographics 2004;24(6):1637–53.

52. Saraf R, Shrivastava M, Kumar N, et al. Embolization of cranial dural arteriovenous fistulae with Onyx: indications, techniques, and outcomes. Indian J Radiol Imaging 2010;20(1):26–33.

53. Yang HC, Kano H, Kondziolka D, et al. Stereotactic radiosurgery with or without embolization for intracranial dural arteriovenous fistulas. Neurosurgery 2010;67(5):1276–83.

54. Yeh PS, Wu TC, Tzeng WS, et al. Endovascular angioplasty and stent placement in venous hypertension related to dural arteriovenous fistulas and venous sinus thrombosis. Clin Neurol Neurosurg 2010;112(2):167–71.

55. Cognard C, Casasco A, Toevi M, et al. Dural arteriovenous fistulas as a cause of intracranial hypertension due to impairment of cranial venous outflow. J Neurol Neurosurg Psychiatr 1998;65(3):308–16.

56. Pollock BE, Flickinger JC, Lunsford LD, et al. Factors associated with successful arteriovenous malformation radiosurgery. Neurosurgery 1998; 42(6):1239–44.

57. Flickinger JC, Kondziolka D, Maitz AH, et al. An analysis of the dose-response for arteriovenous malformation radiosurgery and other factors affecting obliteration. Radiother Oncol 2002;63(3): 347–54.

58. Yashar P, Amar A, Giannotta S, et al. Cerebral arteriovenous malformations: issues of the interplay between stereotactic radiosurgery and endovascular surgical therapy. World Neurosurg 2011;75 638–47.

59. Natarajan SK, Born D, Ghodke B, et al. Histopathological changes in brain arteriovenous malformations after embolization using Onyx or N-butyl cyanoacrylate Laboratory investigation. J Neurosurg 2009; 111(1):105–13.

60. Akakin A, Ozkan A, Akgun E, et al. Endovascular treatment increases but Gamma Knife radiosurgery decreases angiogenic activity of arteriovenous malformations: an in vivo experimental study using a rat cornea model. Neurosurgery 2010;66(1):121–9.

61. Spetzler RF, Hargraves RW, McCormick PW, et al. Relationship of perfusion-pressure and size to risk of hemorrhage from arteriovenous-malformations. J Neurosurg 1992;76(6):918–23.

62. Inoue HK, Ohye C. Hemorrhage risks and obliteration rates of arteriovenous malformations after gamma knife radiosurgery. J Neurosurg 2002;97: 474–6.

63. Zipfel GJ, Bradshaw P, Bova FJ, et al. Do the morphological characteristics of arteriovenous malformations affect the results of radiosurgery? J Neurosurg 2004;101(3):393–401.

64. Andrade-Souza YM, Zadeh G, Ramani M, et al. Testing the radiosurgery-based arteriovenous malformation score and the modified Spetzler-Martin grading system to predict radiosurgical outcome. J Neurosurg 2005;103(4):642–8.

65. Borden JA, Wu JK, Shucart WA. A proposed classification for spinal and cranial dural arteriovenous fistulous malformations and implications for treatment. J Neurosurg 1995;82(2):166–79.

66. Cognard C, Gobin YP, Pierot L, et al. Cerebral dural arteriovenous-fistulas clinical and angiographic correlation with a revised classification of venous drainage. Radiology 1995;194(3):671–80.

67. Maruyama K, Kawahara N, Shin M, et al. The risk of hemorrhage after radiosurgery for cerebral arteriovenous malformations. N Engl J Med 2005;352(2): 146–53.

68. Pollock BE, Flickinger JC, Lunsford LD, et al. Hemorrhage risk after stereotactic radiosurgery of cerebral arteriovenous malformations. Neurosurgery 1996;38(4):652–9.

69. Zabel-du Bois A, Milker-Zabel S, Huber P, et al. Risk of hemorrhage and obliteration rates of LINAC-based radiosurgery for cerebral arteriovenous malformations treated after prior partial embolisation. Int J Radiat Oncol Biol Phys 2006; 66(3):2537.

70. Chang JH, Chang JW, Park YG, et al. Factors related to complete occlusion of arteriovenous

malformations after Gamma Knife radiosurgery. J Neurosurg 2000;93:96–101.

71. Pollock BE, Kondziolka D, Flickinger JC, et al. Magnetic resonance imaging: an accurate method to evaluate arteriovenous malformations after stereotactic radiosurgery. J Neurosurg 1996; 85(6):1044–9.

72. Karlsson B, Lax I, Soderman M. Can the probability for obliteration after radiosurgery for arteriovenous malformations be accurately predicted? Int J Radiat Oncol Biol Phys 1999;43(2):313–9.

73. Cohen-Gadol AA, Pollock BE. Radiosurgery for arteriovenous malformations in children. J Neurosurg 2006;104(6):388–91.

74. Buis DR, Dirven CM, Lagerwaard FJ, et al. Radiosurgery of brain arteriovenous malformations in children. J Neurol 2008;255(4):551–60.

75. Gerszten PC, Adelson PD, Kondziolka D, et al. Seizure outcome in children treated for arteriovenous malformations using Gamma Knife radiosurgery. Pediatr Neurosurg 1996;24(3):139–44.

76. Vernimmen F, Slabbert JP, Wilson JA, et al. Stereotactic proton beam therapy for intracranial arteriovenous malformations. Int J Radiat Oncol Biol Phys 2005;62(1):44–52.

77. Pan D, Chung W, Guo W, et al. Stereotactic radiosurgery for the treatment of dural arteriovenous fistulas involving the transverse-sigmoid sinus. J Neurosurg 2002;96:823–9.

78. Friedman JA, Pollock BE, Nichols DA, et al. Results of combined stereotactic radiosurgery and transarterial embolization for dural arteriovenous fistulas of the transverse and sigmoid sinuses. J Neurosurg 2001;94(6):886–91.

79. Xiao FR, Gorgulho AA, Lin CS, et al. Treatment of giant cerebral arteriovenous malformation: hypofractionated stereotactic radiation as the first stage. Neurosurgery 2010;67(5):1253–9.

80. Friedman WA, Blatt DL, Bova FJ, et al. The risk of hemorrhage after radiosurgery for arteriovenous malformations. J Neurosurg 1996;84(6):912–9.

81. Fabrikant JI, Levy RP, Steinberg GK, et al. Heavy-charged-particle radiosurgery for intracranial arteriovenous-malformations. Stereotact Funct Neurosurg 1991;57(1–2):50–63.

82. Colombo F, Pozza F, Chierego G, et al. Linear-accelerator radiosurgery of cerebral arteriovenous-malformations: an update. Neurosurgery 1994; 34(1):14–21.

83. Pollock BE, Lunsford LD, Kondziolka D, et al. Patient outcomes after stereotaxic radiosurgery for operable arteriovenous-malformations. Neurosurgery 1994;35(1):1–7.

84. Karlsson B, Lindquist C, Kihlstrom L, et al. Gamma-Knife surgery for AVM offers partial protection from hemorrhage prior to obliteration. J Neurosurg 1995; 82(2):A345.

85. Karlsson B, Lindquist C, Steiner L. Effect of Gamma Knife surgery on the risk of rupture prior to AVM obliteration. Minim Invasive Neurosurg 1996;39(1):21–7.

86. Flickinger JC, Kondziolka D, Pollock BE, et al. Complications from arteriovenous malformation radiosurgery: multivariate analysis and risk modeling. Int J Radiat Oncol Biol Phys 1997;38(3):485–90.

87. Flickinger JC, Kondziolka D, Maitz AH, et al. Analysis of neurological sequelae from radiosurgery of arteriovenous malformations: how location affects outcome. Int J Radiat Oncol Biol Phys 1998;40(2): 273–8.

88. Flickinger JC, Kondziolka D, Lunsford LD, et al. Development of a model to predict permanent symptomatic postradiosurgery injury for arteriovenous malformation patients. Int J Radiat Oncol Biol Phys 2000;46(5):1143–8.

89. Flickinger JC, Kondziolka D, Lunsford LD, et al. A multi-institutional analysis of complication outcomes after arteriovenous malformation radiosurgery. Int J Radiat Oncol Biol Phys 1999;44(1):67–74.

90. Sirin S, Kondziolka D, Niranjan A, et al. Prospective staged volume radiosurgery for large arteriovenous malformations: indications and outcomes in otherwise untreatable patients. Neurosurgery 2006;58(1):17–26.

91. Chung WY, Shiau CY, Wu HM, et al. Staged radiosurgery for extra-large cerebral arteriovenous malformations: method, implementation, and results. J Neurosurg 2008;109:65–72.

92. Asgari S, Bassiouni H, Gizewski E, et al. AVM resection after radiation therapy-clinico-morphological features and microsurgical results. Neurosurg Rev 2010;33(1):53–60.

93. Veznedaroglu E, Andrews DW, Benitez RP, et al. Fractionated stereotactic radiotherapy for the treatment of large arteriovenous malformations with or without previous partial embolization. Neurosurgery 2004;55(3):519–30.

94. Qi XS, Schultz CJ, Li XA. Possible fractionated regimens for image-guided intensity-modulated radiation therapy of large arteriovenous malformations. Phys Med Biol 2007;52:5667–82.

95. Hall EJ, Brenner DJ. The radiobiology of radiosurgery: rationale for different treatment regimes for AVMs and malignancies. Int J Radiat Oncol Biol Phys 1993;25(2):381–5.

96. Douglas JG, Goodkin R. Treatment of arteriovenous malformations using Gamma Knife surgery: the experience at the University of Washington from 2000 to 2005. J Neurosurg 2008;109:51–6.

97. Back AG, Vollmer D, Zeck O, et al. Retrospective analysis of unstaged and staged Gamma Knife surgery with and without preceding embolization for the treatment of arteriovenous malformations. J Neurosurg 2008;109:57–64.

98. Blamek S, Tarnawski R, Miszczyk L. LINAC-based stereotactic radiosurgery for brain arteriovenous malformations. Clin Oncol (R Coll Radiol) 2011; 23(8):525–31.

99. Raffa SJ, Chi YY, Bova FJ, et al. Validation of the radiosurgery-based arteriovenous malformation score in a large linear accelerator radiosurgery experience. J Neurosurg 2009;111(4):832–9.

100. Murray G, Brau RA. 10-year experience of radiosurgical treatment for cerebral arteriovenous malformations: a perspective from a series with large malformations. J Neurosurg 2011;115(2): 337–46.

101. Zabel-Du Bois A, Milker-Zabel S, Huber P, et al. Stereotactic LINAC-based radiosurgery in the treatment of cerebral arteriovenous malformations located deep, involving corpus callosum, motor cortex, or brainstem. Int J Radiat Oncol Biol Phys 2006;64(4):1044–8.

102. Pollock BE, Gorman DA, Brown PD. Radiosurgery for arteriovenous malformations of the basal ganglia, thalamus, and brainstem. J Neurosurg 2004;100(2):210–4.

103. Maruyama K, Kondziolka D, Niranjan A, et al. Stereotactic radiosurgery for brainstem arteriovenous malformations: factors affecting outcome. J Neurosurg 2004;100(3):407–13.

104. Kurita H, Kawamoto S, Sasaki T, et al. Results of radiosurgery for brain stem arteriovenous malformations. J Neurol Neurosurg Psychiatr 2000;68(5): 563–70.

105. Kiran NAS, Kale SS, Kasliwal MK, et al. Gamma Knife radiosurgery for arteriovenous malformations of basal ganglia, thalamus and brainstem: a retrospective study comparing the results with that for AVMs at other intracranial locations. Acta Neurochir (Wien) 2009;151(12):1575–82.

106. Javalkar V, Pillai P, Vannemreddy P, et al. Gamma Knife radiosurgery for arteriovenous malformations located in eloquent regions of the brain. Neurol India 2009;57(5):617–21.

107. Andrade-Souza YM, Zadeh G, Scora D, et al. Radiosurgery for basal ganglia internal capsule, and thalamus arteriovenous malformation: clinical outcome. Neurosurgery 2005;56(1):56–63.

108. Zabel-Du Bois A, Milker-Zabel S, Huber P, et al. Pediatric cerebral arteriovenous malformations: the role of stereotactic LINAC-based radiosurgery. Int J Radiat Oncol Biol Phys 2006;65(4):1206–11.

109. Yeon JY, Shin HJ, Kim JS, et al. Clinico-radiological outcomes following Gamma Knife radiosurgery for pediatric arteriovenous malformations. Childs Nerv Syst 2011;27(7):1109–19.

110. Levy EI, Niranjan A, Thompson TP, et al. Radiosurgery for childhood intracranial arteriovenous malformations. Neurosurgery 2000;47(4):834–41.

111. Reyns N, Blond S, Gauvrit JY, et al. Role of radiosurgery in the management of cerebral arteriovenous malformations in the pediatric age group: data from a 100-patient series. Neurosurgery 2007;60(2):268–76.

112. Yen CP, Monteith SJ, Nguyen JH, et al. Gamma Knife surgery for arteriovenous malformations in children. J Neurosurg Pediatr 2010;6(5):426–34.

113. Smyth MD, Sneed PK, Ciricillo SF, et al. Stereotactic radiosurgery for pediatric intracranial arteriovenous malformations: the University of California at San Francisco experience. J Neurosurg 2002; 97(1):48–55.

114. Maity A, Shu HK, Tan JE, et al. Treatment of pediatric intracranial arteriovenous malformations with linear-accelerator-based stereotactic radiosurgery: the University of Pennsylvania experience. Pediatr Neurosurg 2004;40(5):207–14.

# Occlusive Hyperemia Versus Normal Perfusion Pressure Breakthrough after Treatment of Cranial Arteriovenous Malformations

Brad E. Zacharia, MD[a],*, Samuel Bruce, BA[a],
Geoffrey Appelboom, MD[a], E. Sander Connolly Jr, MD[b]

**KEYWORDS**

- Vascular malformation • Arteriovenous malformation
- Perfusion pressure breakthrough • Occlusive hyperemia

Cerebral vascular malformations occur in 0.1% to 4.0% of the general population.[1] Arteriovenous malformations (AVMs), vascular lesions characterized by direct connections between feeding arteries and draining veins without an intervening capillary network, are some of the most dangerous congenital vascular malformations, and occur in approximately 15 of every 100,000 adults.[2] Patients with AVMs tend to present symptomatically between the ages of 10 and 40, most commonly as a result of intracranial hemorrhage.[3] Complete obliteration of the AVM nidus, which can be accomplished by microsurgical resection, endovascular embolization, or radiosurgery, alone or in combination, eliminates the risk of hemorrhage from these lesions. An infrequent but potentially devastating consequence following excision or occlusion of an intracranial AVM involves hemorrhage into the surrounding parenchyma or edema of the surrounding parenchyma. Two hypotheses, normal perfusion pressure breakthrough (NPPB) and occlusive hyperemia,

prevail in the literature regarding postoperative hemorrhage following AVM resection. Since the occlusive hyperemia hypothesis was first postulated in 1993, a debate has persisted within the cerebrovascular community.[4] This article discusses recent advances in cerebrovascular imaging and analysis that have allowed a more complete evaluation of intracerebral changes following AVM resection.

## CEREBRAL HEMODYNAMICS

Cerebral perfusion pressure (CPP) is the net pressure gradient causing blood flow to the brain, and it is defined as the mean arterial pressure (MAP) minus the intracranial pressure (ICP). Cerebral blood flow (CBF) is dependent on both perfusion pressure and cerebrovascular resistance (CVR), such that:

$$CBF = CPP/CVR$$

Disclosures: None of the authors have a conflict of interest.
Source of Funding: Department of Neurologic Surgery.
[a] Department of Neurological Surgery, Columbia University, 630 West 168th Street, Room 5-454, New York, NY 10032, USA
[b] Department of Neurological Surgery, Columbia University, 710 West 168th Street, New York, NY 10032, USA
* Corresponding author.
E-mail address: bez2103@columbia.edu

Neurosurg Clin N Am 23 (2012) 147–151
doi:10.1016/j.nec.2011.09.005
1042-3680/12/$ – see front matter © 2012 Elsevier Inc. All rights reserved.

In a single vessel level, cerebral blood flow can be summarized according to Hagen-Poiseuille's formula (**Fig. 1**). The magnitude of blood flow is proportional to the vessel resistance, and the blood velocity is directly proportional to the pressure difference along the blood vessel. The resistance in a vessel is inversely related to the fourth power of the vessel diameter. Thus even marginal changes of the vessel's radius result in significant alterations of resistance. The ability of intracranial vessels to alter their radius in response to alterations in CPP is termed cerebrovascular autoregulation and is an essential mechanism by which the brain maintains CBF in the face of changes in systemic blood pressure or ICP.

## BASIC AVM PHYSIOLOGY

A basic knowledge of flow and pressure alterations induced by AVMs is important in understanding the mechanisms dictating postoperative complications following AVM resection. Studies regarding flow in and around AVMs, however, are controversial. While some believe that AVMs lead to impaired autoregulation, others contend that loss of autoregulation may be the root cause of AVM formation. For instance, flow regulation can be impaired when perfusion pressures are above or below the limits of autoregulation. Such is the case with venous hypertension, which is often seen in AVMs. The idea of autoregulatory dysfunction has become common thinking in the physiology of AVMs, yet studies have consistently demonstrated preserved $CO_2$ responsiveness both before and after AVM resection.[5,6] An alternative hypothesis, adaptive autoregulatory displacement, contends that vascular territories adjacent to AVMs shift the autoregulatory curve to the left, thus placing the lower pressure limit at a level lower than that postulated for the normal brain.[7]

# *Hagen-Poiseuille's formula*

Q = flow
Δ P = Pressure difference
r = radius
L = length of the tube
η = viscosity

$$Q = \Delta P \; \pi \, r^4 / 8 \, L \, \eta$$

**Fig. 1.** Hagen-Poiseuille's formula demonstrates the key concepts affecting blood flow through the cerebral vasculature.

Brain AVMs are characterized by low resistance within the nidus secondary to the lack of an interposing capillary bed, thus depriving surrounding parenchyma of blood flow. Vascular steal is a phenomenon often associated with AVMs.[5] Single-photon emission computed tomography (CT) studies have demonstrated decreased flow in areas surrounding the malformation. Local CBF measured on Xenon-CT has also demonstrated impairment in areas surrounding the AVM nidus with improvement following AVM resection.[8,9] Using magnetic resonance (MR) perfusion imaging, Guo and colleagues[10] demonstrated perinidal perfusion abnormalities within AVMs that gradually reversed following radiosurgery. Few individuals appear to suffer ischemic consequences as a result of steal, which may be explained by adaptive autoregulatory displacement.

## *Postresection Hemorrhage and Edema*

### *NPPB*

The pioneering hypothesis attempting to explain the phenomenon of postoperative hemorrhage and edema was offered by Spetzler and colleagues[4] in 1978. The hypothesis, termed normal perfusion pressure breakthrough (NPPB), suggests that the parenchyma surrounding a high-flow AVM is chronically hypoperfused; as a result, it has impaired autoregulation, rendering it vulnerable to the normal perfusion pressure likely to be seen following AVM resection. Thus, following removal of an AVM, the local capillary beds and arterioles in the remaining normal parenchyma experience increased perfusion but lack the ability to vasoconstrict and autoregulate. This could lead, in some cases, to hyperemia, compromise of the capillary beds, and resultant edema and/or hemorrhage.

### *Occlusive hyperemia*

For more than a decade NPPB remained the primary explanation for postoperative hemorrhage and edema following AVM resection. An alternative explanation termed occlusive hyperemia was offered by Al-Rodhan and colleagues[11] in 1993 based on their retrospective review of 295 operative AVM cases and mounting evidence against the NPPB hypothesis. Multiple studies before 1993 had demonstrated decreased perinidal CBF that normalized following excision, suggesting that there was perhaps some mechanism maintaining CBF within the normal range despite increased perfusion pressures.[9,12,13] The ability to autoregulate was tested with $CO_2$ reactivity by multiple groups that almost universally demonstrated restoration of normal reactivity after excision.[13-16] The authors concluded that hemorrhage and edema associated with resection of high-flow AVMs was the result of two interrelated mechanisms. First, stagnant arterial flow in former AVM feeders worsens the existing hypoperfusion and ischemia. Postoperative angiograms have frequently demonstrated reduced or stagnant arterial flow in former AVM-feeding vessels, often leading to retrograde thrombosis.[16–19] Al-Rodhan attributed this stagnation to increased resistance to flow, endothelial abnormalities, and a reflex vasoconstriction compensating for normal or increased perfusion pressures.

Second, obstruction of the venous outflow of surrounding parenchyma leads to passive hyperemia and further arterial stagnation, the end result of which is cerebral edema and possible hemorrhage. Al-Rodhan cites prior studies demonstrating abnormalities of the venous system in AVMs including stenosis, agenesis, or occlusion of major venous sinuses.[14,20,21]

Barnett and colleagues observed rapid reduction in elevated draining vein pressure following excision, changes that likely predispose to increased incidence of thrombotic occlusion.[11,14]

## The Current Debate

The basic assumption of NPPB is that a dramatic increase in perinidal pressure reroutes flow toward territories incapable of vasoconstriction in response to the increase in CBF, and several earlier studies support this hypothesis.[13–15,22–24] For example, Muraszko and colleagues[25] tested resected AVM samples with vasoactive substances in vitro; 4 out 24 AVMs were considered nonreactive and lacked spontaneous activity. They found that patients with nonreactive vessels in vitro developed more frequent postoperative edema and hemorrhage. Moreover, using orthogonal polarization spectral (OPS) imaging in 2 patients, Pennings and colleagues[26] assessed arteriolar pulsatility before surgical resection of an AVM. While visualizing microvessel flow, they observed a significant decrease in arteriolar pulsatility immediately after AVM exclusion. Furthermore, they were also able to show a drastic increase in microvascular flow in the perinidal brain tissue following surgery. In 1997, Chyatte used transcranial Doppler ultrasound in conjunction with acetazolamide and $CO_2$ to challenge vessel reactivity in patients before AVM surgery. While vasomotor paralysis was observed in only 2 of the 35 patients, those patients went on to develop postoperative edema/hemorrhage following surgical resection.[27] De Salles and colleagues[22] used angiographic and transcranial doppler ultrasound imaging and also demonstrated impaired vasoreactivity in response to hyperventilation in AVM feeding vessels.

Though the previously mentioned studies using various methodologies have offered evidence in support of NPPB, the hypothesis has been the subject of significant controversy. More recent investigations have contradicted many aspects of the NPPB hypothesis, casting doubt on the link between impaired autoregulation and postoperative complications.[28] As discussed previously, multiple studies demonstrated intact $CO_2$ vasoreactivity following AVM resection.[13–16] Young and colleagues[29] demonstrated improved perfusion in the ipsilateral hemisphere following resection, but no increase in CBF in response to increasing MAP, suggesting intact autoregulation. They demonstrated this phenomenon both in cases without postoperative complications and in those with presumed NPPB. The culmination of these findings led Young and colleagues to postulate adaptive autoregulation as a possible explanation for the hemodynamic alterations seen in AVMs.[6,24,29] A condition of the NPPB hypothesis is that complications occur adjacent to the malformation, as these are the areas placed under chronic stress from the AVM. Barnett and colleagues demonstrated that the worst vascular steal effect actually occurs 2 to 4 cm distal to the malformation, and Young and colleagues demonstrated global increases in CBF following resection, suggesting that focal mechanisms may not predominate.[14,30]

Recent studies have also shed doubt on the mechanisms implicated in the occlusive hyperemia hypothesis. The occlusive hyperemia hypothesis suggests that arterial stagnation leads to hypoperfusion and ischemia in surrounding brain tissue. Meyer and colleagues first noted that arterial stagnation is a common observation following AVM resection. They also noted that stagnating flow is often seen in former feeding arteries, but not their smaller branches. Additionally, they noted that slow transit within the vessels likely reflects a reduction in flow velocity rather than a linear reduction in blood flow. Meyer and colleagues[31] went on to show that postoperative brain tissue oxygenation levels are highest in patients with excessive angiographically confirmed stagnation of flow. Asgari and colleagues[32] confirmed these significant elevations in oxygen saturation in patients with postoperative hyperemic complications, and they felt this finding was significant enough to dispute the possibility of a venous mechanism for postoperative hemorrhagic complications.

As an increasing number of AVMs are being treated with radiosurgery, reports are slowly beginning to come out of similar hemorrhagic complications after treatment. Pollock described 2 patients with abrupt neurologic deterioration within months of AVM radiosurgery, and in both instances, there was radiographic evidence of venous outflow occlusion.[33] Chapman and colleagues[34] followed this with a report of 2 patients who suffered edema and hemorrhagic complications after radiosurgery and demonstrated evidence of venous occlusion. Chapman concluded that a venous occlusive mechanism was likely causative in all 4 cases. Celix and colleagues[35] added further to the evidence regarding postradiosurgery venous occlusion in a 57-year-old man who experienced hemorrhage within 9 days of treatment and had radiographic evidence of a thrombus in the primary draining vein.

## SUMMARY

The pathophysiology underlying the swelling, hemorrhage, and edema that can manifest after AVM resection remains a matter of debate. Throughout the literature, one can find evidence in favor and against the two prevailing hypotheses used to explain postoperative hemorrhage and edema following AVM obliteration, namely NPPB and occlusive hyperemia. As new advances develop in imaging modalities, analysis of oxygenation and CBF, and real-time probing of interstitial biochemical makeup using multimodality monitoring and microdialysis, the mechanism responsible for postoperative complications will continue to be revisited. The authors believe that ultimately these hypotheses are not mutually exclusive and perhaps exist in a spectrum of hemodynamic alteration following AVM resection. Understanding the characteristics of an individual malformation will be crucial in understanding the propensity for postoperative complications and how to optimize treatment to prevent these complications.

## REFERENCES

1. el-Gohary EG, Tomita T, Gutierrez FA, et al. Angiographically occult vascular malformations in childhood. Neurosurgery 1987;20:759.
2. Al-Shahi R, Fang JS, Lewis SC, et al. Prevalence of adults with brain arteriovenous malformations: a community based study in Scotland using capture–recapture analysis. J Neurol Neurosurg Psychiatry 2002;73:547.
3. Fullerton HJ, Achrol AS, Johnston SC, et al. Long-term hemorrhage risk in children versus adults with brain arteriovenous malformations. Stroke 2005;36: 2099.
4. Spetzler RF, Wilson CB, Weinstein P, et al. Normal perfusion pressure breakthrough theory. Clin Neurosurg 1978;25:651.
5. Moftakhar P, Hauptman JS, Malkasian D, et al. Cerebral arteriovenous malformations. Part 2: physiology. Neurosurg Focus 2009;26:E11.
6. Young WL, Pile-Spellman J, Prohovnik I, et al. Evidence for adaptive autoregulatory displacement in hypotensive cortical territories adjacent to arteriovenous malformations. Columbia University AVM Study Project. Neurosurgery 1994;34:601.
7. Kader A, Young WL. The effects of intracranial arteriovenous malformations on cerebral hemodynamics. Neurosurg Clin N Am 1996;7:767.
8. Homan RW, Devous MD Sr, Stokely EM, et al. Quantification of intracerebral steal in patients with arteriovenous malformation. Arch Neurol 1986;43:779.
9. Okabe T, Meyer JS, Okayasu H, et al. Xenon-enhanced CT CBF measurements in cerebral AVMs before and after excision. Contribution to pathogenesis and treatment. J Neurosurg 1983;59:21.
10. Guo WY, Wu YT, Wu HM, et al. Toward normal perfusion after radiosurgery: perfusion MR imaging with independent component analysis of brain arteriovenous malformations. AJNR Am J Neuroradiol 2004; 25:1636.
11. al-Rodhan NR, Sundt TM Jr, Piepgras DG, et al. Occlusive hyperemia: a theory for the hemodynamic complications following resection of intracerebral arteriovenous malformations. J Neurosurg 1993;78:167.
12. Batjer HH, Devous MD Sr, Seibert GB, et al. Intracranial arteriovenous malformation: relationship between clinical factors and surgical complications. Neurosurgery 1989;24:75.
13. Young WL, Prohovnik I, Ornstein E, et al. The effect of arteriovenous malformation resection on cerebrovascular reactivity to carbon dioxide. Neurosurgery 1990;27:257.
14. Barnett GH, Little JR, Ebrahim ZY, et al. Cerebral circulation during arteriovenous malformation operation. Neurosurgery 1987;20:836.
15. Batjer HH, Devous MD Sr, Meyer YJ, et al. Cerebrovascular hemodynamics in arteriovenous malformation complicated by normal perfusion pressure breakthrough. Neurosurgery 1988;22:503.
16. Hassler W, Steinmetz H. Cerebral hemodynamics in angioma patients: an intraoperative study. J Neurosurg 1987;67:822.
17. Miyasaka Y, Yada K, Ohwada T, et al. Retrograde thrombosis of feeding arteries after removal of arteriovenous malformations. J Neurosurg 1990; 72:540.
18. Petty GW, Massaro AR, Tatemichi TK, et al. Transcranial Doppler ultrasonographic changes after treatment for arteriovenous malformations. Stroke 1990; 21:260.
19. Solomon RA, Stein BM. Surgical management of arteriovenous malformations that follow the tentorial ring. Neurosurgery 1986;18:708.

20. Nornes H, Grip A. Hemodynamic aspects of cerebral arteriovenous malformations. J Neurosurg 1980;53:456.

21. Vinuela F, Nombela L, Roach MR, et al. Stenotic and occlusive disease of the venous drainage system of deep brain AVMs. J Neurosurg 1985;63:180.

22. De Salles AA, Manchola I. $CO_2$ reactivity in arteriovenous malformations of the brain: a transcranial Doppler ultrasound study. J Neurosurg 1994;80:624.

23. Massaro AR, Young WL, Kader A, et al. Characterization of arteriovenous malformation feeding vessels by carbon dioxide reactivity. AJNR Am J Neuroradiol 1994;15:55.

24. Young WL, Solomon RA, Prohovnik I, et al. 133Xe blood flow monitoring during arteriovenous malformation resection: a case of intraoperative hyperperfusion with subsequent brain swelling. Neurosurgery 1988;22:765.

25. Muraszko K, Wang HH, Pelton G, et al. A study of the reactivity of feeding vessels to arteriovenous malformations: correlation with clinical outcome. Neurosurgery 1990;26:190.

26. Pennings FA, Ince C, Bouma GJ. Continuous real-time visualization of the human cerebral microcirculation during arteriovenous malformation surgery using orthogonal polarization spectral imaging. Neurosurgery 2006;59:167.

27. Chyatte D. Normal pressure perfusion breakthrough after resection of arteriovenous malformation. J Stroke Cerebrovasc Dis 1997;6:130.

28. Alexander MD, Connolly ES, Meyers PM. Revisiting normal perfusion pressure breakthrough in light of hemorrhage-induced vasospasm. World J Radiol 2010;2:230.

29. Young WL, Kader A, Prohovnik I, et al. Pressure autoregulation is intact after arteriovenous malformation resection. Neurosurgery 1993;32:491.

30. Young WL, Kader A, Ornstein E, et al. Cerebral hyperemia after arteriovenous malformation resection is related to "breakthrough" complications but not to feeding artery pressure. The Columbia University Arteriovenous Malformation Study Project. Neurosurgery 1996;38:1085.

31. Meyer B, Urbach H, Schaller C, et al. Is stagnating flow in former feeding arteries an indication of cerebral hypoperfusion after resection of arteriovenous malformations? J Neurosurg 2001;95:36.

32. Asgari S, Rohrborn HJ, Engelhorn T, et al. Intraoperative measurement of cortical oxygen saturation and blood volume adjacent to cerebral arteriovenous malformations using near-infrared spectroscopy. Neurosurgery 2003;52:1298.

33. Pollock BE. Occlusive hyperemia: a radiosurgical phenomenon? Neurosurgery 2000;47:1178.

34. Chapman PH, Ogilvy CS, Loeffler JS. The relationship between occlusive hyperemia and complications associated with the radiosurgical treatment of arteriovenous malformations: report of two cases. Neurosurgery 2004;55:228.

35. Celix JM, Douglas JG, Haynor D, et al. Thrombosis and hemorrhage in the acute period following gamma knife surgery for arteriovenous malformation. Case report. J Neurosurg 2009;111:124.

# Anesthesia Considerations and Intraoperative Monitoring During Surgery for Arteriovenous Malformations and Dural Arteriovenous Fistulas

Christina Miller, MD*, Marek Mirski, MD, PhD

## KEYWORDS

- Arteriovenous malformation • Dural arteriovenous fistula
- Intraoperative monitoring • Anesthesia

## CEREBRAL VASCULAR PHYSIOLOGY OF ARTERIOVENOUS MALFORMATIONS AND DURAL ARTERIOVENOUS FISTULAS

Brain arteriovenous malformations (AVMs) are anatomically characterized by a tangle of thin-walled vessels that connect the high-pressure arterial circulation to the low-pressure venous system, without an intervening capillary network. Dural arteriovenous fistulas (DAVFs), by comparison, are simpler lesions typically described as either direct or indirect. Direct DAVFs (nonsinus type) have a well-defined arteriovenous shunt and involve only a few vessels. Indirect DAVFs (sinus type) are more complex lesions with numerous, small arterial feeders that travel in the dura and drain into a venous sinus. DAVFs are found outside the pia and involve the dura. The abnormal vasculature of AVMs and, to a lesser degree DAVFs, has several major physiologic effects. Steal phenomenon results when there is high flow across a low-resistance shunt, directly from arterial to venous circulation. The shunt results in decreased pressure in feeding arteries (lower than systemic pressure) and elevated pressure in draining veins. The arterial feeders and venous drainers of the AVM are derived from normal cerebral circulation, and the normal brain tissue adjacent to the nidus that they supply suffers from reduced cerebral perfusion pressure (CPP). Giant AVMs or DAVFs can steal flow from remote vascular territories.[1] The degree of hypotension may result in cerebral blood flow that falls below the normal range of autoregulation.[2] However, studies suggest that vascular reactivity to $CO_2$ is preserved, indicating intact autoregulation that has been shifted to the left rather than completely abolished.[3] The tissue adjacent to the AVM has a lower tissue $Po_2$ than normal, but normal pH and $Pco_2$, suggesting an adaptive capillary exchange mechanism to maintain normal $CO_2$ clearance despite chronic hypoxia. During AVM

Department of Anesthesiology and Critical Care Medicine, Johns Hopkins University School of Medicine, 600 North Wolfe Street, Baltimore, MD 21287, USA
* Corresponding author.
E-mail address: cmill106@jhmi.edu

Neurosurg Clin N Am 23 (2012) 153–164
doi:10.1016/j.nec.2011.09.014
1042-3680/12/$ – see front matter © 2012 Elsevier Inc. All rights reserved.

resection, the tissue $PO_2$ and pH increase while the $Pco_2$ falls.[4] Another type of pathophysiology characteristic of AVMs is the development of diffuse bleeding and brain edema intraoperatively or postoperatively. One proposed mechanism, normal perfusion pressure breakthrough (NPPB), postulates that elimination of the AVM shunt redistributes blood flow to vasculature accustomed to chronic hypotension.[5] The "occlusive hyperemia" hypothesis attributes brain edema to the occlusion of normal venous drainage of tissue adjacent to the AVM during surgery, resulting in vascular engorgement.[6] These phenomena are discussed in detail by Miller and Mirski elsewhere in this issue.

Although less has been reported regarding the pathophysiology of DAVFs, there seems to be less of a concern for physiologic steal and resetting of autoregulation than that which may occur in larger cortical AVMs. Likewise, there is less of an issue with perfusion "breakthrough" edema. However, resection attempts of large DAVFs still pose an anesthetic concern with respect to sudden acute blood loss, venous air embolism, and postoperative seizures. Hence, many of the major anesthetic considerations for resection of parenchymal AVMs are applicable to craniotomies for other indications such as DAVFs.

## MAIN ANESTHETIC CONSIDERATIONS
### Targeted Cerebral Perfusion Pressure

#### Normotension versus induced hypotension
Under normal physiologic conditions, cerebral blood flow (CBF) is controlled by autoregulation over a range of mean arterial pressures (MAPs), traditionally 50 to 150 mm Hg. The introduction of an AVM, which functions as a low-pressure, high-flow shunt, can result in arterial hypotension in territories adjacent to the AVM. Under conditions of chronic hypoperfusion, the lower limit of autoregulatory pressure range (LAR) may be less than normal (shifted to the left) (**Fig. 1**). At pressures below this lower limit, despite maximal vasodilation, these penumbral areas may become ischemic. Larger, more vascular AVMs place a more extensive penumbral area at risk for ischemia. The deliberate use of hypotension as a technique for minimizing blood loss prior to treatment of the AVM must be used with caution and serious consideration given to the impact of a further drop in pressure to a chronically hypoperfused area. If autoregulation is impaired because of chronic hypoperfusion, therapeutic interventions may result in an abnormal increase in CBF, hyperemia, cerebral edema, or hemorrhage. With progressive occlusion of the AVM and increase in

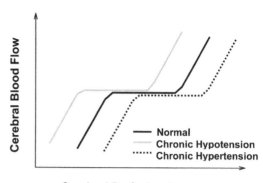

**Cerebral Perfusion Pressure**

**Fig. 1.** Normal blood pressure parameters for cerebral vascular autoregulation. Chronic hypotension secondary to AVM shunting causes the normal curve to shift to the left. Chronic hypertension results in the normal curve shifting to the right. (*From* Serrador JM, Wood SJ, Picot PA, et al. Effect of acute exposure to hypergravity (GX vs. GZ) on dynamic cerebral autoregulation. J Appl Physiol 2001;91(5):1987; with permission.)

perfusion pressure to the surrounding tissue, it may be beneficial to lower the mean arterial pressure to prevent hyperemia, and at the very least prevent elevation of the pressure above baseline.

#### Treatment of hypertension
Careful management of hemodynamic parameters is a consideration during general anesthesia for nearly any type of surgery, but avoidance of hemodynamic lability resulting in either ischemia or hyperemia is even more crucial with surgery for intracranial vascular malformations. Large variations in blood pressure are associated with induction of general anesthesia, direct laryngoscopy, placement of Mayfield pins, and surgical incision, and should be managed aggressively.

#### Required hypertension during ischemia
Certain interventions or complications of treatment for AVM may necessitate induced hypertension to prevent ischemia. The brain tissue adjacent to the AVM that is subject to chronic hypoperfusion may be exquisitely sensitive to interruption of normal blood flow. Thrombosis, embolization, compression from retraction, or temporary mechanical occlusion of feeding vessels may compromise already meager blood flow to penumbral areas, making may it necessary to increase CPP and promote flow through collateral means. Changes in the visual appearance of the brain tissue, attenuation of evoked potential signals, or poor or delayed flow seen on intraoperative angiography may alert the surgeon and anesthesiologist to the possibility that a higher pressure is required to perfuse vulnerable areas. Drugs with

α1-agonist effects such as phenylephrine, ephedrine, norepinephrine, and epinephrine do not alter CBF in primates and humans,[7] though they do cause cerebral vasoconstriction in other animal models. If autoregulation is intact, augmentation of MAP and thus CPP does not result in a change in CBF within the limits of autoregulation. In cases where the blood-brain barrier (BBB) is defective, norepinephrine may cause vasodilation. β-Adrenergic agonists in small doses have minimal effect on cerebral vasculature, but at higher doses can increase cerebral metabolic rate for $O_2$ ($CMRO_2$) with accompanying increase in CBF.

## Hemorrhage Risk

Postoperative intracerebral hemorrhage after excision of an AVM may be caused by insufficient hemostasis and/or inadequate blood pressure control, incomplete resection with residual AVM nidus, NPPB, or venous thrombosis.

## Blood product transfusion: packed red blood cells, fresh frozen plasma, platelets

The need for perioperative transfusion is affected by the patient's starting hematocrit, cardiovascular status, and intraoperative blood loss. Surgically induced blood loss is dependent on several important factors: the size and location of the AVM, surgical expertise, and history of preoperative embolization or radiotherapy to minimize the number and caliber of feeding vessels. Blood loss can also be influenced by operative patient position and intraoperative manipulation of blood pressure. In one retrospective, nonrandomized study, embolization was performed for AVM in 168 patients, 124 of whom had embolization as an adjunct to surgery. Thirty-one percent of the surgical patients required a blood transfusion with a mean of 1.4 units of packed red blood cells per surgical patient with a range of 0 to 18 units.[8] In cases where ongoing surgical blood loss is modest, transfusion of red cells, fresh frozen plasma (FFP), and platelets should be based on serial measures of hematocrit, coagulation studies, and platelet count and function, respectively. In the event of massive hemorrhage, current data from trauma literature supports a more empiric transfusion formulation with a high proportional target ratio of red cells/plasma/platelets of 1:1:1.[9] It is reasonable to have several units typed and crossed at the start of the case; if the AVM is complex or technically difficult to approach, blood loss may be sudden and massive, and a cooler of stored blood should be available in the room and checked in advance for immediate use.

The threshold for transfusion of red cells is a subject of long-standing debate. General guidelines from the American Society of Anesthesiologists (ASA) state that "transfusion is indicated if the hemoglobin concentration is less than 6 g/dL and not indicated if >10 g/dL."[10] However, it is readily accepted that such guidelines must be modified in cases of high-risk procedures where there may be ongoing and substantial blood loss, such as AVM resection. Many guidelines, in addition, promote the consideration of organ ischemia (especially cerebral), ongoing bleeding, intravascular volume status, and patient's risk factors in addition to the hemoglobin threshold.

Other considerations in addition to hemoglobin concentrations alone should assist in dictating optimal transfusion triggers during AVM resection surgery. Early canine studies, for example, demonstrated that hemodilution to a hematocrit of 30% resulted in limiting infarct volume following induction of focal cerebral ischemia as compared with either a higher or lower hematocrit.[11] Thus, this hematocrit level was thought to strike the optimal balance between oxygen-carrying capacity and hemorheology or blood viscosity by decreasing cerebrovascular resistance and enhancing cerebral perfusion. Without definitive clinical support, the 30% blood hematocrit goal has nonetheless been a relative standard in neurosurgical cases over many years. Additional evidence in support of a more generous hemoglobin level during AVM cases comes from studies demonstrating that ischemic areas of the brain often lose their capacity for vascular autoregulation, in which case viscosity has a more significant impact on cerebral perfusion. Dhar and colleagues[12] used positron emission topography scanning to demonstrate an increase in cerebral oxygen delivery and reduced oxygen extraction fraction after blood transfusion in patients with subarachnoid hemorrhage and a hemoglobin of less than 10 g/dL. When hemoglobin is less than 10 g/dL, the investigators concluded that the benefit of increased oxygen-carrying capacity outweighs the concern of increased viscosity, thereby increasing oxygen delivery and augmenting cerebral reserve.

There are additional infectious, immunologic, metabolic, and hemodynamic risks associated with transfusion, and the anesthesiology and neurosurgery teams must weigh all considerations in formulating their blood component targets. In light of the evidence presented it is reasonable, and also the authors' physiologic strategy, to use a transfusion threshold of hemoglobin less than 10 g/dL in the intraoperative and postoperative patient undergoing AVM resection. The risk of sudden hemorrhage invoking critical cerebral ischemia requires a more liberal strategy than a stable, critically ill, nonneurologic patient.

### Disseminated intravascular coagulation

Disseminated intravascular coagulation (DIC) is rare after an uncomplicated craniotomy. Cortical brain tissue has a high concentration of thrombo-plastins, and release of such compounds normally serves to stimulate coagulation. In certain patho-logic states such as traumatic brain injury, brain tumor, or extensive surgical manipulation, the extrinsic coagulation cascade may be robustly triggered, resulting in extensive clotting (mainly in the microcirculation), activation of fibrinolysis, consumption of platelets and coagulation factors, and subsequent bleeding. In 3164 patients who underwent primary craniotomy at the Mayo Clinic, the investigators estimate the incidence of devel-oping DIC within 72 hours of surgery to be between 0.13% and 0.44%, with a mortality rate ranging from 43% to 75%.[13] Treatment is aimed at reversing the underlying cause of DIC and trans-fusing platelets, FFP, or fibrinogen-rich cryopreci-pitate as indicated.

### Intraoperative Monitoring of Evoked Potentials

Intraoperative cortical mapping has been used for AVMs located in particularly eloquent regions, such as the language (under awake anesthesia) or motor (under general anesthesia) cortex to facil-itate its preservation.[14] Many commonly used anesthetic agents affect evoked potentials. All volatile anesthetics, and to a lesser extent high-dose opioids, benzodiazepines, and sedative-hypnotic agents (propofol), cause an increase in latency and decrease in amplitude, although the effect is dose dependent and likely minimal in neurologically intact patients during surgery under routine anesthetic requirements. Nitrous oxide has a more substantial effect, decreasing signal amplitude. Because motor evoked potentials are more sensitive to anesthetics than somatosensory evoked potentials, their employment may warrant the use of intravenous anesthetic agents in place of volatiles or nitrous oxide, but these consider-ations must be weighed with each anesthetic's effect on hemodynamics, cerebral metabolism and blood flow, and impact on postoperative neurologic assessment.

### Postoperative Neurologic Assessment

Postoperative neurologic assessment is of crucial importance following AVM resection, and the anesthesiologist must facilitate a smooth emer-gence from anesthesia in order for the patient to be thoroughly evaluated. A comprehensive preop-erative neurologic examination that documents any baseline deficits is obligatory. The anesthetic plan at the conclusion of the case should consist of rapidly titratable agents that permit fast recovery from general anesthesia; this can be achieved with a total intravenous anesthetic, vola-tile anesthetics, or a combination of agents. Drugs that may be helpful in this regard include nitrous oxide, fentanyl, and remifentanil. When intraopera-tive neuromonitoring signals are of concern, it is common practice to use multiple agents for main-tenance to minimize the impact of any single agent on signal strength.

## ADDITIONAL COMPLICATIONS AND RISKS

### Hyperperfusion Syndrome

Whether true hyperperfusion or NPPB occurs, the regions of the brain adjacent to the AVM experience profound hemodynamic alterations. Following the occlusion of feeder arteries, blood flow that was initially shunted through the low-resistance AVM is progressively diverted to neigh-boring brain tissue that previously experienced chronic relative hypoperfusion. The acute change in blood flow can result in hyperemia, edema, and punctate hemorrhages, due to local capillary breakthrough. Chronic hypoperfusion results in modified or impaired autoregulation, and a return to normal perfusion has a pathologic impact.

Intraoperatively, hyperperfusion syndrome can be caused by inadequate blood pressure control, occlusion of venous drainage before complete resection of arterial feeders, or insufficient hemo-static control of distended capillaries receiving arterial flow. Intraoperative hyperperfusion may be minimized by preoperative embolization. The risk of NPPB is higher with larger, high-flow AVMs, decreased flow through normal cerebral arteries, steal from remote vascular territories such as the vertebrobasilar or contralateral carotid system, extensive contribution from the external carotid artery, and progressive or fluctuating neurologic deficits thought to be due to ischemic rather than hemorrhagic etiology.[1] Attempts have been made using acetazolamide, a known cere-bral vasodilator, to evaluate vasoreactivity and changes in regional cerebral blood flow (rCBF) with various imaging modalities to predict risk of hyperemic complications. Several patterns emerged in regions adjacent to the AVM when compared with distant or contralateral regions: decreased, normal, and hyperaugmentation of rCBF. Areas of decreased augmentation (inter-preted as decreased cerebral reserve)[15] and excessively high augmentation (impaired vaso-constriction) both have been correlated with post-operative hyperemic complications.[16]

## Acute Venous Thrombosis

Spontaneous acute venous thrombosis associated with AVM is rare. Case reports illustrate progressive neurologic decline associated with AVMs and venous thrombosis in patients with hypercoagulability from prothrombin or Factor V Leiden mutations.[17,18] Interventions (surgical or radiosurgical) that result in incomplete resection of the AVM may be complicated by acute venous thrombosis of residual draining veins, venous congestion, brain edema, neurologic decline, and risk of hemorrhage.

## Acute Venous Air Embolism

Venous air embolism (VAE) is always a concern in intracranial surgery, especially when the patient is in a sitting position or in reverse Trendelenburg position.[19] In neurosurgical AVM cases, where potential exposure of venous drainage vessels to air is coupled with high-volume blood flow, substantial risk exists for VAE to occur (**Fig. 2**). There is one case report of a VAE resulting in pulmonary edema in an otherwise healthy 35-year-old patient undergoing craniotomy for AVM in the semi-sitting position.[20]

Precordial Doppler, placed along the right heart border over the right ventricular outflow tract, is the most sensitive noninvasive monitor, detecting as little as 0.05 mL/kg of air in dogs.[21] Hence, this technology is the method of choice by most neuroanesthesiologists for monitoring high-risk surgical cases. Once air embolism is suspected, the goals of treatment include eliminating the source of entrained air, minimizing the volume of the embolus, and hemodynamic support. Further

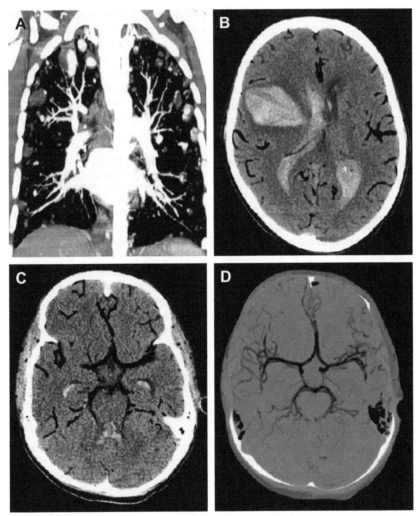

**Fig. 2.** (A–D) Massive cerebral air embolism as negative contrast angiogram. (*From* Andrade CS, Lucato LT, da Costa Leite C. Neurological picture. Massive fatal cerebral air embolism as a negative contrast angiogram. J Neurol Neurosurg Psychiatry 2008;79(12):1358; with permission.)

entrainment of air can be prevented by flooding the surgical field, placing the patient in Trendelenburg position, and applying pressure to the jugular veins bilaterally to promote retrograde venous flow. The use of 100% $Fio_2$ to aid nitrogen elimination from the air bolus, cessation of nitrous oxide, and aspiration blood from the right atrium of a central venous catheter are indicated to minimize the volume of embolus.

## PREOPERATIVE CONSIDERATIONS AND PREPARATIONS
### Prior Embolization: Flow Reduction

Embolization can, in some instances, be the definitive treatment for certain amenable AVMs with favorable angioarchitectural features, but typically it is used preoperatively to reduce the expected intraoperative bleeding and postoperative edema. Strategic placement of embolization material at the margins of the hypervascular nidus aids in subsequent resection of the brittle embolized AVM from normal tissue.[22] Embolization may be performed in multiple stages to decrease the risk of complications and allow the brain to adapt to circulatory changes. The endovascular procedure itself has an associated risk of morbidity and mortality. Many articles report the successful use of a combined approach in large cohorts of patients, but no randomized data exist to suggest that a combined approach is superior to surgery or embolization alone in terms of morbidity and mortality.

### Preoperative Chronic Hypertension

In a 1988 retrospective study of the natural history of 168 patients with intracerebral AVMs, only 9 (5%) had a history of hypertension; of the 31 patients who experienced intracranial hemorrhage, 6 (19%) had a history of hypertension, yet the investigators concluded that the presence of untreated or treated hypertension was of no value in predicting rupture.[23] The evidence for hypertension as a risk factor for AVM rupture is not convincing, and no controlled trials comparing the impact of treated versus untreated hypertension on risk of AVM rupture are available. Untreated hypertension results in a well-described rightward shift of autoregulation to higher MAP values, an effect that is partly reversible with chronic antihypertensive treatment. With the risk of spontaneous AVM rupture being low (2%–4% per year), it would seem wise to treat hypertension and achieve adequate blood pressure control prior to an elective AVM resection. In addition to the benefit to the cardiovascular system, preoperative treatment of hypertension and the option of safely maintaining a lower MAP value (within the range of autoregulation) intraoperatively and postoperatively may reduce surgical bleeding, hyperemia, and hyperperfusion syndrome. Patients should take their antihypertensive medicines on the day of surgery, especially β-blockers and α2 agonists for which acute withdrawal may cause rebound tachycardia or hypertension.

### Systemic Considerations: Cardiac Disease

AVM resection is typically nonemergent, and preexisting medical conditions should be optimized before surgery. In most cases AVM resection should be considered an intermediate-risk procedure; despite major vascular involvement and potential for hemorrhage and large fluid shifts, atherosclerosis is not part of the primary pathology. In nonemergent cases, a careful history and physical examination should be used to elicit evidence of active cardiac conditions (unstable coronary syndromes, severe valvular disease, decompensated heart failure, or significant arrhythmias), functional capacity, and clinical risk factors (history of heart disease, heart failure, cerebrovascular disease, diabetes mellitus, or renal insufficiency). These factors are incorporated into an algorithm to determine whether further preoperative noninvasive testing is warranted.[24]

## ANESTHETIC PLAN
### Invasive and Noninvasive Monitors

Standard ASA monitors (electrocardiography, noninvasive blood pressure, pulse oximeter, oxygen sensor, end-tidal $CO_2$, and temperature probe) are mandatory. Direct arterial pressure monitoring is also a requirement to monitor hemodynamic responses during an intracranial procedure, maintain strict blood pressure control, and draw labs to evaluate adequacy of oxygenation and ventilation, electrolytes, and hematologic parameters. Large-bore intravenous access is necessary because blood loss may be large and precipitous. Positioning should be reviewed with the surgical team, as arm position may inhibit intravenous flow or access to the extremities. Central access should be considered for resection of larger lesions for which it may be necessary to induce hypotension with vasoactive agents, or if large intravascular volume changes may be expected as a consequence of potential serious blood loss. Offering induced hypotension for short periods of time to permit improved visualization and to diminish blood flow may assist the surgeon during periods of uncontrolled bleeding. Blood losses of several liters may occur over a span of a few minutes in such dramatic cases, and the anesthesiologist must be prepared for such occasions with adequate vascular access and resuscitation with blood products.

Jugular bulb venous oxygen saturation ($Sjo_2$) monitoring may be useful for both embolization[25] and surgical resection.[26] As the AVM shunt flow ratio is reduced, continuous $Sjo_2$ falls, providing real-time information on the progress of embolization. In addition, the risk of severe hyperemic complications appeared greatly diminished if a $Sjo_2$ of less than 80% is achieved. However, the complications associated with jugular bulb catheterization, such as acute venous thrombosis, render this technique impractical and even dangerous in the management of AVM patients.

## Induction

The goals of induction include hemodynamic stability, control of the airway, and adequate oxygenation and ventilation. Induction can be achieved with a variety of intravenous or inhalational agents, but adequate depth of anesthesia should be achieved before laryngoscopy. Pretreatment with lidocaine, 1 mg/kg intravenously, may help in blunting airway reflexes and response to sympathetic stimulation. If intracranial hypertension is of primary concern, it may be best to avoid inhaled anesthetics entirely and use intravenous agents such as propofol to lower intracranial pressure (ICP) to the greatest extent possible and maintain CPP. Succinylcholine may increase ICP and should be avoided in patients with underlying motor deficits, but may be indicated if concerns about airway management prevail. Nondepolarizing muscle relaxants have no effect on CBF or ICP.

Hypertension has been implicated as a risk factor for spontaneous rupture of intracranial aneurysms, although the risk of rupture with acutely labile blood pressure is lower with AVMs.[27] Observational studies infer that moderate hypertension does not precipitate rupture of intracranial AVM.[27] It seems prudent to use direct arterial pressure monitoring and meticulously control hemodynamic lability.

## Maintenance

### Physiologic goals

Goals for anesthetic maintenance include hemodynamic stability, cerebral perfusion, control of intracranial pressure, facilitation of neuromonitoring signals, brain relaxation for improved surgical exposure, and resuscitation of intravascular fluid loss. In the authors' practice, maintenance is usually achieved with a combination of sub-minimum alveolar concentration values of isoflurane, nitrous oxide (unless contraindicated), and opioid (bolus or infusion). This combination of agents generally permits adequate neuromonitoring signals and is maintained in stable concentrations to prevent signal-quality fluctuation. If signals are inadequate, propofol may be used to supplement the anesthetic and reduce the nitrous oxide and/or volatile concentration. During periods of intense stimulation, boluses of opioid and/or propofol can be used to control hemodynamic response. If normotensive blood pressure control remains inadequate, antihypertensives may be used; agents where the effect is rapidly terminated in cases of precipitous blood loss are preferred.

Meticulous control of hemodynamic parameters is essential during the surgical process, and MAP goals may vary during the course of the procedure as resection proceeds and flow is shifted from the AVM to neighboring tissues. Communication with the surgeon regarding the appearance of the brain tissue, neuromonitoring signals, and target MAP is important. Drugs that vasodilate the cerebral vasculature, raise ICP, and exacerbate steal phenomena (nitroglycerin, nitroprusside, volatile anesthetic in high concentrations) should be avoided in favor of those that do not. Preferred agents include esmolol, labetalol, and nicardipine. Esmolol is rapidly titratable, as is the calcium-channel blocker nicardipine, which does cause cerebral vasodilation but does not appear to increase ICP. β-Blockers may be less than ideal in the patients with bradycardia, bronchospasm, or chronic obstructive pulmonary disease, in which case nicardipine is favorable. Augmentation of the blood pressure is best achieved with drugs with $\alpha$1 agonism (phenylephrine, ephedrine, norepinephrine, high-dose dopamine) that do not alter CBF.

Brain relaxation is achieved through several methods. Positioning with the head up and avoidance of extreme flexion, extension, or rotation of the neck promotes venous drainage. Moderate hyperventilation and hypocapnia reduce CBF, cerebral blood volume, ICP prior to dural opening, and brain bulk, thus enhancing surgical exposure. Prolonged hyperventilation has fallen out of favor in patients with traumatic brain injury because of evidence suggesting it may expand ischemic areas and compromise neurologic outcome.[28] Hyperventilation does improve operating conditions,[29] and moderate hyperventilation ($Paco_2$ 25–30 mm Hg) for relatively brief periods to facilitate surgical exposure is probably not detrimental. Osmotic diuretics such as mannitol or hypertonic saline may be administered for the purpose of reducing brain water, promoting brain relaxation, and minimizing postoperative edema.

Hypothermia has been shown to reduce $CMRo_2$ by approximately 6% per degree,[30] which reduces

CBF and should theoretically be neuroprotective if ischemic tissues are at risk. However, evidence is lacking for neurologic insults of differing etiology. More profound hypothermia presents the adverse effects of bacteremia, wound infection, hyperglycemia, prolonged drug clearance, coagulopathy, and arrhythmias. In the large controlled trial sponsored by the National Institutes of Health, the Intraoperative Hypothermia for Aneurysm Surgery Trial (IHAST), the investigators found no difference in neurologic outcome but noted a slight increase in bacteremia in the hypothermic group.[31] The results of this trial, however, contradict extensive animal data regarding moderate hypothermia.

### Fluid and blood product management

Fluid restriction is a common practice to prevent brain edema in neurosurgical cases, but it is imperative to maintain adequate intravascular volume and stable systemic hemodynamics. Normal plasma osmolality ranges from 275 to 300 mOsm/kg, averaging 290 mOsm/kg with [$Na^+$] being the most important determinant. The BBB when intact, in contrast to other capillary beds throughout the body, is impermeable to most hydrophilic solutes including $Na^+$ (as well as mannitol). In the brain where $Na^+$ does not cross the BBB freely, osmotic pressure has a far greater impact than oncotic pressure. An increase in 1 mEq/L of $Na^+$ results in an increase of 19.3 mm Hg of osmotic pressure at $37°C$. $Na^+$ is paired with an anion, doubling the impact on osmotic pressure. At 285 mOsm/kg, the osmotic pressure is approximately 5500 mm Hg, compared with an oncotic pressure of about 25 mm Hg from protein. Thus small changes in [$Na^+$] across an intact BBB can generate substantial osmotic pressure gradients and have a clinically significant impact on brain water content. To minimize brain edema, serum tonicity must be maintained. Hypotonic fluids should be avoided, and some anesthesiologists prefer to avoid lactated Ringer's as well, which may exacerbate brain swelling in large quantities. Colloid has no proven benefit over crystalloid. Infusion of hydroxyethyl starches (Hetastarch) can result in progressive hemodilution, impair hemostasis in a dose-dependent manner, and interfere with fibrin polymerization, causing a coagulopathy that is not reversed by fibrin administration.

There is no consensus on the glycemic goals for neurosurgery patients. Although hyperglycemia has long been recognized as a factor in worsened cerebral metabolism and adverse neurologic outcomes in experimental models, recent prospective, large-scale, randomized controlled trials have shown deleterious results regarding tight glucose control and mortality. The Normoglycemia in

Intensive Care Evaluation — Survival Using Glucose Algorithm Regulation (NICE-SUGAR) trial demonstrated increased mortality in the intensive (blood glucose 80–108 mg/dL) versus conventional (blood glucose <144–180 mg/dL) group.[32] Another controlled trial compared two extremes of the spectrum, intensive insulin (blood glucose goal 80–110 mg/dL) and conventional therapy (blood glucose goal <215 mg/dL), in 483 critical neurosurgical patients for elective or emergent craniotomy. The incidence of iatrogenic hypoglycemia (glucose <50 mg/dL) was threefold higher in the intensive group (94% had at least one episode of hypoglycemia, average 8 episodes) than the conventional group (63%, average 3), an alarmingly high incidence in both groups. The patients in the intensive group had statistically significantly shorter intensive care unit (ICU) stays and decreased infection rate. The Glasgow Outcome Scores (GOS) and overall survival at 6 months were similar in the two groups.[33] A moderate target for glucose such as that proposed by the NICE-SUGAR trial (blood glucose 140–180 mg/dL) with efforts to prevent hypoglycemia and minimize glucose variability is probably sensible.[34] Insulin administration requires serial blood glucose measurements, and a conservative dosing approach should be used during surgery when general anesthesia will mask symptoms of hypoglycemia.

### Emergence: neurologic assessment

The goals for emergence include hemodynamic stability, minimal increases in ICP from coughing, bucking, or vomiting, and adequate neurologic assessment before extubation. Neuromuscular blockade (at least partial) is typically maintained until the patient is out of Mayfield pins and will not cause serious injury with movement. The patient should be normothermic (or only mildly hypothermic). Electrolyte abnormalities, acid-base disturbances, and anemia should be corrected. Prophylactic antiemetics should be administered before emergence. Carefully titrated opioid, regional techniques such as a scalp block with a long-acting local anesthetic, or anticonvulsants such as gabapentin comprise a multimodal approach to postoperative pain control and help facilitate a smooth emergence. In general, a brief neurologic examination is performed while the patient is awake and still intubated, checking pupil size and reactivity, gag reflex, gross motor function, and the ability to follow commands. If the patient meets criteria (adequate oxygenation and ventilation, strength, airway patency and protection, consciousness, and the ability to follow commands), extubation is ideal and permits minimization of sedation as well as more accurate, continuous neurologic assessment. If concerns about capability of the patient to meet these criteria exist, it may be prudent to transition to the ICU intubated with titratable sedation (eg, propofol infusion) after the best assessment of postoperative neurologic function has been ascertained in the operating room. Delayed emergence can be attributable to many factors: residual anesthesia, hemodynamic instability, aforementioned laboratory derangements, cerebral edema, hemorrhage, hematoma, pneumocephalus, stroke, or seizure.

## SPECIAL CONDITIONS
### Embolization for AVM

Embolization procedures are performed in interventional radiology suites that are generally remote from the operating room and available resources in the event of an emergency the precision required for these procedures generally dictates that the patient be under general anesthesia, intubated, paralyzed, and mechanically ventilated so that ventilation can be paused during crucial portions of the procedure. In addition to standard ASA monitors for general anesthesia, direct arterial pressure monitoring is required for intracranial interventions. During angiography radiopaque, hyperosmolar contrast is injected to visualize the vascular system. This contrast remains sequestered in the vasculature until it is renally excreted. Transient increases in intravascular volume due to osmotic activity can occur, followed by osmotic diuresis and dehydration. In addition, the sheath used for arterial access requires frequent flushing with heparinized saline to prevent thromboembolism. The volume of flush (frequently several liters) is not easily quantified until the end of the procedure. These factors can conspire to create potentially large shifts in intravascular volume and hemodilutional anemia, which may be poorly tolerated by patients with cardiac disease or renal insufficiency. Despite a minimally invasive approach, embolization may cause dramatic changes in distribution of CBF, and the potential for cerebral edema and hemorrhage is still significant. The anesthesiologist should be vigilant for hemodynamic signs of intracranial hypertension, and agents to acutely lower ICP such as mannitol and hypertonic saline should be readily available. A thorough neurologic examination and assurance that the patient is awake and able to protect their airway is essential before extubation.

### Pregnancy

Retrospective data indicate that the rate of hemorrhage from AVM rupture is similar in pregnant women and nonpregnant women of childbearing age; the risk of rupture is not increased in pregnancy.[35] One study identified ruptured AVM as the cause of 36% of cases of hemorrhagic stroke during pregnancy or the puerperium; the majority of events occurred in the third trimester or first week of the postpartum period,[36] a time of great hemodynamic fluctuation. Presentation during pregnancy is usually the result of hemorrhage following rupture, though some patients may present with seizures, headache, or focal neurologic signs. In most cases these patients have no prior diagnosis of cerebral AVM. If known prior to delivery, Caesarean section under general anesthesia has been used successfully to minimize increases in ICP associated with labor and delivery.

## POSTOPERATIVE CARE PLAN

After surgical resection of an AVM, the patient is admitted for neurologic intensive care monitoring for at least 48 hours. The goals of the postoperative period include strict blood pressure control with continuous arterial pressure monitoring to prevent hypotension or ischemia and hypertension, NPPB, hyperemia, edema, or hemorrhage. Patients at high risk for postoperative NPPB (larger, high-flow AVMs) may require induced hypotension to prevent hyperemia in areas that were chronically underperfused before surgery. Rapidly titratable agents such as esmolol or nicardipine may be useful in achieving this goal. Patients undergoing craniotomy experience moderate to severe pain postoperatively. Traditionally, short-acting opioids were administered on an as-needed basis by the nurse for fear that sedating effects would interfere with the neurologic examination, a practice that frequently results in the inadequate treatment of pain. There is evidence in neurosurgical patients that intravenous patient-controlled analgesia is effective at controlling postcraniotomy pain with no untoward effects,[37] and ongoing research is aimed at validating the safety of this approach.

Sedation is often required to tolerate intubation and mechanical ventilation, but comfort must be balanced against the need for frequent neurologic assessment. Short-acting agents such as opioids, benzodiazepines, and propofol are frequently used for sedation, but effects can accumulate over time and contribute to reduced consciousness, impaired cognition, and delirium. Dexmedetomidine provides sedation with fewer adverse effects, a trait that is desirable in a critically ill population and especially those with neurologic issues. The Acute Neurological ICU Sedation Trial (ANIST), a double-blinded, randomized, controlled crossover study, demonstrated improvement in cognition with dexmedetomidine when compared with propofol during sedation in neurologic patients.[38]

The risk of seizure as the presenting symptom of an AVM is approximately 15% to 40%, independent of hemorrhage. Risk factors for seizure include male gender, age less than 65 years, AVM greater than 3 cm, and temporal lobe location.[39] Patients who present with seizure should be optimized on anticonvulsant medications before surgery. If patients are not on preoperative anticonvulsants, a loading dose may be given intraoperatively. Levetiracetam, phenytoin, and fosphenytoin are common perioperative intravenous anticonvulsants. The latter two can cause substantial hypotension and may delay emergence; loading doses should be given as a slow infusion well in advance of anticipated emergence. Intracranial blood (intraparenchymal or subarachnoid) may induce convulsions caused by high iron levels. In patients with head trauma, there is evidence that prophylactic phenytoin reduces seizure risk in the first week, but has no additional benefit beyond that point.[40] It is probably reasonable to continue anticonvulsant therapy for 1 week after AVM resection and then discontinue it if there is no evidence of epileptic activity.

Other goals of postoperative critical care are not unique to neurosurgical patients. Perioperative antibiotics are usually given for 24 hours postoperatively to prevent wound infection. Deep venous thrombosis prophylaxis should be started in nonambulatory patients; generally mechanical methods are used in neurosurgery patients to avoid increasing the risk of bleeding. Stress ulcer prophylaxis is routine. When the patient is able to tolerate oral intake, a transition from intravenous to oral home medications should be started if indicated. Anticoagulation is generally safe 12 to 24 hours after a craniotomy if indicated, but should be started with caution using conservative doses; unfractionated or low molecular weight heparin may be given in more frequent divided doses to minimize the risk of bleeding.

## SUMMARY

AVMs and DAVFs are an abnormal conduit between the arterial and venous systems. Hemorrhage, usually intraventricular or intraparenchymal, is the most concerning sequela; prior AVM or DAVF rupture is the biggest risk factor for rebleeding. Resection of AVMs or DAVFs is generally an elective procedure except in cases of acute hemorrhage where emergent hematoma evacuation is required. The anesthetic considerations for surgical resection of AVMs and DAVFs incorporate many principles that are common to craniotomies for other indications, specifically: tightly controlled hemodynamic parameters; manipulation of

systemic blood pressure and CPP; control of ICP facilitation of surgical exposure to minimize blood loss and injury to the brain; selection of anesthetic agents that will aid neuroprotection, neuromonitoring signals, and neurologic assessment on emergence; blood and fluid management to optimize oxygen delivery and minimize edema; preparation for and early recognition of acute massive blood loss and VAE; careful consideration of suitability for extubation; and postoperative pain control The vascular pathophysiology of AVMs, and to a lesser extent that of DAVFs, increases the complexity of anesthetic management. A high-flow, low-resistance shunt decreases the perfusion pressure to neighboring brain tissue that develops an adaptive response to chronic hypoperfusion and is exquisitely sensitive to ischemia. As a result of resection of arterial flow to the AVM or DAVF, blood is redistributed to this adjacent tissue, and acute increases in flow have the potential to cause hyperemia and hemorrhage, complications that may be reduced with aggressive management of blood pressure. A comprehensive understanding of AVM and DAVF pathophysiology and rapidly titratable anesthetic and vasoactive agents allow the anesthesiologist to alter blood pressure targets as resection evolves, so as to optimize patient outcome. This intensive management is continued postoperatively in the ICU until stability is achieved and the brain acclimatizes to new parameters.

## REFERENCES

1. Spetzler RF, Martin NA, Carter LP, et al. Surgical management of large AVM's by staged embolization and operative excision. J Neurosurg 1987;67(1):17–28.
2. Fogarty-Mack P, Pile-Spellman J, Hacein-Bey L, et al. The effect of arteriovenous malformations on the distribution of intracerebral arterial pressures. AJNR Am J Neuroradiol 1996;17(8):1443–9.
3. Young WL, Prohovnik I, Ornstein E, et al. The effect of arteriovenous malformation resection on cerebrovascular reactivity to carbon dioxide. Neurosurgery 1990;27(2):257–66.
4. Charbel FT, Hoffman WE, Misra M, et al. Increased brain tissue oxygenation during arteriovenous malformation resection. Neurol Med Chir (Tokyo) 1998; 38(Suppl):171–6.
5. Spetzler RF, Wilson CB, Weinstein P, et al. Normal perfusion pressure breakthrough theory. Clin Neurosurg 1978;25:651–72.
6. al-Rodhan NR, Sundt TM Jr, Piepgras DG, et al. Occlusive hyperemia: a theory for the hemodynamic complications following resection of intracerebral arteriovenous malformations. J Neurosurg 1993; 78(2):167–75.

7. Rogers AT, Stump DA, Gravlee GP, et al. Response of cerebral blood flow to phenylephrine infusion during hypothermic cardiopulmonary bypass: influence of $PaCO_2$ management. Anesthesiology 1988;69(4):547–51.

8. Ledezma CJ, Hoh BL, Carter BS, et al. Complications of cerebral arteriovenous malformation embolization: multivariate analysis of predictive factors. Neurosurgery 2006;58(4):602–11.

9. Zink KA, Sambasivan CN, Holcomb JB, et al. A high ratio of plasma and platelets to packed red blood cells in the first 6 hours of massive transfusion improves outcomes in a large multicenter study. Am J Surg 2009;197(5):565–70 [discussion: 570].

10. American Society of Anesthesiologists Task Force on Perioperative Blood Transfusion, Adjuvant Therapies. Practice guidelines for perioperative blood transfusion and adjuvant therapies: an updated report by the American Society of Anesthesiologists Task Force on Perioperative Blood Transfusion and Adjuvant Therapies. Anesthesiology 2006;105(1): 198–208.

11. Lee SH, Heros RC, Mullan JC, et al. Optimum degree of hemodilution for brain protection in a canine model of focal cerebral ischemia. J Neurosurg 1994;80(3):469–75.

12. Dhar R, Zazulia AR, Videen TO, et al. Red blood cell transfusion increases cerebral oxygen delivery in anemic patients with subarachnoid hemorrhage. Stroke 2009;40(9):3039–44.

13. Pasternak JJ, Hertzfeldt DN, Stanger SR, et al. Disseminated intravascular coagulation after craniotomy. J Neurosurg Anesthesiol 2008;20(1):15–20.

14. Gabarrós A, Young WL, McDermott MW, et al. Language and motor mapping during resection of brain arteriovenous malformations: indications, feasibility, and utility. Neurosurgery 2011;68(3): 744–52.

15. Ogasawara K, Yoshida K, Otawara Y, et al. Cerebral blood flow imaging in arteriovenous malformation complicated by normal perfusion pressure breakthrough. Surg Neurol 2001;56(6):380–4.

16. Batjer HH, Devous MD Sr. The use of acetazolamide-enhanced regional cerebral blood flow measurement to predict risk to arteriovenous malformation patients. Neurosurgery 1992;31(2):213–7.

17. Taha M, Patel U, Wharton SB, et al. Fatal spontaneous thrombosis of a cerebral arteriovenous malformation in a young patient with a rare heterozygous prothrombin gene mutation. Case report. J Neurosurg 2007;106(Suppl 2):143–6.

18. Link MJ, Schermerhorn TC, Fulgham JR, et al. Progressive neurological decline after partial spontaneous thrombosis of a Spetzler-Martin Grade 5 arteriovenous malformation in a patient with Leiden factor V mutation: management and outcome. J Neurosurg 2004;100(5):940–5.

19. Mirski MA, Lele AV, Fitzsimmons L, et al. Diagnosis and treatment of vascular air embolism. Anesthesiology 2007;106(1):164–77.

20. Ishida K, Hishinuma M, Miyazawa M, et al. Pulmonary edema due to venous air embolism during craniotomy: a case report. Masui 2008;57(10): 1257–60 [in Japanese].

21. Furuya H, Suzuki T, Okumura F, et al. Analysis and comparison of venous air embolism detection methods. Neurosurgery 1980;7(2):135–41.

22. Nagashima H, Okudera H, Muraoka S, et al. Strategic embolisation for successful resection of a large cerebral arteriovenous malformation. J Clin Neurosci 2000;7(Suppl 1):86–7.

23. Brown RD Jr, Wiebers DO, Forbes G, et al. The natural history of unruptured intracranial arteriovenous malformations. J Neurosurg 1988;68(3):352–7.

24. Fleisher LA, Beckman JA, Brown KA, et al. ACC/AHA 2007 Guidelines on Perioperative Cardiovascular Evaluation and Care for Noncardiac Surgery: Executive Summary: A Report of the American College of Cardiology/American Heart Association Task Force on Practice Guidelines (Writing Committee to Revise the 2002 Guidelines on Perioperative Cardiovascular Evaluation for Noncardiac Surgery) Developed in Collaboration With the American Society of Echocardiography, American Society of Nuclear Cardiology, Heart Rhythm Society, Society of Cardiovascular Anesthesiologists, Society for Cardiovascular Angiography and Interventions, Society for Vascular Medicine and Biology, and Society for Vascular Surgery. J Am Coll Cardiol 2007;50(17):1707–32.

25. Katayama Y, Tsubokawa T, Hirayama T, et al. Continuous monitoring of jugular bulb oxygen saturation as a measure of the shunt flow of cerebral arteriovenous malformations. J Neurosurg 1994; 80(5):826–33.

26. Wilder-Smith OH, Fransen P, de Tribolet N, et al. Jugular venous bulb oxygen saturation monitoring in arteriovenous malformation surgery. J Neurosurg Anesthesiol 1997;9(2):162–5.

27. Szabo MD, Crosby G, Sundaram P, et al. Hypertension does not cause spontaneous hemorrhage of intracranial arteriovenous malformations. Anesthesiology 1989;70(5):761–3.

28. Muizelaar JP, Marmarou A, Ward JD, et al. Adverse effects of prolonged hyperventilation in patients with severe head injury: a randomized clinical trial. J Neurosurg 1991;75(5):731–9.

29. Gelb AW, Craen RA, Rao GS, et al. Does hyperventilation improve operating condition during supratentorial craniotomy? A multicenter randomized crossover trial. Anesth Analg 2008;106(2): 585–94.

30. Croughwell N, Smith LR, Quill T, et al. The effect of temperature on cerebral metabolism

and blood flow in adults during cardiopulmonary bypass. J Thorac Cardiovasc Surg 1992;103(3): 549–54.

31. Todd MM, Hindman BJ, Clarke WR, et al, Intraoperative Hypothermia for Aneurysm Surgery Trial (IHAST) Investigators. Mild intraoperative hypothermia during surgery for intracranial aneurysm. N Engl J Med 2005;352(2):135–45.

32. NICE-SUGAR Study Investigators, Finfer S, Chittock DR, Su SY, et al. Intensive versus conventional glucose control in critically ill patients. N Engl J Med 2009;360(13):1283–97.

33. Bilotta F, Caramia R, Paoloni FP, et al. Safety and efficacy of intensive insulin therapy in critical neurosurgical patients. Anesthesiology 2009; 110(3):611–9.

34. Bilotta F, Rosa G. Glucose management in the neurosurgical patient: are we yet any closer? Curr Opin Anaesthesiol 2010;23(5):539–43.

35. Horton JC, Chambers WA, Lyons SL, et al. Pregnancy and the risk of hemorrhage from cerebral arteriovenous malformations. Neurosurgery 1990; 27(6):867–71.

36. Skidmore FM, Williams LS, Fradkin KD, et al. Presentation, etiology, and outcome of stroke in pregnancy and puerperium. J Stroke Cerebrovasc Dis 2001; 10(1):1–10.

37. Morad AH, Winters BD, Yaster M, et al. Efficacy of intravenous patient-controlled analgesia after supratentorial intracranial surgery: a prospective randomized controlled trial. Clinical article. J Neurosurg 2009;111(2):343–50.

38. Mirski MA, Lewin JJ 3rd, Ledroux S, et al. Cognitive improvement during continuous sedation in critically ill, awake and responsive patients: the Acute Neurological ICU Sedation Trial (ANIST). Intensive Care Med 2010;36(9):1505–13.

39. Hoh BL, Chapman PH, Loeffler JS, et al. Results of multimodality treatment for 141 patients with brain arteriovenous malformations and seizures: factors associated with seizure incidence and seizure outcomes. Neurosurgery 2002;51(2):303–9.

40. Temkin NR, Dikmen SS, Wilensky AJ, et al. A randomized, double-blind study of phenytoin for the prevention of post-traumatic seizures. N Engl J Med 1990;323:497–502.

# Vein of Galen Malformations: Epidemiology, Clinical Presentations, Management

Pablo F. Recinos, MD[a,b], Gazanfar Rahmathulla, MD[b],
Monica Pearl, MD[c], Violette Renard Recinos, MD[d],
George I. Jallo, MD[a], Philippe Gailloud, MD[c],
Edward S. Ahn, MD[a,*]

## KEYWORDS

- Vein of galen malformation • Arteriovenous malformation
- Clinical presentation • Management

The vein of Galen aneurysmal malformation (VGAM) is a congenital vascular malformation that comprises 30% of the pediatric vascular and 1% of all pediatric congenital anomalies.[1-3] Abnormal development causes shunting of arterial blood into the median prosencephalic vein (MProsV) of Markowski, which is the ectatic vessel. Although this vein is a precursor of the vein of Galen, it is a separate entity, making the term vein of Galen malformation a misnomer.[4-6] The rare nature of these lesions, along with differences in their evolution, presentation, angioarchitecture, and effects on systemic physiology, makes their management a formidable challenge.

## HISTORICAL OVERVIEW

The first published description of a presumed VGAM was in 1895 by Steinheil.[7] However, this was an arteriovenous malformation (AVM) that

drained into the vein of Galen and not a true VGAM.[8] At the time, there was no distinction between a VGAM and an AVM that drained into the vein of Galen. In 1949, Boldrey and Miller[9] treated 2 patients with "arteriovenous fistula of the cerebral vein of Galen" with carotid artery ligation. Of these 2 patients, the second patient likely represented a true VGAM.[8,9] In 1955, Silverman and colleagues[10] described 2 neonates who had died of cardiac failure without a primary cardiovascular disorder and were also found to have an AVM involving the vein of Galen. They were the first to suggest that a cerebral AVM could be the cause of cardiac failure. In 1964, Gold and colleagues[2] were the first to classify patients with a VGAM into 3 different groups based on their presenting features. It was the first correlation between age of presentation, hemodynamic manifestations, and angioarchitecture of the lesion.

Disclosures: The authors have nothing to disclose.
[a] Division of Pediatric Neurosurgery, The Johns Hopkins Hospital, 600 North Wolfe Street, Harvey 811, Baltimore, MD 21287, USA
[b] Department of Neurosurgery, Rosa Ella Burkhardt Brain Tumor and Neuro-Oncology Center, Cleveland Clinic, 9500 Euclid Avenue, S73, Cleveland, OH 44195, USA
[c] Division of Interventional Neuroradiology, The Johns Hopkins Hospital, 600 North Wolfe Street, Baltimore, MD 21287, USA
[d] Department of Neurosurgery, Cleveland Clinic, 9500 Euclid Avenue, S60, Cleveland, OH 44195, USA
* Corresponding author.
E-mail address: eahn4@jhmi.edu

1042-3680/12/$ – see front matter © 2012 Elsevier Inc. All rights reserved.

neurosurgery.theclinics.com

Treatment of VGAMs was initially surgical, but surgical results were associated with a high morbidity and mortality.[2,11,12] In 1982, Hoffman and colleagues[11] reported a series of 29 patients with VGAM. Of 29 patients, 16 were managed operatively, making it the largest reported surgical series at the time. They reported 56% mortality in patients treated with surgery. Based on their results and reported literature, they concluded that only surgical occlusion of the fistulous tracts, rather than resection of the lesion, was necessary. This differed from surgical management of other AVMs in which resection of the nidus was the operative goal.

With advances in imaging, microcatheters, and angiographic techniques, it has become possible to better define the angiographic anatomy of the VGAM. The ability to superselectively occlude vessels using coils and liquid embolic agents (in particular, n-butyl cyanoacrylate [n-BCA]; Trufill, Codman Neurovascular, NJ, USA), has made it technically feasible to perform an endovascular approach to previously inaccessible, deep-seated lesions. In addition, selective vessel occlusion could be performed with improved mortality and morbidity compared with open surgical techniques. Lasjaunias and colleagues[3] pioneered treatment of this condition and classified vein of Galen malformations in detail.[13–16] In 1989, his group reported on the results of 36 patients treated via the transfemoral route with no morbidity and a 13% mortality.[17] Thus, endovascular treatment became the primary treatment option for patients with a VGAM.

## ANATOMY AND EMBRYOLOGY OF THE VEIN OF GALEN

In normal neurovascular development, the choroid plexus becomes responsible for fluid circulation within the neural tube after closure of the anterior and posterior neuropores between gestational weeks 6 and 10. At this stage, the telencephalon is supplied by multiple choroidal arteries that arise from the choroid plexus. Concurrently, the MProsV of Markowski develops on the roof of the diencephalon and is responsible for the venous drainage.[18] Between gestational weeks 10 and 11, the arterial network of the cortex matures and the choroidal arteries lose their central role in cerebral vascularization. Paired internal cerebral veins develop and drain the choroid plexus. The internal cerebral veins terminate in the posterior portion of the MProsV of Markowski, which at this point has begun to involute. Remnants of the caudal portion of the median prosencephalic vein then join the internal cerebral veins to form the vein of Galen.[6,19]

When a VGAM develops, arteriovenous shunts form between the choroidal circulation and the MProsV of Markowski. The presence of these shunts keeps the MProsV of Markowski patent and promotes its enlargement, which forms the VGAM. It also prevents the normal formation of the vein of Galen. Raybaud and colleagues[6] noted that the anterior choroidal arteries, posterior choroidal arteries, and anterior cerebral arteries drained directly into the VGAM. In addition, the circumferential, mesencephalic, meningeal, and, rarely, subependymal arteries anastomosed on the VGAM, although these are not usually a dominant feature of this malformation.[3,20]

The deep cerebral venous anatomy of VGAMs is of particular importance and has been the subject of considerable debate. VGAMs may drain through a normal straight sinus and/or through a falcine sinus, a persistent embryonic sinus that joins to the posterior third of the superior sagittal sinus. Variations in drainage include hypoplastic or absent straight sinuses and multiple or sinuous falcine sinuses.[21] The presence of a straight sinus does not preclude the existence of a VGAM.[21] More important is the concept that, rather than being separate from the deep venous drainage system, a VGAM may maintain connections with the galenic system.[22,23] This concept is critical in determining an endovascular treatment plan, because these drainage pathways may only be visible on follow-up imaging studies after endovascular treatment.[21]

In contrast with the VGAM, adjacent parenchymal AVMs can cause aneurysmal dilatation of the vein of Galen. These dilatations are known as vein of Galen aneurysmal dilatations or varicosities and are different from VGAMs. Previously, no distinction existed between these 2 entities, which resulted in imprecise descriptions of the anatomic features and natural history of a VGAM.[8]

## CLASSIFICATION

Various classification systems have been proposed for VGAMs. The 2 most clinically used systems are those of Lasjaunias and Yaşargil. Lasjaunias and colleagues[24] described 2 angiographic types of aneurysmal malformations: a primary or true vein of Galen malformation and a secondary type resulting from a deep AVM that drains into the vein of Galen. The primary type was further subdivided into a mural type and a choroidal type. The mural type has 1 or many direct arterial connections into the wall of the MProsV of Markowski. The choroidal type has many choroidal feeders that form a nidal network that drains into the MProsV of Markowski.

Yaşargil proposed 4 types of aneurysmal malformations based on the arterial feeder patterns of drainage into the vein of Galen[12,25]:

1. Type I is made up of 1 or more direct fistulas between the pericallosal and posterior cerebral arteries and the vein of Galen (**Fig. 1**).
2. Type II consists of a thalamoperforator network that lies between the arterial feeders and the vein of Galen (**Fig. 2**).
3. Type III has multiple fistulous connections from different vessels having characteristics of type I and II malformations (**Fig. 3**).
4. Type IV have adjacent AVMs that drain into the vein of Galen and cause a secondary aneurysmal venous dilatation (**Fig. 4**).

Only a primary vein of Galen malformation (Lasjaunias classification) and types I to III malformations (Yaşargil classification) represent true VGAMs, in which the MProsV of Markowski is the pathologic vessel. Secondary vein of Galen malformations (Lasjaunias classification) and type IV malformations (Yaşargil classification) are AVMs that produce secondary dilatation of the vein of Galen.

## CLINICAL FEATURES AND PATHOPHYSIOLOGY

Patients with a VGAM most commonly present with cardiac and neurologic complications. The clinical presentation depends on the age of presentation. Neonates tend to present with high-output cardiac failure, pulmonary hypertension, and, in more severe cases, multiorgan system failure. Infants commonly present with hydrocephalus, seizures, or neurocognitive delay. Older children and adults usually present with headaches or intracranial hemorrhage. If cardiac failure presents outside the neonatal period, it is usually mild to moderate and can be medically controlled.

## Cardiac Manifestations and Associated Systemic Complications

The high-flow, low-resistance arteriovenous connection that is present in a VGAM causes a compensatory increase in blood volume and cardiac output. As a result, cerebral blood flow can comprise as much as 80% of the cardiac output in these cases.[26] In utero, the placenta is also a low-resistance system that competes with the VGAM for blood flow and limits the blood flow that passes through the VGAM. However, postpartum blood flow greatly increases through the VGAM.[4]

There are several factors that lead to worsening cardiac function. Increased venous return because of the VGAM can lead to pulmonary hypertention.[27,28] The presence of a patent ductus arteriosus (PDA) and/or patent foramen ovale

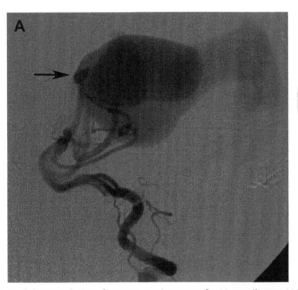
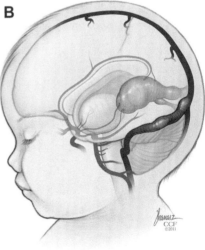

**Fig. 1.** (*A*) Lateral view from an angiogram of a Yaşargil type I VGAM. The black arrow points to the direct arteriovenous shunt between choroidal arteries and the vein of Galen (median prosencephalic vein of Markowski). (*B*) Yaşargil type I VGAM. Direct arterial feeders from the anterior and posterior circulation drain into the enlarged MProsV of Markowski. In addition, a persistent falcine sinus drains blood from the VGAM into the superior sagittal sinus, which can cause the straight sinus to be hypoplastic (as in this figure) or completely absent. (Part [*A*] *Courtesy of* Gailloud P, MD. The Johns Hopkins Hospital.)

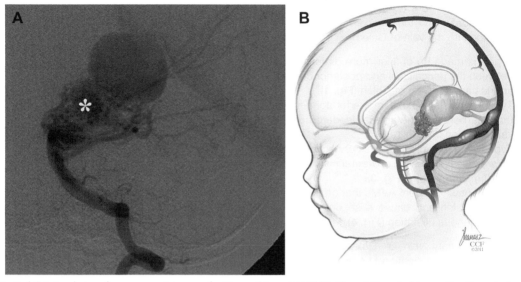

**Fig. 2.** (A) Lateral view from an angiogram of a Yaşargil type II VGAM. The white asterisk overlies the arterioarterial posterior thalamoperforator network supplying the VGAM. (B) Yaşargil type II VGAM. Arterial feeders are seen entering an arterioarterial niduslike network, which subsequently drain into the enlarged MProsV of Markowski. (Part (A) *Courtesy of* Gailloud P, MD. The Johns Hopkins Hospital.)

increases the volume of venous return, which worsens pulmonary hypertension. In addition, these right-to-left shunts decrease coronary blood flow, which can result in myocardial ischemia.[26,29–31] Diastolic flow reversal can occur in the descending aorta, which can lead to hepatic and renal insufficiency.[4,30]

### Neurologic Manifestations

Normal cerebral development requires normal fluid balance among the extracellular, intracellular, and intravascular spaces. When a VGAM is present, the efferent flow from the torcula is directed medially given the persistent occipital and marginal

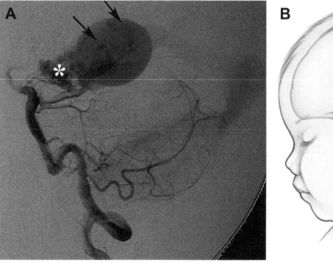
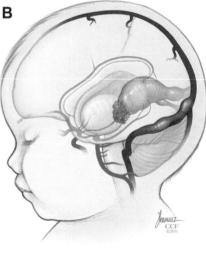

**Fig. 3.** (A) Lateral view from an angiogram of a Yaşargil type III VGAM. The black arrows denote the direct arteriovenous shunts and the white asterisk overlies the arterioarterial network supplying the VGAM. (B) Yaşargil type III VGAM. Direct arterial feeders from the anterior and posterior circulation and feeders from the arterioarterial niduslike network drain into the enlarged MProsV of Markowski. (Part (A) *Courtesy of* Gailloud P, MD. The Johns Hopkins Hospital.)

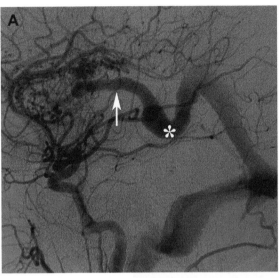
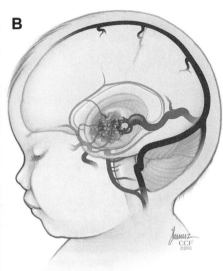

**Fig. 4.** (*A*) Lateral view from an angiogram of a Yaşargil type IV VGAM. A corpus callosum AVM is present draining into an enlarged internal cerebral vein (*white arrow*) and a dilated vein of Galen (*white asterisk*). (*B*) Yaşargil type IV VGAM with a deep AVM draining into an enlarged vein of Galen. In contrast with Yaşargil types I to III, the venous system has otherwise developed normally. (Part (*A*) *Courtesy of* Gailloud P, MD. The Johns Hopkins Hospital.)

sinuses.[8] In turn, flow is directed away from the dural sinuses, which can lead to hypoplastic or thrombosed jugular bulbs as well as enlarged facial veins.[4,27] Venous congestion and intracranial venous hypertension can develop, which disrupt the fluid balance among the intracranial spaces, leading to impaired cortical development.[27]

Cerebral atrophy and irreversible brain damage can occur as a result of persistent venous congestion. When they are detected in the antepartum or neonatal period, they are associated with a poor prognosis.[32] In severe cases, there may be rapid parenchymal loss, which is known as melting brain.[5] Infants and children who are initially neurologically normal can still experience progressive neurologic and cognitive decline manifested by the development of calcifications, subependymal atrophy, and epilepsy.[8,27,30] Restoring a hemodynamic balance by correcting the venous hypertension after endovascular treatment can lead to regression of the cerebral calcifications.[33] Neurologic deficits usually occur from vascular steal caused by high flow through the VGAM, whereas developmental retardation is caused by venous congestion.[30]

Hydrocephalus and macrocrania are typical presenting signs of infants. Obstructive hydrocephalus can occur from compression of the cerebral aqueduct by the VGAM (**Fig. 5A**).[18,34] However, the predominant cause seems to be communicating hydrocephalus that occurs from decreased cerebrospinal fluid (CSF) absorption as a result of the intracranial venous hypertension, caused by disruption of the hydrovenous equilibrium.[34,35] In both cases, hydrocephalus is a secondary phenomenon that results from the VGAM.

Headaches and seizures are common presenting symptoms in older children with a VGAM.[5,27,30] In addition, subarachnoid, and intraparenchymal hemorrhage can also be the cause of presentation in older children with a VGAM.[2,5,36,37] Although the VGAM tends to be smaller with a more limited arteriovenous shunting in older patients, the angiomatous network supplying the VGAM can produce microaneurysms.[4]

## DIAGNOSTIC WORKUP

Most patients with a VGAM are diagnosed in the neonatal period. A thorough evaluation of the neonate being managed for a suspected VGAM begins with a bedside clinical examination and a battery of diagnostic tests to determine the management strategy. The neonatal evaluation should include a complete clinical evaluation of the neonate including weight and head circumference. An echocardiogram provides baseline data for patients without cardiac insufficiency and helps quantify the severity of cardiac failure in symptomatic patients. Renal and liver function tests should be obtained to screen for renal and hepatic insufficiency, especially when cardiac insufficiency is

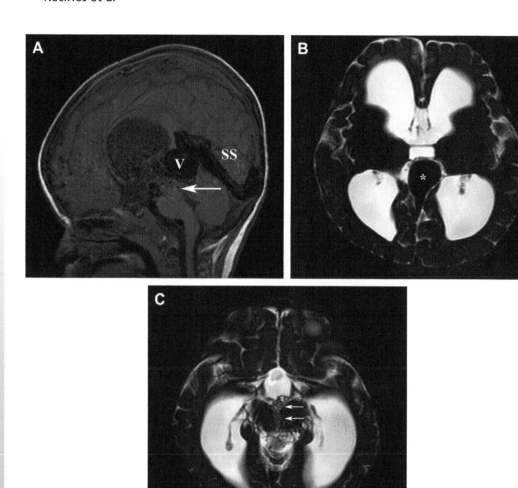

**Fig. 5.** (*A*) Midline sagittal T1-weighted magnetic resonance imaging (MRI) shows the VGAM (V) draining into a straight sinus (SS) with compression of the cerebral aqueduct (*arrow*) and resultant hydrocephalus. Note the pulsation artifact across the image in the phase encoding direction. (*B*) Axial T2-weighted MRI of the same patient with a VGAM (*asterisk*) that causes hydrocephalus. (*C*) Axial T2-weighted MRI showing multiple transmesencephalic feeders (*white arrows*) in an Yaşargil type II VGAM.

present.[30] A transfontanelle ultrasound can be performed at the bedside to assess the brain parenchyma, evaluate the VGAM, and assess the ventricular size. Magnetic resonance imaging (MRI) of the brain can help confirm the diagnosis of VGAM and detect cerebral changes such as infarcts, atrophy, and hydrocephalus (see **Fig. 5**).[38,39] An electroencephalogram should be performed on patients in the intensive care unit setting to rule out seizure activity.

Computed tomography (CT) is a useful screening tool and is often the imaging modality that detects a mass in older patients (**Fig. 6**).[29] CT angiography is a useful, noninvasive imaging modality that provides a clear map of the arteries and veins. It has better spatial resolution and can be obtained faster than magnetic resonance angiography (MRA).[40,41] Conventional angiography is the gold standard imaging modality to evaluate the VGAM angioarchitecture. However, it should be performed as part of a planned endovascular intervention rather than for diagnostic purposes because the VGAM can be initially evaluated by MRI/MRA.[8]

## MANAGEMENT STRATEGIES

The management of VGAMs is divided into medical, endovascular, and surgical modalities. Appropriate management depends on the patient's age

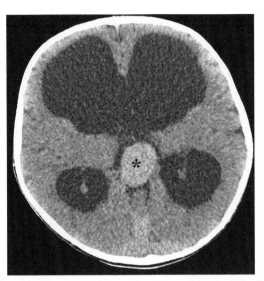

**Fig. 6.** Axial noncontrast head CT shows marked hydrocephalus and a midline hyperdense VGAM (*asterisk*).

at presentation and on the patient's clinical picture. In addition, a multidisciplinary team approach (including neurology, neurosurgery, interventional neuroradiology, cardiology, and neonatal intensive care) is recommended given the high degree of complexity these patients often present.

## Medical Management

The primary goal of medical management in VGAM treatment is to stabilize cardiac and systemic complications until endovascular intervention can be performed.[42] In neonates, high-output cardiac failure can lead to renal insufficiency, hepatic insufficiency, and myocardial ischemia. Increased flow can also prevent closure of the ductus arteriosus, which exacerbates hypoxemia.[30] By decreasing flow to the VGAM, perfusion to the kidneys and heart improves, venous hypertension in the pulmonary circulation can be decreased, and persistent right-to-left shunts can close. Management options to decrease flow include diuretics, inotropic agents, and vasodilators.[4,18] However, no optimal management paradigm has been established. The success of medical management is directly related to how severe the patient's symptoms are on presentation. Neonates typically have more severe heart failure and subsequently worse outcomes. When heart failure is present in infants and children, it tends to be mild and can be managed with greater success.[8,18]

## Endovascular Treatment

The development of endovascular techniques has greatly improved the poor prognosis of patients

with a VGAM. The overall endovascular treatment goal is to restore hemodynamic balance and achieve a physiologic, rather than anatomic, cure that leads to favorable neurologic and developmental outcomes.[21] The treatment should be performed using a stepwise approach to avoid rapid hemodynamic changes, which can lead to parenchymal hemorrhage from a perfusion breakthrough phenomenon[43] or massive venous thrombosis.[18] Partial embolization can decrease flow through the VGAM sufficiently to control cardiac failure, while minimizing the risk of complications.[8,18,44] Stepwise embolization also allows for gradual fluid hemodynamic adjustments, which minimizes the risk to cerebral development.[18,29,45]

The timing of intervention is also critical. Lasjaunias and colleagues[8] described an optimal therapeutic window for initiating endovascular treatment. The first treatment is recommended at 4 to 5 months of age to maximize efficacy of the intervention and minimize the risk of delay in cerebral maturation.[21] If treatment is deferred longer, correction of hydrocephalus may not be possible by treating the VGAM and neurologic and cognitive sequelae can become permanent.[8,18,21] After the first treatment, subsequent treatments are performed using a routine interval of 6 to 8 weeks or a shorter interval of 4 weeks for more complex lesions.[21] Emergent embolization is sometimes necessary in neonates. In these cases, the primary goal is to decrease flow through the VGAM to normalize systemic physiology. In addition, reducing flow through a VGAM in a neonate can help recreate conditions to allow maturation of the cerebral venous system.[8]

Technically, the VGAM may be targeted either through a transarterial or transvenous approach. Several investigators advocate the primary use of the transarterial route, reserving transvenous embolization for instances in which transarterial embolization has been exhausted.[8,18,21,27] Despite being technically less challenging than the transarterial approach, transvenous VGAM treatment offers less hemodynamic control than transarterial embolization in staged devascularization. Care must be taken with endovenous coiling to minimize the risk of deep venous thrombosis.

The route of access depends on the age of the patient. In neonates, the umbilical artery can be used for access if treatment is required during the first 3 days of life.[4,21] Otherwise, femoral access is preferred. When a transvenous approach is considered, the femoral vein is typically used. In rare cases, a transjugular or even transtorcular approach via direct puncture may be used.

The 2 currently available liquid embolic agents in the United States are *n*-butyl cyanoacrylate (n-BCA; Trufill, Codman Neurovascular, NJ) and ethylene vinyl alcohol copolymer (Onyx, Micro Therapeutics, CA).[8,18,46] Several investigators preferred the embolic agent n-BCA because of its reliability and safety.[4,8,18] It can be used with or without the adjunct use of microcoils, which are not recommended as the sole endovascular occlusion agent because they do not offer sufficient penetration of the feeding branches.[21]

## Surgery

Although microsurgery was historically the primary treatment strategy, it is no longer a first-line option. However, surgery does play several adjunct roles. Hydrocephalus can be treated with CSF diversion either through shunting or by endoscopic third ventriculostomy. However, hydrocephalus can significantly improve with embolization of the VGAM, therefore embolization should always precede hydrocephalus treatment, if possible. In rare cases of transtorcular embolization, a surgical window is created to provide venous access. Surgery is also used for evacuation of intracranial hematomas. In addition, surgery remains a last-resort option when embolization attempts have failed.[18,47,48]

## CLINICAL PRESENTATION AND TIMING OF INTERVENTION
### Antepartum

Routine ultrasound screening in prenatal care can lead to identification of a VGAM. Fetal MRI is becoming increasingly prevalent for a more detailed evaluation in the antepartum period (**Fig. 7**). Structurally, a dilated venous sac can be seen posterior to the third ventricle. The sac can then be differentiated from other cystic structures based on the pulsatile flow located within the venous sac.[29,49,50] Associated sequelae, such as cardiac dysfunction and hydrocephalus, can also be identified.[4,29]

When a VGAM is diagnosed in the antepartum period, it is critical to appropriately evaluate the patient for secondary sequelae before counseling the mother of the patient. The presence of a VGAM is not an indication for termination of the pregnancy, early delivery, or delivery via cesarean section.[8] However, a VGAM associated with antenatal cardiac failure carries an 80% mortality.[38] In addition, the presence of severe cerebral damage in the antenatal or neonatal period has been associated with irreversible multiorgan failure. The extremely poor outcome in these patients is not improved with radiological obliteration of the VGAM.[8,42] Therefore, cardiac failure and severe cerebral damage in the antenatal period are

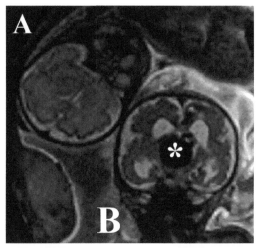

**Fig. 7.** T2-weighted image from a prenatal MRI shows a twin gestation. Note the VGAM (*white asterisk*) in twin B, which causes hydrocephalus and white matter changes. Contrast this appearance with the age-appropriate myelination pattern and normal-sized ventricles in twin A. (*Courtesy of* Gailloud P, MD. The Johns Hopkins Hospital.)

appropriate indications for termination of the pregnancy or for withholding further treatment after birth.[8]

### Neonate

There are 3 management categories for neonates with a VGAM: (1) those who are not offered endovascular treatment, (2) those in whom endovascular treatment can be deferred, and (3) those who require emergent endovascular intervention.[42] The degree of cardiac and systemic manifestations dictates the management strategy that is selected. Patients with mild cardiac overload can be medically managed until embolization is performed at 4 to 5 months of age.[8,18,21,27] Patients with severe cardiogenic shock, multisystem organ failure, and/or irreversible brain damage have a very poor prognosis and are not candidates for endovascular intervention. A subset of patients requires emergent endovascular embolization. Lasjaunias and colleagues[8] proposed a 21-point score (Bicêtre neonatal evaluation score) to help guide management of VGAM in neonates. The score is based on cardiac function, cerebral function, respiratory function, hepatic function, and renal function (**Table 1**). Patients who score less than 8 are recommended no treatment. Patients who score between 8 and 12 are recommended emergent endovascular treatment. Patients who score greater than 12 are recommended medical management initially and are ideally treated endovascularly at 5 months of age.[8]

**Table 1**
**The Bicêtre neonatal valuation score**

| Points | Cardiac Function | Cerebral Function | Respiratory Function | Hepatic Function | Renal Function |
|---|---|---|---|---|---|
| 5 | Normal | Normal | Normal | — | — |
| 4 | Overload, no medical treatment | Subclinical, isolated EEG abnormalities | Tachypnea, finishes bottle | — | — |
| 3 | Failure; stable with medical treatment | Nonconvulsive intermittent neurologic signs | Tachypnea, does not finish bottle | No hepatomegaly, normal hepatic function | Normal |
| 2 | Failure; not stable with medical treatment | Isolated convulsion | Assisted ventilation, normal saturation $Flo_2 < 25\%$ | Hepatomegaly, normal hepatic function | Transient anuria |
| 1 | Ventilation necessary | Seizures | Assisted ventilation, normal saturation $Flo_2 > 25\%$ | Moderate or transient hepatic insufficiency | Unstable diuresis with treatment |
| 0 | Resistant to medical therapy | Permanent neurologic signs | Assisted ventilation, desaturation | Abnormal coagulation, elevated enzyme levels | Anuria |

Maximum score = 5 (cardiac) + 5 (cerebral) + 5 (respiratory) + 3 (hepatic) + 3 (renal) = 21.
*Abbreviations:* EEG, electroencephalogram; $Flo_2$, fractional inspired oxygen.
*From* Lasjaunias PL, Chng SM, Sachet M, et al. The management of vein of Galen aneurysmal malformations. Neurosurgery 2006;59:S184; with permission.

Although the Bicêtre neonatal evaluation score is a useful guide in determining the management and timing of intervention in neonates with a VGAM, exceptions to the scoring system have been reported. For example, McSweeney and colleagues[51] noted 1 patient with an initial Bicêtre score of 6 who had endovascular therapy and was neurologically intact after more than 2.5 years of follow-up. In addition, 2 patients with an initial maximum Bicêtre score of 21 had a subsequent precipitous decline and died before endovascular treatment.[51,52] Therefore, treatment should be guided by the Bicêtre score but ultimately individualized according to each patient's presentation.

### Infants

The management of infants depends on their age on presentation, the severity of symptoms, and the angiographic appearance of the VGAM. If an infant presents before the age of 6 months, endovascular treatment can still be performed in the optimal therapeutic window as previously described.[18,45]

Symptomatic infants typically present with seizures, hydrocephalus, or neurocognitive delay. Although cardiac failure can also be a presenting symptom, it is typically less severe than in neonates. When symptoms are present in older infants and children, intervention is warranted. The goal of treatment in these patients is to reestablish the hydrovenous equilibrium by decreasing flow and increasing resistance through the VGAM.[8] Incomplete occlusion of the VGAM can reverse neurologic symptoms and improve the patient's quality of life.[8]

When hydrocephalus is present, its pathophysiology must be carefully considered before proceeding with treatment. Given that hydrocephalus is a secondary phenomenon, treatment of the VGAM will address the cause of the hydrocephalus. In addition, CSF diversion in patients with hydrocephalus secondary to a VGAM can have a deleterious effect.[34,53] In a series of 43 patients with VGAM, Zerah and colleagues[34] noted that 66% of nonshunted patients were neurologically and cognitively normal, compared with 33% in the shunted group. In addition, 5% of nonshunted patients had significant mental retardation, compared with 15% in the shunted group. In addition, development of epilepsy and new intracranial hemorrhage can occur as a result of shunt placement.[34]

### Older Children and Adults

Older children and adults commonly present with mild headaches or a hemorrhagic event. The goal of intervention is to prevent future neurologic deficits from vascular steal and to prevent psychomotor retardation from venous congestion.[30] In patients who present with mild headaches, their symptoms may be related to the VGAM or be incidental in nature.[30] These patients are more challenging to treat because the intervention risks must be weighed against a perceived benefit. Previously, it was thought that asymptomatic patients or patients with minor symptoms could be managed conservatively because the VGAM would eventually thrombose spontaneously. Spontaneous VGAM thrombosis has subsequently been shown to be a rare event, occurring in only 2.5% of patients.[8] In addition, the natural history of untreated VGAM is that patients eventually experience neurocognitive delay. Thus, a detailed a neurocognitive assessment should be performed as part of the evaluation. If the patient is truly asymptomatic, the risks of treatment versus observation must be clearly discussed with the patient's family with the understanding that the treatment may eventually be required. Asymptomatic patients must be closely monitored for neurocognitive changes. If changes are detected, endovascular intervention must be revisited.

## PROGNOSIS

Before the advent of endovascular techniques, surgery was the primary treatment modality although it had an exceptionally high mortality. Many series reported mortality reaching 100% in the neonatal population.[2,4,11] Although there are select reports of good outcomes following surgery,[47,48] the outcomes of larger series do not compare with the results obtained with endovascular treatment. In 1991, Friedman and colleagues[54] reported a mortality of 50% and mental retardation rate of 37%. With improvement in endovascular techniques and neonatal intensive care, mortality significantly decreased. In 1993, the same group reported a series of 11 patients with no mortality and a 55% rate of functionally normally patients.[55]

Early reports focused on the technical aspects of treating a VGAM with endovascular therapy without emphasis on the neurologic outcome.[26,56,57] In select reports, complete radiographic obliteration was considered a successful outcome, even if the patient subsequently died. In more recent reports, the shift has focused on survival and neurocognitive outcome. In 2006, Lasjaunias and colleagues[8] reported a series of 233 patients with VGAM treated with embolization, which is currently the largest reported experience. They reported a 10.6% overall mortality. Neonates had a mortality of 52%, which was significantly higher than the mortality in infants

(7.2%) and children (0%). In addition, 74% of surviving patients were neurologically normal, 15.6% were moderately retarded, and 10.4% experienced severe mental retardation during a median follow-up time of 4.4 years. Between 90% and 100% obliteration was achieved in 55% of patients, further emphasizing that complete obliteration of a VGAM is not necessary in all cases to achieve clinical improvement.

## SUMMARY

A VGAM is a congenital vascular malformation that is defined by direct and/or indirect arterial feeders flowing into the MProsV of Markowski. It can be detected in the antepartum period on screening ultrasound and further visualized on MRI. In the postpartum period, a VGAM classically presents with cardiac failure in neonates, with seizures, hydrocephalus, or neurocognitive delay in infants, and with headaches or intracranial hemorrhage in older children and adults.

Endovascular therapy is the first-line treatment of a VGAM and its associated sequelae. Ideally, the first intervention is performed at 4 to 5 months of age, although some cases require emergent endovascular treatment. Patient selection and the timing of intervention in the neonatal period are guided by the 21-point Bicêtre score. Medical management is used to stabilize the patient until endovascular intervention can be performed. Surgery is used as an adjunct to treat hydrocephalus, intracranial hemorrhages, and as a last resort when endovascular interventions have failed. Given the complex nature of treating patients with a VGAM, a multidisciplinary approach is recommended. Endovascular therapy combined with a multidisciplinary management strategy to treat a VGAM has significantly lowered mortality and can result in normal neurologic development in surviving patients.

## ACKNOWLEDGMENTS

The authors are grateful to Joseph Kanasz (Medical Illustrator, Cleveland Clinic) for providing the illustrations for this article.

## REFERENCES

1. Casasco A, Lylyk P, Hodes JE, et al. Percutaneous transvenous catheterization and embolization of vein of Galen aneurysms. Neurosurgery 1991;28:260.
2. Gold A, Ransohoff J, Carter S. Vein of Galen malformation. Acta Neurol Scand Suppl 1964;40(Suppl 11):1.
3. Lasjaunias P, Terbrugge K, Piske R, et al. Dilatation of the vein of Galen. Anatomoclinical forms and endovascular treatment apropos of 14 cases explored and/or treated between 1983 and 1986. Neurochirurgie 1987;33:315 [in French].
4. Hoang S, Choudhri O, Edwards M, et al. Vein of Galen malformation. Neurosurg Focus 2009;27:E8.
5. Khullar D, Andeejani AM, Bulsara KR. Evolution of treatment options for vein of Galen malformations. J Neurosurg Pediatr 2010;6:444.
6. Raybaud CA, Strother CM, Hald JK. Aneurysms of the vein of Galen: embryonic considerations and anatomical features relating to the pathogenesis of the malformation. Neuroradiology 1989;31:109.
7. Dandy W. Arteriovenous aneurysm of the brain. Arch Surg 1928;17:190.
8. Lasjaunias PL, Chng SM, Sachet M, et al. The management of vein of Galen aneurysmal malformations. Neurosurgery 2006;59:S184.
9. Boldrey E, Miller ER. Arteriovenous fistula (aneurysm) of the great cerebral vein (of Galen) and the circle of Willis; report on two patients treated by ligation. Arch Neurol Psychiatry 1949;62:778.
10. Silverman BK, Breckx T, Craig J, et al. Congestive failure in the newborn caused by cerebral A-V fistula; a clinical and pathological report of two cases. AMA Am J Dis Child 1955;89:539.
11. Hoffman HJ, Chuang S, Hendrick EB, et al. Aneurysms of the vein of Galen. Experience at the hospital for sick children, Toronto. J Neurosurg 1982;57:316.
12. Yaşargil MG, Antic J, Laciga R, et al. Arteriovenous malformations of vein of Galen: microsurgical treatment. Surg Neurol 1976;(3):195.
13. Burrows PE, Lasjaunias PL, Ter Brugge KG, et al. Urgent and emergent embolization of lesions of the head and neck in children: indications and results. Pediatrics 1987;80:386.
14. Lasjaunias P. Vein of Galen malformations. Neurosurgery 1989;25:666.
15. Lasjaunias P, Ter Brugge K, Lopez Ibor L, et al. The role of dural anomalies in vein of Galen aneurysms: report of six cases and review of the literature. AJNR Am J Neuroradiol 1987;8:185.
16. Rodesch G, Lasjaunias P, Terbrugge K, et al. Intracranial arteriovenous vascular lesions in children. Role of endovascular technics apropos of 44 cases. Neurochirurgie 1988;34:293 [in French].
17. Lasjaunias P, Rodesch G, Terbrugge K, et al. Vein of Galen aneurysmal malformations. Report of 36 cases managed between 1982 and 1988. Acta Neurochir (Wien) 1989;99:26.
18. Gailloud P, O'Riordan DP, Burger I, et al. Diagnosis and management of vein of Galen aneurysmal malformations. J Perinatol 2005;25:542.
19. Horowitz MB, Jungreis CA, Quisling RG, et al. Vein of Galen aneurysms: a review and current perspective. AJNR Am J Neuroradiol 1994;15:1486.
20. Johnston IH, Whittle IR, Besser M, et al. Vein of Galen malformation: diagnosis and management. Neurosurgery 1987;20:747.

21. Pearl M, Gomez J, Gregg L, et al. Endovascular management of vein of Galen aneurysmal malformations. Influence of the normal venous drainage on the choice of a treatment strategy. Childs Nerv Syst 2010;26(10):1367–79.

22. Gailloud P, O'Riordan DP, Burger I, et al. Confirmation of communication between deep venous drainage and the vein of Galen after treatment of a vein of Galen aneurysmal malformation in an infant presenting with severe pulmonary hypertension. AJNR Am J Neuroradiol 2006;27:317.

23. Levrier O, Gailloud PH, Souei M, et al. Normal galenic drainage of the deep cerebral venous system in two cases of vein of Galen aneurysmal malformation. Childs Nerv Syst 2004;20:91.

24. Lasjaunias P, Rodesch G, Pruvost P, et al. Treatment of vein of Galen aneurysmal malformation. J Neurosurg 1989;70:746.

25. Yaşargil MG. AVM of the brain, clinical considerations, general and special operative techniques, surgical results, nonoperated cases, cavernous and venous angiomas, neuroanesthesia, vol. III B. New York: Thieme; 1988.

26. King WA, Wackym PA, Vinuela F, et al. Management of vein of Galen aneurysms. Combined surgical and endovascular approach. Childs Nerv Syst 1989;5:208.

27. Alvarez H, Garcia-Monaco R, Rodesch G, et al. Vein of Galen aneurysmal malformations. Neuroimaging Clin N Am 2007;17:189.

28. Chevret L, Durand P, Alvarez H, et al. Severe cardiac failure in newborns with VGAM. Prognosis significance of hemodynamic parameters in neonates presenting with severe heart failure owing to vein of Galen arteriovenous malformation. Intensive Care Med 2002;28:1126.

29. Gupta AK, Varma DR. Vein of Galen malformations: review. Neurol India 2004;52:43.

30. Krings T, Geibprasert S, Terbrugge K. Classification and endovascular management of pediatric cerebral vascular malformations. Neurosurg Clin N Am 2010;21:463.

31. Pellegrino PA, Milanesi O, Saia OS, et al. Congestive heart failure secondary to cerebral arterio-venous fistula. Childs Nerv Syst 1987;3:141.

32. Norman MG, Becker LE. Cerebral damage in neonates resulting from arteriovenous malformation of the vein of Galen. J Neurol Neurosurg Psychiatry 1974;37:252.

33. Bansal A, Gailloud P, Jordan L, et al. Regression of cerebral calcifications after endovascular treatment in a case of vein of Galen arteriovenous malformation. J Neurosurg Pediatr 2009;4:17.

34. Zerah M, Garcia-Monaco R, Rodesch G, et al. Hydrodynamics in vein of Galen malformations. Childs Nerv Syst 1992;8:111.

35. Mickle JP, Quisling RG. The transtorcular embolization of vein of Galen aneurysms. J Neurosurg 1986;64:731.

36. Amacher AL, Shillito J Jr. The syndromes and surgical treatment of aneurysms of the great vein of Galen. J Neurosurg 1973;39:89.

37. Gupta AK, Rao VR, Varma DR, et al. Evaluation management, and long-term follow up of vein of Galen malformations. J Neurosurg 2006;105:26.

38. Rodesch G, Hui F, Alvarez H, et al. Prognosis of antenatally diagnosed vein of Galen aneurysmal malformations. Childs Nerv Syst 1994;10:79.

39. Seidenwurm D, Berenstein A, Hyman A, et al. Vein of Galen malformation: correlation of clinical presentation, arteriography, and MR imaging. AJNR Am J Neuroradiol 1991;12:347.

40. Gatscher S, Brew S, Banks T, et al. Multislice spiral computed tomography for pediatric intracranial vascular pathophysiologies. J Neurosurg 2007 107:203.

41. Muneuchi J, Joo K, Higashiyama K, et al. Multislice spiral computed tomography in a neonate with vein of Galen aneurysmal malformation. J Pediatr 2007;150:323.

42. Garcia-Monaco R, De Victor D, Mann C, et al. Congestive cardiac manifestations from cerebrocranial arteriovenous shunts. Endovascular management in 30 children. Childs Nerv Syst 1991;7:48.

43. Spetzler RF, Wilson CB, Weinstein P, et al. Normal perfusion pressure breakthrough theory. Clin Neurosurg 1978;25:651.

44. Long DM, Seljeskog EL, Chou SN, et al. Giant arteriovenous malformations of infancy and childhood. J Neurosurg 1974;40:304.

45. Nangiana J, Lim M, Silva R, et al. Vein of Galen malformations: part II management contemporary. Neurosurgery 2008;30:1.

46. Jankowitz BT, Vora N, Jovin T, et al. Treatment of pediatric intracranial vascular malformations using Onyx-18. J Neurosurg Pediatr 2008;2:171.

47. Hernesniemi J. Arteriovenous malformations of the vein of Galen: report of three microsurgically treated cases. Surg Neurol 1991;36:465.

48. Moriarity JL Jr, Steinberg GK. Surgical obliteration for vein of Galen malformation: a case report. Surg Neurol 1995;44:365.

49. Nuutila M, Saisto T. Prenatal diagnosis of vein of Galen malformation: a multidisciplinary challenge. Am J Perinatol 2008;25:225.

50. Vintzileos AM, Eisenfeld LI, Campbell WA, et al. Prenatal ultrasonic diagnosis of arteriovenous malformation of the vein of Galen. Am J Perinatol 1986;3:209.

51. McSweeney N, Brew S, Bhate S, et al. Management and outcome of vein of Galen malformation. Arch Dis Child 2010;95:903.

52. Cherif A, Néji K, Sebaï L, et al. Vein of Galen aneurysmal malformation: a neonatal case with unusual evolution. Arch Pediatr 2007;14:893 [in French].

53. Jea A, Bradshaw TJ, Whitehead WE, et al. The high risks of ventriculoperitoneal shunt procedures for

hydrocephalus associated with vein of Galen malformations in childhood: case report and literature review. Pediatr Neurosurg 2010;46:141.

54. Friedman DM, Madrid M, Berenstein A, et al. Neonatal vein of Galen malformations: experience in developing a multidisciplinary approach using an embolization treatment protocol. Clin Pediatr (Phila) 1991;30:621.

55. Friedman DM, Verma R, Madrid M, et al. Recent improvement in outcome using transcatheter embolization techniques for neonatal aneurysmal malformations of the vein of Galen. Pediatrics 1993;91:583.

56. Ciricillo SF, Edwards MS, Schmidt KG, et al. Interventional neuroradiological management of vein of Galen malformations in the neonate. Neurosurgery 1990;27:22.

57. Dowd CF, Halbach VV, Barnwell SL, et al. Transfemoral venous embolization of vein of Galen malformations. AJNR Am J Neuroradiol 1990;11:643.

# Dural Carotid-Cavernous Fistulas: Epidemiology, Clinical Presentation, and Management

Neil R. Miller, MD

## KEYWORDS

- Dural carotid-cavernous sinus fistula • Endovascular
- Superior ophthalmic vein • Arterialization

A carotid-cavernous sinus fistula (CCF) is an abnormal communication between the cavernous sinus and the carotid arterial system. CCFs can be classified by cause (traumatic vs spontaneous), velocity of blood flow (high vs low flow), and anatomy (direct vs dural, internal carotid vs external carotid vs both).[1,2]

Some fistulas are characterized by a direct connection between the cavernous segment of the internal carotid artery and the cavernous sinus. These fistulas are usually of the high-flow type. They are called direct CCFs and are most often caused by a single, traumatic tear in the arterial wall or at times by the rupture of an intracavernous aneurysm.[1,2] Other CCFs are dural.[2,3] Many of these lesions are actually congenital arteriovenous fistulas that develop spontaneously, often in the setting of atherosclerosis, systemic hypertension, connective tissue disease, and during or after childbirth. Dural CCFs consist of a communication between the cavernous sinus and 1 or more meningeal branches of the internal carotid artery (**Fig. 1**), the external carotid artery (**Fig. 2**), or both (**Fig. 3**).[1] Of these, fistulas involving branches from both the internal and external carotid arteries are the most common. These fistulas usually have low rates of arterial blood flow. In this article, the author discusses the pathogenesis, causes, clinical manifestations, diagnosis, treatment, and prognosis of dural CCFs.

## PATHOGENESIS

Dural CCFs usually become symptomatic spontaneously. The pathogenesis of these fistulas is somewhat controversial.[4] One hypothesis is that spontaneous dural CCFs form after the rupture of 1 or more of the thin-walled dural arteries that normally traverse the cavernous sinus.[5] According to this hypothesis, after rupture, extensive preformed dural arterial anastomoses not directly involved in the fistula dilate and contribute collateral blood supply, resulting in an angiographic appearance indistinguishable from that of a congenital vascular malformation. Indeed, sequential arteriography demonstrates that the feeder vessels of dural CCFs change with time as the vessels spontaneously open and close.[6] Although this theory is favored by some investigators,[1] it fails to explain why spontaneous dural CCFs are more common in elderly women than in men. A second theory for the origin of dural CCFs is that most develop in response to spontaneous venous thrombosis in the cavernous sinus and represent an attempt to provide a pathway for collateral venous outflow.[7] Most investigators favor this theory because it also explains the pathogenesis of arteriovenous fistulas that develop in the sigmoid and other dural sinuses.[4]

Although many patients who develop a dural CCF are otherwise perfectly healthy, certain factors

The author has nothing to disclose.
Wilmer Eye Institute, Johns Hopkins Hospital, Woods 458, 600 North Wolfe Street, Baltimore, MD 21287, USA
*E-mail address:* nrmiller@jhmi.edu

Neurosurg Clin N Am 23 (2012) 179–192
doi:10.1016/j.nec.2011.09.008
1042-3680/12/$ – see front matter © 2012 Elsevier Inc. All rights reserved.

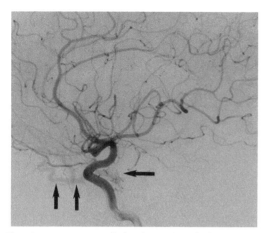

Fig. 1. Appearance of dural CCF in which the only contribution is from extradural branches of the internal carotid artery (type B of Barrow and colleagues). A selective left internal carotid arteriogram shows a fistula at the posterior portion of the cavernous carotid artery (*arrow*). Note a faintly opacified superior ophthalmic vein (*double arrows*). The left external carotid arteriogram was normal. (*Data from* Barrow DL, Spector RH, Braun IF, et al. Classification and treatment of spontaneous carotid-cavernous sinus fistulas. J Neurosurg 1985;62:248–56.)

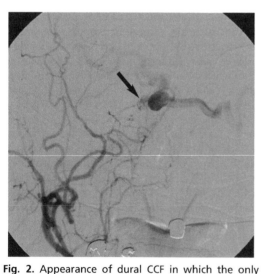

Fig. 2. Appearance of dural CCF in which the only contribution is from extradural branches of the external carotid artery (type C of Barrow and colleagues) (*arrow*). The fistula is fed by extradural branches of the left external carotid artery, particularly the internal maxillary artery. There was no contribution from the ipsilateral internal carotid artery or from the contralateral internal or external carotid arteries. (*Data from* Barrow DL, Spector RH, Braun IF, et al. Classification and treatment of spontaneous carotid-cavernous sinus fistulas. J Neurosurg 1985;62:248–56.)

seem to be predisposed to the development of this lesion. These factors include pregnancy, systemic hypertension, atherosclerotic vascular disease, connective tissue disease (eg, Ehlers-Danlos syndrome type IV), and minor trauma (**Fig. 4**).[8–10]

## CLINICAL MANIFESTATIONS

Dural CCFs usually occur in middle-aged or elderly women, but they may produce symptoms in either gender at any age, even in childhood or infancy.[11] The symptoms and signs produced by these lesions are influenced by several factors, including the size of the fistula, the location within the cavernous sinus, the rate of flow, and especially the drainage pattern.[12–14]

### Posteriorly Draining Fistulas

When dural CCFs drain posteriorly into the superior and inferior petrosal sinuses, they are usually asymptomatic. In some cases, however, such fistulas produce a cranial neuropathy, such as a trigeminal neuropathy,[15] facial nerve paresis,[16] or an ocular motor nerve paresis.[17] In most of these cases, there is no evidence of orbital congestion.[2,3]

In most cases of ocular motor nerve paresis caused by a posteriorly draining dural CCF, the onset of the paresis is sudden, and only one of the ocular motor nerves is affected. The oculomotor nerve is most often affected, and the resulting paresis may be complete with the involvement of the pupil, incomplete with pupil involvement, or incomplete with pupil sparing (**Fig. 5**). In almost all cases, the paresis is associated with ipsilateral orbital or ocular pain, a presentation that initially suggests an intracranial aneurysm.[18,19] The correct diagnosis in such cases is not evident until cerebral angiography is performed. In other cases, the posteriorly draining fistula produces an abducens or trochlear nerve paresis, again usually associated with ocular or orbital pain.[5,18,20,21]

The cranial neuropathies that are caused by a posteriorly draining dural CCF usually are the initial sign of the fistula. In many of these cases, failure to diagnose and treat the fistula leads eventually to a change in the direction of the flow of blood in the fistula. The flow becomes anterior, and patients develop evidence of orbital congestion. In other cases, the blood flow in the fistula is initially anterior, producing orbital manifestations. With time, however, the anterior drainage ceases, and posterior flow is associated with the development of the cranial neuropathy.

Dural fistulas that drain posteriorly sometimes cause brainstem congestion that may be associated with neurologic deficits.[22] In addition,

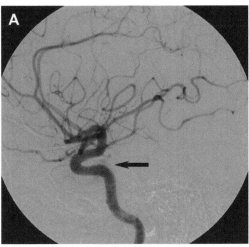
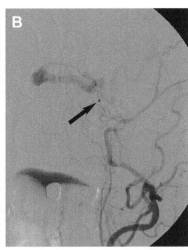

**Fig. 3.** Appearance of a dural CCF fed by extradural branches from *both* the internal and external carotid arteries (type D of Barrow and colleagues). (*A*) Selective left internal carotid arteriogram, lateral view, shows a large collection of contrast material in the cavernous sinus (*arrow*). The fistula drains anteriorly into the left superior ophthalmic vein, which is markedly enlarged (*arrow*). (*B*) Selective left external carotid arteriogram, lateral view, shows multiple contributions from extradural branches of the left external carotid artery (*arrow*). (*Data from* Barrow DL, Spector RH, Braun IF, et al. Classification and treatment of spontaneous carotid-cavernous sinus fistulas. J Neurosurg 1985;62:248–56.)

such fistulas rarely may produce intracranial hemorrhage.[23]

## Anteriorly Draining Fistulas

Dural CCFs that drain anteriorly usually produce visual symptoms and signs.[3] In the mildest cases, there is redness of one or, rarely, both eyes caused by dilation and arterialization of both conjunctival and episcleral veins (**Fig. 6**). In these cases, the appearance may suggest a primary ocular disorder, such as conjunctivitis, episcleritis, or thyroid eye disease; however, a careful examination of the

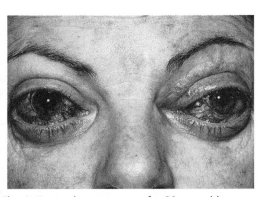

**Fig. 4.** External appearance of a 39-year-old woman with Ehlers-Danlos syndrome who developed spontaneous bilateral dural CCF. The fistulas were successfully closed using an endovascular approach, but the patient died several months later of unrelated vascular complications of the underlying disease.

dilated vessels usually demonstrates a typical tortuous corkscrew appearance that is virtually pathognomonic of a dural CCF (**Fig. 7**).[3,24,25] There also may be minimal eyelid swelling, conjunctival chemosis, proptosis, or a combination of these findings. Diplopia from abducens nerve paresis may be present (**Fig. 8**). The ocular fundus may seem normal, or there may be mild dilation of retinal veins.

In more advanced dural CCFs, particularly those with a high rate of flow, the symptoms and signs are identical with those in patients with a direct CCF.[3,12,13,26–28] In these cases, signs of orbital congestion, including proptosis, chemosis, and the dilation of conjunctival vessels, are obvious and severe (**Fig. 9**).[29–31] Diplopia may result from ophthalmoparesis caused by ocular motor nerve pareses, orbital congestion, or both mechanisms, and there may be significant periorbital or retro-ocular discomfort or pain, initially suggesting an inflammatory process or even the Tolosa-Hunt syndrome.[32,33] Some patients develop facial pain, facial weakness, or both.[34] Raised episcleral venous pressure may produce increased intraocular pressure that occasionally is quite high.[24,27,35,36] Angle-closure glaucoma may develop from elevated orbital venous pressure, congestion of the iris and choroid, and forward displacement of the iris-lens diaphragm.[28,37] In other cases, chronic ischemia produces neovascular glaucoma. Ophthalmoscopic abnormalities include venous stasis retinopathy with retinal hemorrhages, central retinal vein occlusion, proliferative

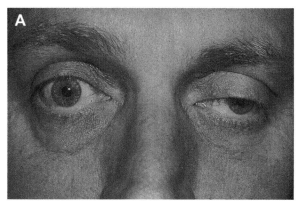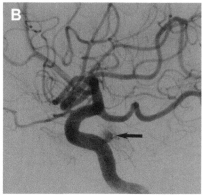

Fig. 5. Oculomotor nerve paresis caused by a posteriorly draining dural CCF. The patient was a 58-year-old man who developed an acute left-sided fronto-orbital headache. Four weeks later, he developed diplopia, and 7 days afterwards, he developed right ptosis and a dilated right pupil. He was thought to have an intracranial aneurysm, and an arteriogram was performed. (A) The patient has a left ptosis and exotropia consistent with a left oculo-motor nerve paresis. (B) Selective left internal carotid arteriogram, lateral view, shows a left-sided posteriorly draining dural carotid-cavernous sinus fistula (arrow). The patient's oculomotor nerve paresis resolved after the fistula was closed.

retinopathy, retinal detachment, vitreous hemor-rhage, choroidal folds, choroidal effusion, choroidal detachment, or optic disk swelling (**Fig. 10**).[38–43]

Visual loss, although less frequent than in patients with direct CCFs, occurs in up to 30% of patients with dural CCFs.[5,30,31,44] It may be caused by ischemic optic neuropathy, chorioreti-nal dysfunction, or uncontrolled glaucoma.[28,35,41]

The ocular manifestations of unilateral dural CCFs are almost always ipsilateral to the fistula, but they may be solely contralateral or bilateral (**Fig. 11**).[3,12,13,45] When unilateral fistulas cause bilateral manifestations, there is a high probability that the fistula is draining into cortical veins (**Fig. 12**).[13]

Although most dural fistulas are unilateral, bilat-eral spontaneous dural fistulas do occur. Patients with bilateral dural CCFs often have severe systemic hypertension, atherosclerosis, or some type of systemic connective tissue disease, such as Ehlers-Danlos syndrome type IV. Most patients with bilateral dural CCFs have bilateral findings; however, some patients with bilateral fistulas have only unilateral signs.[3]

In some instances, dural CCFs drain both ante-riorly and posteriorly. In most of these cases, the only manifestations are those related to the ante-rior drainage; however, some patients develop manifestations from the posterior drainage, such as facial nerve paresis or acute hemiparesis asso-ciated with neuroimaging evidence of brainstem congestion.[16,46]

## DIAGNOSIS

The diagnosis of a dural CCF should be consid-ered in any patient who spontaneously develops a red eye, chemosis of the conjunctiva, abducens nerve paresis, or mild orbital congestion with prop-tosis. Auscultation of the orbit may disclose a bruit, but this is uncommon.

When a dural CCF is suspected, computed tomographic (CT) scanning, CT angiography, magnetic resonance (MR) imaging, MR angiog-raphy, orbital ultrasonography, transorbital and transcranial color Doppler imaging, or a combina-tion of these tests may be of benefit in confirming the diagnosis (**Fig. 13**).[2,3] The gold standard diag-nostic test, however, remains a catheter angio-gram. Because many dural CCFs are fed either

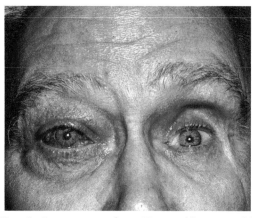

Fig. 6. Appearance of a 61-year-old man with moderate proptosis and redness of the right eye caused by a right-sided dural CCF. This appearance is often mistaken for episcleritis or dysthyroid orbitopathy.

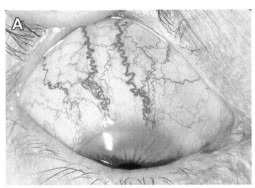
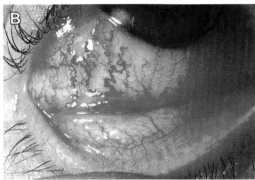

**Fig. 7.** (*A*, *B*) Appearance of conjunctival and episcleral vessels in 2 patients with spontaneous dural CCF. Note dilation, tortuosity, and corkscrew appearance of the veins in both cases.

by meningeal branches of the external carotid artery or by meningeal branches of both the internal and external carotid arteries, and others are fed by arteries from both sides or are fed by unilateral arteries but produce bilateral symptoms and signs, selective angiography of both internal and external carotid arteries on both sides should always be performed.[47] When performed by an experienced neuroradiologist, catheter angiography has a morbidity of less than 1% and virtually no mortality, except in patients with connective tissue disorders, such as Ehlers-Danlos syndrome, in whom the risks are much greater because of the excessive fragility of the extracranial and intracranial vessels.[9]

## NATURAL HISTORY

Most patients with a dural CCF have no difference in mortality from that of the normal population because the lesion usually affects only the eyes. Spontaneous intracranial hemorrhage is exceptionally rare.[23] Thus, when one considers the natural history of a dural CCF, one usually is dealing with ocular morbidity.

Regardless of whether they drain anteriorly or posteriorly and whether they are high-flow or low-flow fistulas, 20% to 50% of dural CCFs, even those associated with significant congestive orbital signs, close spontaneously (**Fig. 14**).[28] In some cases, the symptoms and signs begin to resolve within days to weeks after symptoms

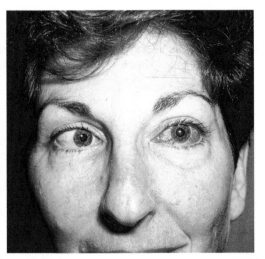

**Fig. 8.** Abducens nerve paresis in a 34-year-old woman with a left-sided dural CCF. When the patient attempts to look to the left, the left eye abducts only to just beyond the midline. Note the mild left proptosis and the markedly dilated conjunctival veins of the left eye.

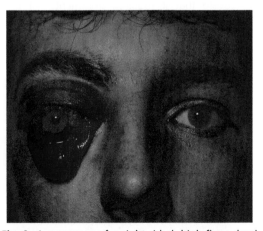

**Fig. 9.** Appearance of a right-sided, high-flow, dural CCF in a 21-year-old man. The right eye is proptotic, and there is significant chemosis of the conjunctiva. The appearance of this patient is indistinguishable from that of a patient with a high-flow, direct CCF.

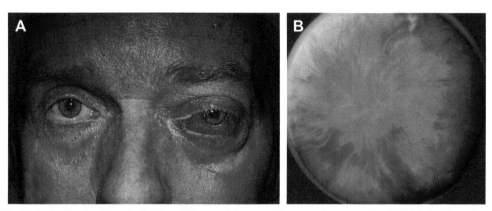

**Fig. 10.** Central retinal vein occlusion in a 52-year-old man with a spontaneous, dural CCF. (*A*) External appearance shows moderate proptosis of the left eye, associated with conjunctival chemosis and arterialization of conjunctival and episcleral vessels. The patient noted progressive visual loss in the left eye over several days. (*B*) Ophthalmoscopic appearance of left ocular fundus shows changes consistent with a severe central retinal vein occlusion.

develop; in others, they do not resolve until months to years after the fistula has become symptomatic. Other dural CCFs close after angiography, after air flight travel, or after incomplete treatment.[48,49]

It is appropriate to follow clinically patients who have mild ocular manifestations to see if the fistula will close spontaneously. During the waiting period, patients need not alter their lifestyle. They should, however, be examined at regular intervals so that their visual function, intraocular pressure, and ophthalmoscopic appearance can be monitored. In the meantime, exposure keratopathy caused by proptosis can be treated with ocular lubrication, and persistent, bothersome diplopia can be treated with prism therapy or occlusion of one eye. Increased intraocular pressure is rarely so severe that it requires treatment.[27] If it is substantially elevated, one can try to lower it with one of the many topical agents that reduce the production of aqueous humor; however, because the cause of the elevated intraocular pressure in most cases is raised episcleral venous pressure, such agents may not be helpful. In the final analysis, however, the best treatment of severely increased intraocular pressure is closure of the fistula.

Patients with a dural CCF may experience acute worsening of ocular manifestations. The clinical deterioration results from an increase in blood flow through the fistula in some cases, but in others, it is caused by spontaneous or posttreatment thrombosis of the superior ophthalmic vein.[49–51] Patients in whom spontaneous progressive thrombosis of the superior ophthalmic vein causes initial worsening of symptoms and signs usually begin to improve within several weeks.

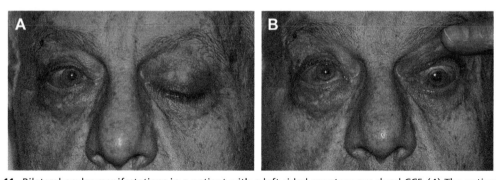

**Fig. 11.** Bilateral ocular manifestations in a patient with a left-sided spontaneous dural CCF. (*A*) The patient has redness of the right eye caused by dilated conjunctival and episcleral vessels. There is also a significant left ptosis. (*B*) The left eye also has dilated conjunctival and episcleral vessels, and there is a left exotropia and a dilated left pupil consistent with a left oculomotor nerve paresis.

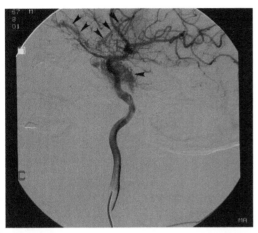

**Fig. 12.** Cortical venous drainage from a dural CCF. Selective left internal carotid arteriogram shows a dural CCF (*single arrowhead*) with drainage into the superior ophthalmic vein (*double arrowheads*) and also into several cortical veins (*triple arrowheads*).

and most eventually experience complete resolution of symptoms and signs (**Fig. 15**). Systemic corticosteroids given when deterioration occurs may lessen the severity of symptoms and signs

and perhaps reduce the length of time until recovery occurs.[50]

## TREATMENT

The visual manifestations of a dural CCF usually do not require local treatment. Occasionally, as previously noted, increased intraocular pressure requires treatment with topical or oral pressure-lowering agents. Although pressure-lowering ocular surgery has been advocated for patients in whom medical therapy does not reduce the intraocular pressure to an acceptable level,[35,52] if intraocular pressure remains unacceptably elevated despite maximum medical therapy, the definitive treatment of the fistula should be performed instead of ocular surgery. Ocular surgery should only be considered if the treatment of the fistula cannot be performed or is unsuccessful or if the intraocular pressure remains elevated despite closure of the fistula.[38] Similarly, although the proliferative retinopathy that may occasionally accompany a severe, high-flow dural CCF can be treated successfully with photocoagulation,[38,53] it is best to treat the fistula producing the retinopathy whenever possible. Again, if the fistula cannot be

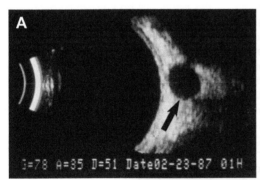

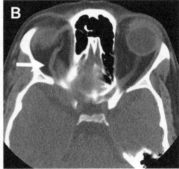

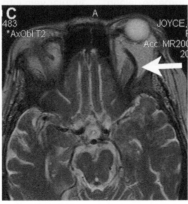

**Fig. 13.** Noninvasive methods of diagnosing a CCF. (*A*), Ultrasonography of the orbit in a patient with an ipsilateral dural CCF. Note large round void (*arrow*) representing cross-section of an enlarged superior ophthalmic vein. (*B*) CT axial image in a patient with a right-sided dural CCF. Note enlarged superior ophthalmic vein (*arrow*). (*C*) MR axial image in a patient with a left-sided dural CCF. Note enlarged left superior ophthalmic vein (*arrow*).

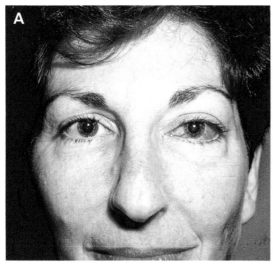
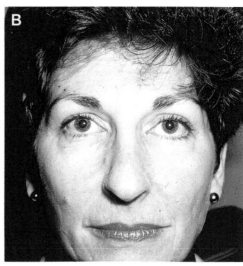

**Fig. 14.** Spontaneous closure of the left-sided dural CCF that caused the left abducens nerve paresis in the patient whose external appearance is depicted in **Fig. 8**. (A) Before closure, the left eye is injected and a left esotropia is present; (B) After closure, the redness, proptosis, and left abducens nerve paresis have completely resolved.

treated or treatment is unsuccessful, photocoagulation may be needed to preserve vision.

Dural CCFs may be treated by direct surgery,[54] conventional radiation therapy,[55] stereotactic radiosurgery,[49,56] intermittent manual self-compression of the affected internal carotid artery with the contralateral hand,[57,58] or occlusion of the ipsilateral internal carotid artery.[59] However, endovascular procedures, including transarterial embolization, transvenous embolization, or a combination of these techniques, usually are the optimum treatment of those lesions that produce progressive or unacceptable symptoms and signs, including visual loss, diplopia, an intolerable bruit, severe proptosis, and, most importantly, cortical venous drainage.[60] Several synthetic and natural materials can be used for embolization. Platinum coils are most often used, but other materials include absorbable gelatin (Gelfoam, Pharmacia & Upjohn, New York, NY, USA); Silastic (Dow Corning, Midland, MI, USA); low-viscosity silicone rubber; autogenous clot, muscle, or dura; tetradecyl sulfate (a sclerosing agent); polyvinyl alcohol particles (Ivalon, Unipoint Laboratory, High Point, NC, USA); ethanol; ethylene vinyl alcohol copolymer (Onyx, ev3, Irvine, CA, USA), oxidized cellulose (Oxycel, Worcester, UK); various preparations of cyanoacrylate glue, or a combination of these.[30,31,45,58,61–79]

In patients with a fistula fed only by meningeal branches of the external carotid artery, the embolization material is introduced via a microcatheter placed in the external carotid artery and passed into the specific branch or branches that feed the fistula. In this setting, successful closure of the fistula is almost always possible, resulting in rapid resolution of all symptoms and signs. When the fistula is fed by meningeal branches from both the external and internal carotid arteries, only the branches from the external carotid artery are usually embolized in the hopes that the flow to the fistula will be sufficiently decreased to result in its subsequent closure. The internal carotid artery is usually not embolized in this setting unless the interventionalist can successfully catheterize the meningohypophyseal trunk or other meningeal feeders from the artery. If the fistula does not close with this technique, the fistula often can be treated subsequently via a transvenous route. In this setting as well as in patients whose fistulae are fed only by meningeal branches from the internal carotid artery, the favored transvenous approach is usually via the femoral or internal jugular vein into the ipsilateral or rarely the contralateral inferior or superior petrosal sinus and from there into the cavernous sinus,[31,62,64–66,73,77] but if this approach fails, a variety of other approaches may be used, most of which involve the cannulation of the superior or inferior ophthalmic veins (**Fig. 16**).[3,45,61,64,65,67,70,71,73,76,78] In some cases, more than one session and more than one approach is needed, and in rare cases, the cavernous sinus can be cannulated directly via an orbital approach.[70,79] Using currently available techniques, successful closure of dural CCFs can be achieved in 80% to 100% (**Fig. 17**).[26,31,45,69,77,80]

Complications from endovascular treatment of dural CCFs are uncommon except in patients with connective-tissue disorders, such as Ehlers-Danlos syndrome.[9,81] Nevertheless, significant

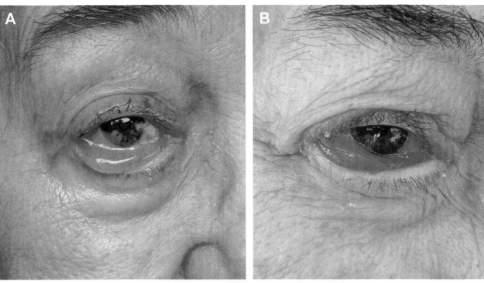

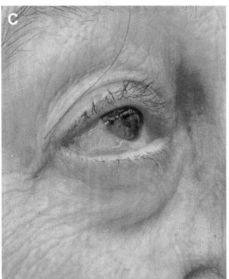

**Fig. 15.** Spontaneous closure of a dural CCF after cerebral angiography. The patient was a 75-year-old woman who developed progressive conjunctival chemosis and injection of the right eye. (*A*) The patient's right eye is swollen and chemotic. Cerebral angiography confirmed a right-sided dural CCF fed by branches of the right internal and external carotid arteries. It was elected to follow the patient without intervention. (*B*) Two weeks after the angiogram, the patient developed more severe swelling, injection, and conjunctival chemosis. Repeat angiography revealed that the superior ophthalmic vein had thrombosed and the fistula was closed. One week after the onset of worsening, the patient began to experience reduction in swelling and redness of the right eye. (*C*) Two months later, the patient has minimal swelling and redness of the right eye.

complications have been reported, including hemorrhage at the catheter site, in the orbit from perforation of the superior or inferior ophthalmic vein, or even intracranially; damage to orbital structures, such as the trochlea when the superior ophthalmic vein is used for access to the cavernous sinus; local infection; sepsis; ophthalmic artery occlusion; and both transient and permanent neurologic deficits, particularly facial pain and ocular motor nerve pareses but also brainstem infarction.[30,31,45,64,69,71–73,75,77,82–84] An analysis of 4 large series of patients with dural CCFs treated endovascularly revealed that of a total of 339 patients, there were complications in 35 (10.3%).[30,31,45,77] Thus, because the embolization techniques used to close dural CCFs can be associated with vision-threatening and even life-threatening complications, physicians performing such procedures should explain to patients not only the benefits but also the risks of these

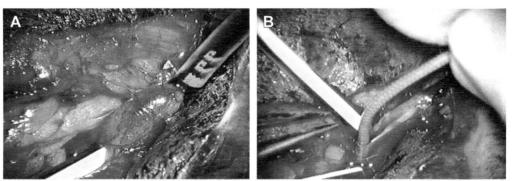

**Fig. 16.** Isolation (*A*) and cannulation (*B*) of the superior ophthalmic vein in a patient with an ipsilateral dural CCF.

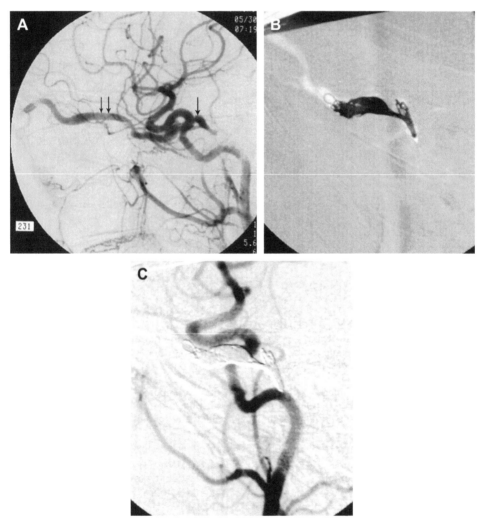

**Fig. 17.** Successful endovascular closure of a dural CCF using a superior ophthalmic vein approach. (*A*) Before treatment, common carotid angiogram shows the fistula, which drains both anteriorly (*double arrows*) and posteriorly (*single arrow*). (*B*) Roadmap image shows multiple platinum coils within the fistula. (*C*) Postprocedure common carotid angiogram shows obliteration of the fistula with preservation of the flow through the ipsilateral internal carotid artery.

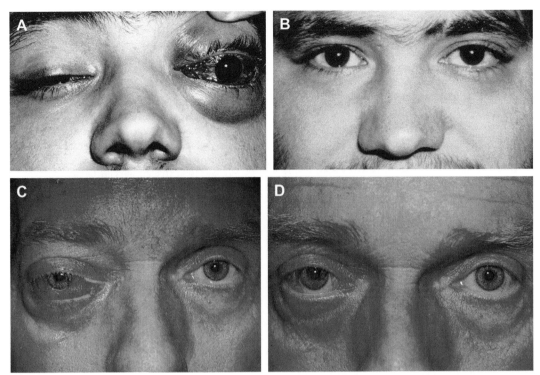

**Fig. 18.** Results of transvenous occlusion of dural CCF in 2 patients. (*A*) Preoperative appearance of a 28-year-old man with a left-sided fistula. Note proptosis, chemosis, and redness of the left eye. (*B*) Four months after successful endovascular occlusion of the fistula, the patient's appearance is almost normal. (*C*) Preoperative appearance of a 36-year-old man with a right-sided dural CCF. Note chemosis, redness, and proptosis of the right eye. (*D*) Six months after successful endovascular occlusion of the fistula, the patient's appearance is almost normal.

procedures and must be prepared to deal with them should they occur.[83–85]

## PROGNOSIS AFTER TREATMENT

It is not unusual for dural CCFs to recanalize or form new abnormal vessels after transarterial embolization with particles or other material.[75] Recurrence of ocular symptoms and signs herald the recurrence of the fistula, and patients in whom manifestations recur require repeat angiography and consideration of further treatment. Symptoms and signs usually begin to improve within hours to days after the successful closure of a dural CCF (**Fig. 18**).[3] Any preexisting bruit immediately disappears, and intraocular pressure immediately returns to normal. Proptosis, conjunctival chemosis, redness of the eye, and ophthalmoparesis (whether caused by orbital congestion or an ocular motor nerve paresis) usually resolve completely within weeks to months, and most patients have a normal or near-normal external appearance within 6 months. At the same time, patients with visual loss caused by choroidal effusion or detachment usually experience substantial, if not complete, recovery of visual function. Unfortunately, patients with visual loss caused by retinal damage (eg, central retinal vein occlusion) usually have persistently poor visual function.

Patients whose dural CCFs are treated with techniques other than endovascular closure, such as stereotactic radiosurgery, often take longer to improve than patients whose fistulas are closed by endovascular techniques.[56,86] Nevertheless, these techniques may provide excellent results over time.

## SUMMARY

The diagnosis and management of dural CCFs have improved substantially in recent years. The widespread availability of noninvasive imaging techniques combined with improvements in catheter angiography permit rapid and accurate diagnosis in most cases, and new endovascular and other therapeutic techniques allow most patients with these lesions to be treated successfully with little or no morbidity and mortality and with the resolution of most, if not all, clinical manifestations.

## REFERENCES

1. Barrow DL, Spector RH, Braun IF, et al. Classification and treatment of spontaneous carotid-cavernous sinus fistulas. J Neurosurg 1985;62:248–56.
2. Miller NR. Carotid-cavernous fistulas. In: Miller NR, Newman NJ, Biousse V, Kerrison JB, editors. 6th edition, Walsh and Hoyt's clinical neuro-ophthalmology, vol. 2. Baltimore (MD): Lippincott-Williams & Wilkins; 2005. p. 2263–96.
3. Miller NR. Diagnosis and management of dural carotid-cavernous sinus fistulas. Neurosurg Focus 2007;23:1–15.
4. Debrun GM, Viñuela F, Fox AJ, et al. Indications for treatment and classification of 132 carotid-cavernous fistulas. Neurosurgery 1988;22:285–9.
5. Newton TH, Hoyt WF. Dural arteriovenous shunts in the region of the cavernous sinus. Neuroradiology 1970;1:71–81.
6. Takahashi M, Nakano Y. Magnification angiography of dural carotid-cavernous fistulae, with emphasis on clinical and angiographic evolution. Neuroradiology 1980;19:249–56.
7. Houser OW, Campbell JK, Campbell RJ, et al. Arteriovenous malformation affecting the transverse dural sinus: an acquired lesion. Mayo Clin Proc 1979;54:651–61.
8. Mironov A. Classification of spontaneous dural arteriovenous fistulas with regard to their pathogenesis. Acta Radiol 1995;36:582–92.
9. Schievink WI, Piepgras DG, Earnest F 4th, et al. Spontaneous carotid-cavernous fistulae in Ehlers-Danlos syndrome type IV. J Neurosurg 1991;74:991–8.
10. Taki W, Nakahara I, Nishi S, et al. Pathogenetic and therapeutic considerations of carotid-cavernous sinus fistulas. Acta Neurochir 1994;127:6–14.
11. Lau FH, Yuen HK, Rao SK, et al. Spontaneous carotid cavernous fistula in a pediatric patient: case report and review of literature. J AAPOS 2005;9:292–4.
12. Stiebel-Kalish H, Setton A, Nimii Y, et al. Cavernous sinus dural arteriovenous malformations: patterns of venous drainage are related to clinical signs and symptoms. Ophthalmology 2002;109:1685–91.
13. Stiebel-Kalish H, Setton A, Berenstein A, et al. Bilateral orbital signs predict cortical venous drainage in cavernous sinus dural AVMs. Neurology 2002;58:1521–4.
14. Suh DC, Lee JH, Kim SJ, et al. New concepts in cavernous sinus dural arteriovenous fistula. Correlation with presenting symptom and venous drainage patterns. Stroke 2005;36:1134–9.
15. Rizzo M, Bosch EP, Gross CE. Trigeminal sensory neuropathy due to dural external carotid-cavernous sinus fistula. Neurology 1982;32:89–91.
16. Moster ML, Sergott RC, Grossman RI. Dural carotid-cavernous sinus vascular malformation with facial nerve paresis. Can J Ophthalmol 1988;23:27–9.
17. Eggenberger E. A brutal headache and double vision. Surv Ophthalmol 2000;45:147–53.
18. Hawke SH, Mullie MA, Hoyt WF, et al. Painful oculomotor nerve palsy due to dural-cavernous sinus shunt. Arch Neurol 1989;46:1252–5.
19. Lee AG. Third nerve palsy due to a carotid cavernous fistula without external eye signs. Neuro-ophthalmology 1996;16:183–7.
20. Kishi S, Sawada A, Mori T, et al. Three cases of carotid cavernous sinus fistulas where the main ocular manifestation was restricted ocular motility. J Jpn Ophthalmol Soc 1999;103:597–603 [in Japanese].
21. Selky AK, Purvin VA. Isolated trochlear nerve palsy secondary to dural carotid-cavernous sinus fistula. J Neuroophthalmol 1994;14:52–4.
22. Kai Y, Hamada JI, Morioka S, et al. Brain stem venous congestion due to dural arteriovenous fistulas of the cavernous sinus. Acta Neurochir 2004;146:1107–12.
23. Harding AE, Kendall B, Leonard TJ, et al. Intracerebral haemorrhage complicating dural arteriovenous fistula: a report of two cases. J Neurol Neurosurg Psychiatry 1984;47:905–11.
24. Keltner JL, Gittinger JW Jr, Miller NR, et al. A red eye and high intraocular pressure. Surv Ophthalmol 1986;31:328–36.
25. Bhatti MT, Peters KR. A red eye and then a really red eye. Surv Ophthalmol 2003;48:224–9.
26. Meyers PM, Halbach VV, Dowd CF, et al. Dural carotid cavernous fistula: definitive endovascular management and long-term follow-up. Am J Ophthalmol 2002;134:85–92.
27. Ishijima K, Kashiwagi K, Nakano K, et al. Ocular manifestations and prognosis of secondary glaucoma in patients with carotid-cavernous fistula. Jpn J Ophthalmol 2003;47:603–8.
28. Bujak M, Margolin E, Thompson A, et al. Spontaneous resolution of two dural carotid-cavernous fistulas presenting with optic neuropathy and marked congestive ophthalmopathy. J Neuro-Ophthalmol 2010;30:220–7.
29. de Keizer R. Carotid-cavernous and orbital arteriovenous fistulas: ocular features, diagnostic and hemodynamic considerations in relation to visual impairment and morbidity. Orbit 2003;22:121–42.
30. Kim DJ, Kim DI, Suh SH, et al. Results of transvenous embolization of cavernous dural arteriovenous fistula: a single-center experience with emphasis on complications and management. AJNR Am J Neuroradiol 2006;27:2078–82.
31. Kirsch M, Henkes H, Liebig T, et al. Endovascular management of dural carotid-cavernous sinus fistulas in 141 patients. Neuroradiology 2006;48:486–90.
32. Brazis PW, Capobianco DJ, Chang FL, et al. Low flow dural arteriovenous shunt: another cause of "sinister" Tolosa-Hunt syndrome. Headache 1994;34:523–5.

33. Procope JA, Kidwell ED Jr, Copeland RA Jr, et al. Dural cavernous sinus fistula: an unusual presentation. J Natl Med Assoc 1994;86:363–4.

34. Jensen RW, Chuman H, Trobe JD, et al. Facial and trigeminal neuropathies in cavernous sinus fistulas. J Neuroophthalmol 2004;24:31–8.

35. Phelps CD, Thompson HS, Ossoinig KC. The diagnosis and prognosis of atypical carotid-cavernous fistula (red-eyed shunt syndrome). Am J Ophthalmol 1982;93:423–6.

36. Zito E, Biton C, Abada S, et al. Carotid-cavernous fistulas: regarding a case. Bull Soc Ophtalmol Fr 1998;98:436–41 [in French].

37. Talks SJ, Salmon JF, Elston JS, et al. Cavernous-dural fistula with secondary angle-closure glaucoma. Am J Ophthalmol 1997;124:851–3.

38. Fiore PM, Latina MA, Shingleton BJ, et al. The dural shunt syndrome. I. Management of glaucoma. Ophthalmology 1990;97:56–62.

39. Gonshor LG, Kline LB. Choroidal folds and dural cavernous sinus fistula. Arch Ophthalmol 1991;109:1065–6.

40. Kojima H, Urakawa Y, Sato Y, et al. Central retinal vein occlusion associated with spontaneous carotid cavernous fistula. Folia Ophthalmol Jpn 1991;42:1869–74.

41. Kupersmith MJ, Marino Vargas E, Warren F, et al. Venous obstruction as the cause of retinal/choroidal dysfunction associated with arteriovenous shunts in the cavernous sinus. J Neuroophthalmol 1996;16:1–6.

42. Moldovan SM, Borderie V, Francais-Maury C, et al. Dural carotid-cavernous fistula with uveal effusion syndrome. J Fr Ophtalmol 1997;20:217–20 [in French].

43. Saitou M, Matsuhashi H, Yoshimoto H. Central retinal vein occlusion in a patient with spontaneous carotid cavernous sinus fistula. Folia Ophthalmol Jpn 1998;49:470–3 [in Japanese].

44. Grove AS Jr. The dural shunt syndrome: pathophysiology and clinical course. Ophthalmology 1984;91:31–44.

45. Yu SC, Cheng HK, Wong GK, et al. Transvenous embolization of dural carotid-cavernous fistulae with transfacial catheterization through the superior ophthalmic vein. Neurosurgery 2007;60:1032–8.

46. Shintani S, Tsuruoka S, Shiigai T. Carotid-cavernous fistula with brainstem congestion mimicking tumor on MRI. Neurology 2000;55:1929–31.

47. Debrun G. Angiographic workup of a carotid cavernous sinus fistula (CCF), or what information does the interventionalist need for treatment? Surg Neurol 1995;44:75–9.

48. Liu HM, Wang YH, Chen YF, et al. Long-term clinical outcome of spontaneous carotid cavernous sinus fistulae supplied by dural branches of the internal carotid artery. Neuroradiology 2001;43:1007–14.

49. Lau LI, Wu HM, Wang AG, et al. Paradoxical worsening with superior ophthalmic vein thrombosis after gamma knife radiosurgery for dural arteriovenous fistula of cavernous sinus: a case report suggesting the mechanism of the phenomenon. Eye 2006;20:1426–8.

50. Sergott RC, Grossman RI, Savino PJ, et al. The syndrome of paradoxical worsening of dural-cavernous sinus arteriovenous malformations. Ophthalmology 1987;94:205–12.

51. Golnik KC, Miller NR. Diagnosis of cavernous sinus arteriovenous fistula by measurement of ocular pulse amplitude. Ophthalmology 1992;99:1146–52.

52. Keltner JL, Satterfield D, Dublin AB, et al. Dural and carotid cavernous sinus fistulas: diagnosis, management, and complications. Ophthalmology 1987;94:1585–600.

53. Harris MJ, Miller NR, Fine SL. Photocoagulation treatment of proliferative retinopathy secondary to a carotid-cavernous sinus fistula. Am J Ophthalmol 1980;90:515–8.

54. Day JD, Fukushima T. Direct microsurgery of dural arteriovenous malformation type carotid-cavernous sinus fistulas: indications, technique, and results. Neurosurgery 1997;41:1119–26.

55. Yen MY, Yen SH, Teng MM, et al. Radiotherapy of dural carotid-cavernous sinus fistulas. Neuroophthalmology 1996;16:133–42.

56. Chong GT, Mukundan S, Kirkpatrick JP, et al. Stereotactic radiosurgery in the treatment of a dural carotid-cavernous fistula. J Neuroophthalmol 2010;30:138–44.

57. Kai Y, Hamada J, Morioka M, et al. Treatment of cavernous sinus dural arteriovenous fistulae by external manual carotid compression. Neurosurgery 2007;60:253–8.

58. Vinh Moreau-Gaudry V, Lefournier V, Descour F, et al. Dural carotid-cavernous fistulas: progression in therapeutic management from 1989 to 2004. A report of ten cases. J Fr Ophtalmol 2009;32:404–10 [in French].

59. Kupersmith MJ, Berenstein A, Choi IS, et al. Management of nontraumatic vascular shunts involving the cavernous sinus. Ophthalmology 1988;95:121–30.

60. Gemmete JJ, Ansari SA, Gandhi D. Endovascular techniques for treatment of carotid-cavernous fistula. J Neuroophthalmol 2009;29:62–71.

61. Venturi C, Bracco S, Cerase A, et al. Endovascular treatment of a cavernous sinus dural arteriovenous fistula through the superior ophthalmic vein via cannulation of a frontal vein. Neuroradiology 2003;45:574–8.

62. Arat A, Cekirge S, Saatci I, et al. Transvenous injection of Onyx for casting of the cavernous sinus for the treatment of a carotid-cavernous fistula. Neuroradiology 2004;46:1012–5.

63. Satomi J, Satoh K, Matsubara S, et al. Angiographic changes in venous drainage of cavernous sinus

dural arteriovenous fistulae after palliative transarterial embolization of observational management: a proposed stage classification. Neurosurgery 2005;56:494–502.

64. Wakhloo AK, Perlow A, Linfante I, et al. Transvenous n-butyl-cyanoacrylate infusion for complex dural carotid cavernous fistulas: technical considerations and clinical outcome. AJNR Am J Neuroradiol 2005;26:1888–97.

65. Suzuki S, Lee DW, Jahan R, et al. Transvenous treatment of spontaneous dural carotid-cavernous fistulas using a combination of detachable coils and Onyx. AJNR Am J Neuroradiol 2006;27:1346–9.

66. Andreou A, Ioannidis I, Psomas M. Transvenous embolization of a dural carotid-cavernous fistula through the contralateral superior petrosal sinus. Neuroradiology 2007;49:259–63.

67. Badillla J, Haw C, Rootman J. Superior ophthalmic vein cannulation through a lateral orbitotomy for embolization of a cavernous dural fistula. Arch Ophthalmol 2007;125:1700–2.

68. San Millán D, Oka M, Fasel JH, et al. Transvenous embolization of a dural arteriovenous fistulas of the laterocavernous sinus through the pterygoid plexus. Neuroradiology 2007;49:665–8.

69. Théaudin M, Saint-Maurice JP, Chapot R, et al. Diagnosis and treatment of dural carotid-cavernous fistulas: a consecutive series of 27 patients. J Neurol Neurosurg Psychiatry 2007;78:174–9.

70. White JB, Layton KF, Evans AJ, et al. Transorbital puncture for the treatment of cavernous sinus dural arteriovenous fistulas. AJNR Am J Neuroradiol 2007;28:1415–7.

71. Lee JW, Kim DJ, Jung JY, et al. Embolisation of indirect carotid-cavernous sinus dural arterio-venous fistulae using the direct superior ophthalmic vein approach. Acta Neurochir 2008;150:557–61.

72. Li MH, Tan HQ, Fang C, et al. Trans-arterial embolisation therapy of dural carotid-cavernous fistulae using low concentration n-butyl-cyanoacrylate. Acta Neurochir 2008;150:1149–56.

73. Bhatia KD, Wang L, Parkinson RJ, et al. Successful treatment of six cases of indirect carotid-cavernous fistula with ethylene vinyl alcohol copolymer (Onyx) transvenous embolization. J Neuro-Ophthalmol 2009;29:3–8.

74. Gandhi D, Ansari SA, Cornblath WT. Successful transarterial embolization of a Barrow type D dural carotid-cavernous fistula with ethylene vinyl alcohol copolymer (Onyx). J Neuro-Ophthalmol 2009;29:9–12.

75. Wakhloo AK. Endovascular treatment of dural carotid cavernous sinus fistulas. J Neuro-Ophthalmol 2009;29:1–2.

76. Wolfe SQ, Cumberbatch NM, Aziz-Sultan MA, et al. Operative approach via the superior ophthalmic vein for the endovascular treatment of carotid cavernous fistulas that fail traditional endovascular access. Neurosurgery 2010;66(ONS Suppl 2):293–9.

77. Yoshida Y, Melake M, Oishi H, et al. Transvenous embolization of dural carotid cavernous fistulas: a series of 44 consecutive patients. AJNR Am J Neuroradiol 2010;31:651–5.

78. Dashti SR, Fiorella D, Spetzler RF, et al. Transorbital endovascular embolization of dural carotid-cavernous fistula: access to cavernous sinus through direct puncture: case examples and technical report. Neurosurgery 2011;68(ONS Suppl 1):75–83.

79. Elhammady MS, Petersen EC, Aziz-Sultan MA. Onyx embolization of a carotid cavernous fistula via direct transorbital puncture. J Neurosurg 2011;114:129–32.

80. Miller NR, Monsein LH, Debrun GM, et al. Treatment of carotid-cavernous sinus fistulas using a superior ophthalmic vein approach. J Neurosurg 1995;83:838–42.

81. Kashiwagi S, Tsuchida E, Goto K, et al. Balloon occlusion of a spontaneous carotid-cavernous fistula in Ehlers-Danlos syndrome type IV. Surg Neurol 1993;39:187–90.

82. Taniguchi I, Kazuo K, Miyazaki D, et al. Ophthalmic artery occlusion after neuroradiological embolization to treat spontaneous carotid-cavernous sinus fistula. Folia Ophthalmol Jpn 1994;45:668–71.

83. Leibovitch I, Modjtahedi S, Duckwiler GR, et al. Lessons learned from difficult or unsuccessful cannulations of the superior ophthalmic vein in the treatment of cavernous sinus dural fistulas. Ophthalmology 2006;113:1220–6.

84. Wladis EJ, Peebles R, Weinberg DA. Management of acute orbital hemorrhage with obstruction of the ophthalmic artery during attempted coil embolization of a dural arteriovenous fistula of the cavernous sinus. Ophthal Plast Reconstr Surg 2007;23:57–9.

85. Devoto MH, Egbert JE, Tomsick TA, et al. Acute exophthalmos during treatment of a cavernous sinus-dural fistula through the superior ophthalmic vein. Arch Ophthalmol 1997;115:823–4.

86. Barcia-Salorio JL, Soler F, Barcia JA, et al. Stereotactic radiosurgery for the treatment of low-flow carotid-cavernous fistulae: results in a series of 25 cases. Stereotact Funct Neurosurg 1994;63:266–70.

# Index

Note: Page numbers of article titles are in **boldface** type.

Neurosurg Clin N Am 23 (2012) 193–197
doi:10.1016/S1042-3680(11)00128-8
1042-3680/12/$ – see front matter © 2012 Elsevier Inc. All rights reserved.

# *Moving?*

## *Make sure your subscription moves with you!*

To notify us of your new address, find your **Clinics Account Number** (located on your mailing label above your name), and contact customer service at:

**Email: journalscustomerservice-usa@elsevier.com**

**800-654-2452** (subscribers in the U.S. & Canada)
**314-447-8871** (subscribers outside of the U.S. & Canada)

**Fax number: 314-447-8029**

**Elsevier Health Sciences Division**
**Subscription Customer Service**
**3251 Riverport Lane**
**Maryland Heights, MO 63043**

*To ensure uninterrupted delivery of your subscription, please notify us at least 4 weeks in advance of move.

Printed and bound by CPI Group (UK) Ltd, Croydon, CR0 4YY

03/10/2024

01040355-0001